THE SURVIVAL MEDICINE HANDBOOK

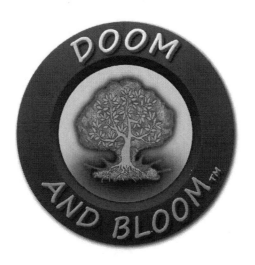

A DOOM AND BLOOM™ GUIDE

THE SURVIVAL MEDICINE HANDBOOK

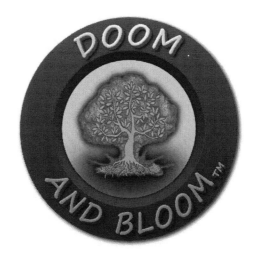

A GUIDE FOR WHEN HELP IS NOT ON THE WAY

JOSEPH ALTON, M.D.

AMY ALTON, A.R.N.P.

DISCLAIMER

The information given and opinions voiced in this volume are for educational and entertainment purposes only and does not constitute medical advice or the practice of medicine. No provider-patient relationship, explicit or implied, exists between the publisher, authors, and readers. This book does not substitute for such a relationship with a qualified provider. As many of the strategies discussed in this volume would be less effective than proven present-day medications and technology, the authors and publisher strongly urge their readers to seek modern and standard medical care with certified practitioners whenever and wherever it is available.

The reader should never delay seeking medical advice, disregard medical advice, or discontinue medical treatment because of information in this book or any resources cited in this book.

Although the authors have researched all sources to ensure accuracy and completeness, they assume no responsibility for errors, omissions, or other inconsistencies therein. Neither do the authors or publisher assume liability for any harm caused by the use or misuse of any methods, products, instructions or information in this book or any resources cited in this book.

No portion of this book may be reproduced by any electronic, mechanical or other means without the written permission of the authors. Any and all requests for such permission should be sent by email to drbonesclass@aol.com.

Most illustrations by Jeff Meyer of anaseer.com

Copyright 2013 Doom and Bloom™, LLC

All rights reserved.

Printed in the United States of America

ISBN-13: 978-0988872530

ISBN: 0988872536

DEDICATIONS

This book is dedicated to my wife Amy, whose positive attitude and sunny disposition truly puts the "Bloom" in "Doom and Bloom". She is the person who first made it clear to me that this book was both possible to write and needed by those who want to be medically prepared in times of trouble.

JOSEPH ALTON, M.D.

I dedicate this book to my husband Joe, whose selfless attitude and compassion for his patients over the years has never wavered. He is unceasing in his efforts to help those who want to learn how to keep their loved ones healthy, in good times or bad.

AMY ALTON, A.R.N.P.

Additionally, we both dedicate this book to those who are willing to take responsibility for the health of their loved ones in times of trouble. We salute your courage in accepting this assignment; have no doubt, you will save lives.

JOSEPH ALTON, M.D. AND AMY ALTON, A.R.N.P.

"DO WHAT YOU CAN, WITH WHAT YOU HAVE, WHERE YOU ARE."

THEODORE ROOSEVELT

ABOUT JOSEPH ALTON, M.D. AND AMY ALTON, A.R.N.P.

Joseph Alton practiced as a board-certified Obstetrician and Pelvic Surgeon for more than 25 years before retiring to devote his efforts to preparing families medically for any scenario. He is a Fellow of the American College of Obstetrics and Gynecology and the American College of Surgeons, served as department chairman at local hospitals and as an adjunct professor at local university nursing schools. He is a contributor to well-known preparedness magazines and is frequently invited to speak at survival and preparedness conferences throughout the country on the subject of medical readiness. A member of MENSA, Dr. Alton collects medical books from the 19th century to gain insight on off-the-grid medical protocols.

Amy Alton is an Advanced Registered Nurse Practitioner and a Certified Nurse-Midwife. She has had years of experience working in large teaching institutions as well as smaller, family-oriented hospitals. Amy has extensive medicinal herb and vegetable gardens and works to include natural remedies into her strategies.

Dr. and Ms. Alton are devoted aqua culturists (currently raising tilapia) and aquaponic, raised bed, and container gardening experts. As "Dr. Bones and Nurse Amy", they host a medical preparedness website at www.doomandbloom.net, and produce video and radio programs under the Doom and Bloom™ label. Dr. and Ms. Alton are firm believers that, to remain healthy in hard times, we must use all the tools in the medical woodshed. Their goal is to promote integrated medicine; in this way, they can offer their readers the most options to keep their loved ones healthy in a long-term survival situation.

PREFACE

+++

THE SECOND EDITION

When we first embarked on the adventure of writing the first edition of this book, "The Doom and Bloom™ Survival Medicine Handbook", we were overwhelmed by the challenge that confronted us. Although there was a wealth of information about the occasional injury on a wilderness hike,

few books considered the possibility of a setting so remote or devastated that NO hope of modern medical care existed for the long term. Even books that were meant for use in third world environments often ended their chapters by exhorting their readers to get to modern medical care as soon as possible.

We realized that we were in uncharted territory. Our concern was the major catastrophe that isolated a family from modern medicine for the long term. Trained personnel would not exist in this scenario, or would be overwhelmed by the demand for their services. What does a mother or father do in this circumstance? How would they deal with injuries or sickness? What could we, as medical professionals, do to improve their family's chances of surviving and staying healthy?

We decided that a how-to manual in plain English was the best option. We had to put together a strategy for each medical issue that we felt a head of household would encounter in times in trouble. It had to be simple. It had to make use of limited resources in a sustainable manner. It had to be realistic.

The last part was the hardest. It's difficult to make people believe that a head injury or a gunshot wound to the chest may not be survivable. No one wants to return to a time when, for example, pregnancy was a major cause of death. It's painful to think about, but we must face the hard truth, sometimes.

So we looked at every individual medical problem we could think of. How could we teach a non-medical person how to approach that problem in simple fashion? We considered what medical supplies they would need, how to use them, and how to replace them, when possible, with natural alternatives. More importantly, we figured out ways to best prevent medical problems.

It wasn't easy. Many times, we had to dig back into our collection of 19th century medical books to find methods that would be useful in grid-down situations. These methods weren't superior to what modern medicine has to offer; as a matter of fact, some are downright obsolete. Despite this, we found a number of ways that our great grandparents used that might be of benefit in a long term survival setting.

When the book was published, we expected that, perhaps, a couple of hundred people might obtain it. A year later, tens of thousands have the book in their possession. The book has received acclaim and it has received criticism; luckily for us, more of the former than the latter.

This 2nd Edition covers more issues that the first book, and covers almost every subject in more detail. The book updates a number of areas of the first book with new strategies that we have devised for various problems. Every section has been amended in some way; some a little, some a lot.

We hope that this book will serve as a useful reference to the average family. The person that will accept responsibility for their family's medical well-being in uncertain times is a very special person. We hope that we have provided a tool for their goal: To succeed, even if everything else fails.

TAKING RESPONSIBILITY

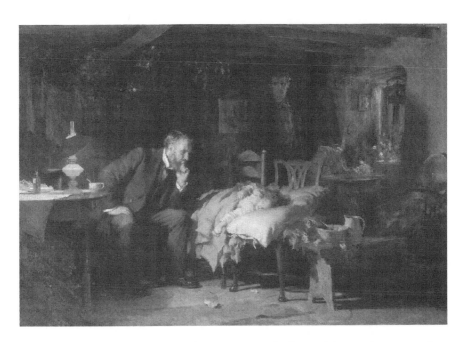

Most outdoor medicine guides are intended to aid you in managing emergency situations in austere and remote locations. Certainly, modern medical care on an ocean voyage or wilderness hike is not readily available; even trips to the cities of underdeveloped countries may fit this category as well.

There are medical strategies for these mostly short term scenarios that are widely published, and they are both reasonable and effective. An entire medical education system exists to deal with limited wilderness or disaster situations, and it is served by a growing industry of supplies and equipment. You expect, not unreasonably, that the rescue helicopter is already on the way.

What is your goal when an emergency occurs in a remote setting? The basic premise of "wilderness" or "disaster" medicine is to:

- Evaluate the injured or ill patient.
- Stabilize their condition.

- Transport the individual to the nearest modern hospital, clinic, or emergency care center.

This series of steps makes perfect sense; you are not a physician and, somewhere, there are facilities that have a lot more technology than you have in your backpack. Your priority is to get the patient out of immediate danger and then ship them off; this will allow you to continue on your wilderness adventure. Transporting the injured person may be difficult to do (sometimes very difficult), but you still have the luxury of being able to "pass the buck" to those who have more knowledge, technology and supplies. And why not? You aren't a medical professional, after all.

One day, however, there may come a time when a pandemic, civil unrest or terrorist event may precipitate a situation where the miracle of modern medicine may be unavailable. Indeed, not only unavailable, but even to the point that the potential for access to modern facilities no longer exists.

We refer to this type of long-term scenario as a "collapse". In a collapse, you will have more risk for illness and injury than on a hike in the woods, yet little or no hope of obtaining more advanced care than you, yourself, can provide. It's not a matter of a few days without modern technology, such as after a hurricane or tornado. Help is NOT on the way; therefore, you have become the place where the "buck" stops for the foreseeable future.

Few are prepared to deal with the harsh reality of a long-term survival situation. To go further, very few are willing to even entertain the possibility that such a tremendous burden might be placed upon them. Even for those stalwarts that are willing, there are few, if any, books that will consider this drastic turn of events. Yet, the likelihood of your exposure to such a situation, at some point in your life, may not be so small. It stands to reason, therefore, that some medical education might be useful in times of trouble.

Almost all handbooks (some quite good) on wilderness or third world medicine will usually end a section with: "Go to the hospital immediately". Although this is excellent advice for modern times, it won't be very helpful in an uncertain future when the hospitals might all be out of commission. We only have to look at Hurricane Katrina in 2005 to know that even modern medical facilities may be useless if they are under-staffed, under-supplied, and overcrowded.

Unwittingly, the majority of the citizens in New Orleans became their own medical care providers in the aftermath of the storm. With medical assistance teams overwhelmed, no one was coming to the aid of one injured or ill individual when thousands needed help at once. Each household became the "end of the line" when it came to its own well-being.

If you become the end of the line with regards to the medical well-being of your family or group, there are certain adjustments that have to be made. Medical supplies must be accumulated to deal with varied emergencies. Medical knowledge must be obtained, shared, and assimilated. These medical supplies and skills must then be adjusted to fit the mindset that you must adopt in a collapse: That things have changed for the long term, and that you are the sole medical resource when it comes to keeping your people healthy.

This is a huge responsibility. Many, when confronted, will decide that they cannot bear the burden of being in charge of the medical care of others. Others, however, will find the fortitude to grit their teeth and wear the badge of survival "medic". These individuals may have some medical experience, but most will simply be fathers and mothers who understand that someone must be appointed to handle things when medical help is NOT on the way.

If this reality first becomes apparent when a loved one becomes deathly ill, the likelihood that you will have the training and supplies needed to be an effective medical provider will be close to zero. This is a sure way to assure that, when everything else fails, you will, too.

This volume is meant to educate and prepare those who want to ensure the health of their loved ones. If you can absorb the information here, you will be better equipped to handle 90% of the emergencies that you will see in a power-down scenario. As well, you will have a realistic view of what medical issues are survivable without modern facilities.

These realities may place you between a rock and a hard place. Over time, you will certainly have to make difficult decisions. With this book, we hope to give you the tools to arrive at choices that will increase your chances of successfully treating injuries and disease.

All the information contained in this book is meant for use in a post-apocalyptic setting, when modern medicine no longer exists. If your leg is broken in five places, it stands to reason that you'll do better in an orthopedic hospital ward than with a splint made out of two sticks and strips of a T-shirt.

The strategies discussed here are not the most effective means of taking care of certain medical problems. In fact, some of them are straight out of the last century. They adhere to the philosophy that something is better than nothing; in a survival situation, that "something" might just get you through the storm. As Theodore Roosevelt once said, "You must do what you can, with what you have, where you are".

Hopefully, societal destabilization will never happen. This book is a weapon against, not an argument for, an end of the world scenario. If we never encounter a long-term survival situation, this book will still have its uses. Natural catastrophes such as Hurricane Katrina will always rear their ugly heads.

These events are inevitable at one point or another, and will tax even the most advanced medical delivery systems. Medical personnel will be unlikely to be readily available to help you if they are overwhelmed by mass casualties.

Even a few days without access to health care may be fatal in an emergency. The information provided here will be valuable while you are waiting for help to arrive. With some medical knowledge and supplies, you may gain precious time for an injured loved one and aid in their recovery.

An important caveat: In most locales, the practice of medicine or dentistry without a license is against the law. None of the recommendations in this book will protect you from liability if you implement them where there is a functioning government and legal system. Consider obtaining formal medical education if you want to become a healthcare provider in a pre-collapse society. All it takes is your time, energy, and dedication.

Although you will not be a physician after reading this volume, you will certainly be more of a medical asset to your family, group, or community than you were before. Among other things, you will have:

- Learned to think about what to do when you become the end of the line in terms of your family's medical well-being.
- Considered preventative medicine and sanitation.
- Looked at your environment to see what plants might have medicinal value.
- Put together a medical kit which, along with standard equipment, includes traditional medications and natural remedies.
- Thought about how to improvise in an austere setting.

Most importantly, you will have become medically prepared to face the very uncertain future; and after all, isn't that what you wanted to accomplish when you first picked up this book?

WHAT THIS BOOK ISNT...

the degree of

Doctor of Medicine

honors and privileges ther
f, the seal of the University
ident and the Dean are herev

The first part of this preface described this and other books that might be helpful in scenarios that might occur as a result of the aftermath of a major disaster or long-term catastrophe. The information in this book will be useful to those preparing for those events. It might also be helpful in a remote setting for those who have to fend for themselves for long periods of time.

This book will not meet the needs of certain people. If you are already a doctor or formally-trained medical professional, you will feel that some of the information in this book is below your pay grade.

You would be right, as this book is not primarily intended for you. It is meant for the non-medical professional who is concerned about keeping their family healthy when trained personnel, such as yourself, are no longer around.

This book might have some use, however, for the flexibly-minded medical pro. In a long-term survival situation, medical personnel will not have the luxury of "Stabilize and Transport" and will have to adjust their mindset. This book is of that mindset already. It might be helpful for some who would ordinarily transport a patient out: It might make them think about how to prepare for when they might be the highest medical resource left.

The book does not claim to be a comprehensive review of every topic covered in it. Don't expect, for example, 50 pages on how to treat Athlete's Foot between its covers.

As well, this book is not meant for the person who expects to perform advanced medical procedures in the wilderness or any other power-down survival setting. You will not learn how to perform a cardiac bypass by reading this book, nor will you be learning how to successfully re-attach an amputated leg.

If nothing else, this book is realistic, and does not claim to cure problems that only modern technology will help. Having said this, you will still be able to deal with the majority of survivable issues you will encounter in an austere setting.

This book is about integrated medicine, so if you are dead set against either conventional or alternative methods of healing, you will not be happy with this book. This book often bucks the conventional medical wisdom; at the same time, it is suspect of alternative claims that a particular substance is a cure-all for every disease. This book looks at what is likely to be of benefit in emergency situations with limited supplies. With it, you'll have the best chance of maintaining the long-term health of a family or community.

TABLE OF CONTENTS

✚✚✚

INTRODUCTION

✚ ✚ ✚

ARE YOU NORMAL?

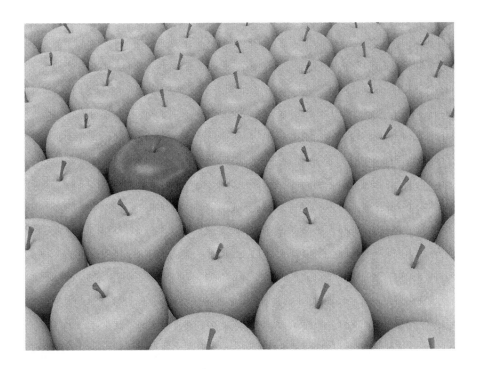

Let's say a man with a microphone comes up to you. He says:

"Excuse me, sir (or madam), may I ask you a question? Are you normal?"

Seems like such a simple question, doesn't it? It's a rare individual who believes that they're not normal. You'd probably give him a strange look and walk on. The truth, however, is that the answer is not as simple as it seems.

Okay, then, let's talk a little about "normal" people. The word "normal" has several definitions, but we'll focus on two:

1. "Standard, average or conforming to the group", and...
2. "Sane".

"Normal" people have certain characteristics that would match the above. You'd agree, I'm sure, that "normal folks" need a level of organization in their life. They don't want a lot of clutter, so they make sure to keep no more than 3 days' supply of food in the pantry. They wait until the gas tank is nearly empty to refill it, and have no medical supplies other than a few Band-Aids and some aspirin in the medicine cabinet.

Whenever there's a crisis, whether it's national (like the 9/11 attacks) or personal (like losing a job), they see before them just a bump on the road. When they stumble, they pick themselves up, brush the dirt off, and continue on their merry way as if nothing had happened.

Normal folk don't feel that there are lessons to be learned by current events. A major storm is just a news story or a chance to play some board games with the kids. This is because they are confident that others will resolve all their problems.

They pay taxes, so they believe the government will step in and give them a helping hand whenever they need it. The help could be in the form of food stamps in hard financial times, in swift emergency responses in natural calamities or in efficient and effective intervention in areas of civil unrest. Most people believe wholeheartedly that help will always be on the way, even if they have personally experienced a disaster situation.

Various surveys prove that this is the "normal" thinking of most people in civilized countries. Given the definition of "normal" listed above, this attitude certainly is "standard" and conforms to the group, but is it "sane"?

Let's take the case of essential personnel for any municipality. This would include police officers, firefighters, emergency medical techs, etc.

These are the emergency responders that "normal" folks expect to get them out of a crisis. But what would really happen?

In surveys performed in several cities' police precincts and fire stations, many public servants we depend upon have indicated that they will NOT report in the case of a truly serious catastrophe. The same goes for various other essential personnel, such as doctors, nurses, and paramedics.

Unthinkable? To some, perhaps; however, the professional that we count on to rescue us in times of trouble also have wives, husbands, parents, and children. Who do you think they will rush to protect in a horrendous emergency, you or their own families? This is just a simple fact of life, and not a criticism of the brave men and women who keep us safe.

In the aftermath of Hurricane Katrina, the New Orleans Police Department surveyed those law enforcement officers who did not report for duty. Although some, indeed, were victims of the catastrophe, most cited their families as the reason for their absence. To expect them to do their duty and, at the same time, leave their own loved ones at risk might be standard and "normal" in our society, but it certainly isn't "sane".

So how do "normal" people become "sane" people? By realizing that society can be fragile and there are events that may occur to send the world into disarray. Once things happen that knock us off-kilter, a downward spiral will make life difficult. Certainly, it will be a challenge for all, but less so for that small minority known as "Preppers" or "The Preparedness Community".

Preppers are what we call people who stockpile food and supplies for use in a societal upheaval. They also take time to re-learn skills largely lost to modern urbanites/suburbanites; skills that would be useful if modern conveniences are no longer available.

What types of events could cause such a collapse to happen? There are various scenarios that could lead to times of trouble: Flu pandemics, terrorist attacks, solar flares, and economic collapse are just some of the possible calamities that could befall a community, a region or even a country. The likelihood of any one of these life-changing occurrences may be very small, but what is the chance that NONE of these events will occur over the course of your lifetime? Your children's lifetimes?

The preparedness community (perhaps 3% of the population) understands that there could be storm clouds on the horizon. Unlike the oblivious majority, they face perilous circumstances with a "can-do" attitude. It can be argued that they are the "normal ones". Even though they are not "conforming to the group", they are more "sane" than their fellow citizens.

Instead of facing an uncertain future with fear and desperation, the preparedness community is using this opportunity to learn new skills that can get them through any catastrophe. Many of these skills were common knowledge to their ancestors, such as growing food and using natural products for medicinal uses.

By learning things that are useful in a power-down situation, they increase the likelihood that they and their loved ones will succeed if, heaven forbid, everything else fails. If a calamitous scenario transpires, they will be prepared for the worst, even while hoping for the best.

Some documentaries have portrayed Preppers as clad in camouflage, armed to the teeth, and hunkered down in some foxhole. For the grand majority of them, this could not be farther from the truth. The self-reliant nation is not eagerly waiting for some terrible series of events to bring society down. They want nothing more than to die at age 100, with their grandchildren whispering in their ear: "Gee, Grandpa, what the heck are we going to do with all these supplies?"

They view their preparations as insurance. You buy health insurance, but that doesn't mean you want to get sick; you buy life insurance, but you certainly don't want to die. Being prepared is insurance as well. Instead of paying money for something that isn't tangible, you're buying food, medical supplies, and other things that will ensure that you and your loved ones will do well regardless of what slings and arrows life may throw at you.

The road to self-reliance is a long and winding one. It will take some of your time and some of your energy to become self-sufficient. It will take some of your money, as well, to accumulate things that will be useful in obtaining a head start to success in dark times. This can be done frugally; a 50 pound bag of rice, for example, is still under $20 at the time of this writing.

Many of the products that will be useful in a collapse scenario can also be improvised. A bandanna and a stick will be almost as good a tourniquet as a high-tech, commercially manufactured one. Look at what you have in your home and consider the ways that an item can be used in a survival situation.

A realistic assessment of your storage will give you a good idea of how prepared you are for an unforeseen event. Where are you deficient? What purchases or improvisations will offer you the best opportunity to be ready? What skills would be useful to learn?

Benjamin Franklin once said: "When the well is dry, we learn the worth of water". The same can be said of many aspects of modern technology. If you are thrown into a situation where there is no electric power, how many items in your house will be useless? Quite a few, I suspect.

Thus, it stands to reason that, among other things, you should consider the ways that you will produce power. For most people, there are a few un-rechargeable batteries in a drawer somewhere. This may get you a few hours' worth of flashlight or radio use, but what then? It's important to have a strategy that will give you a steady supply of at least minimal power. Switch to rechargeable batteries, and get a solar battery charger so that you can keep a renewable power source in your possession at all times. Consider the various other options, such as propane gas, wind power and solid solar panels with marine batteries and inverters.

You don't have to be an industrial engineer or an extremely wealthy person to put these together; just some motivation and perhaps a little elbow grease, and you'll be on your way.

This volume is meant to help you begin your journey to medical preparedness. You won't be a physician after reading this. I promise you, however, that you will know more about assuring your family's medical well-being and be more of an asset than a liability to those you care about.

If you begin to prepare for difficult times, and maintain a positive attitude, you will be an example for others in your family or community to emulate. If they see that preparing just makes good old common sense, they might start to prepare as well. Imagine an entire community, nation or even the world ready to deal with life's untoward events. In that circumstance, "conforming to the group" would actually be "sane", and we would live in a truly "normal" world.

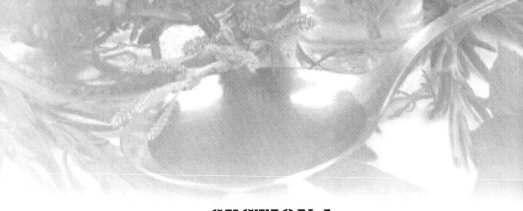

SECTION 1

✚ ✚ ✚

PRINCIPLES OF MEDICAL PREPARDNESS

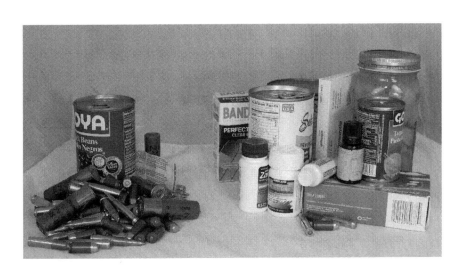

Public Perception of Preparedness (L) vs. Actual Preparedness (R)

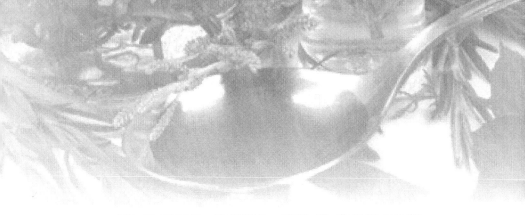

DOOM AND GLOOM VS.
DOOM AND BLOOM

✚✚✚

There are a variety of reasons that the majority of the population chooses not to prepare for hard times. One reason relates to the perception that those that store food and other items are full of "Doom and Gloom". Many in the general public still see the old-time camouflage-clad survivalists when they think of preparedness. Certainly, their portrayal in the media has done little to rehabilitate this image.

The term "Doom and Gloom" itself is full of the worst connotations; synonymous with despair and inaction, very few are willing to identify with what they consider to be a personality flaw. I don't blame them. Placing oneself into a category that always sees the negative in a situation is an unattractive option.

Yet, events are occurring in rapid succession. Our quality of life is being eroded even as we speak. The downward spiral may be starting, and it's difficult for many to escape a negative attitude when they consider the future of our society. The problems are many, and the solutions are few (and they are painful, as well).

It is easy to choose the despair and inaction that goes with being a "Doom and Gloomer"; there's not a lot of sweat involved in sitting in front of a television or computer, bemoaning the ills of modern-day civilization. You don't have to study or learn new skills; you don't have to change your current lifestyle. You can just sit there and watch soap operas and reality shows. Although there's not a lot to like about the term "Doom and Gloom", plenty of people are just fine with the apathetic, do-nothing attitude that goes along with it.

These are dangerous times. There are many (very many) who are in denial of this fact. These people could be cured of this denial simply by examining current events. "Storms of the Century" are occurring with regularity, and our infrastructure and reserves suffer as a result. Even many in the path of a disaster shake it off without a second thought, despite the loss of lives and property.

Besides those in denial, we return to the "Doom and Gloomers", fully aware of the situation but apathetically waiting for the apocalypse in a morose stupor. They will be no better off than the oblivious majority in times of trouble; worse, really, as they have been miserable for a longer time.

Furthermore, their negativity has soured the general public on the idea of preparedness. For the future of our society, this is probably the worst legacy of the "Doom and Gloom" mindset. The less prepared our citizens are for hard times, the more difficult it will be for there to be a future at all.

There is hope, however. The preparedness community understands that there can be rough seas ahead. They see the signs of the deterioration that have begun to erode the civilization that we have enjoyed for so long. Facts do not cease to exist just because they are ignored, and we may be on the brink of a meltdown.

So, why do today's Preppers have an advantage over everyone else in terms of their potential for success in the future? Because, unlike the "Doom and Gloom" crowd, they have evolved a new, more positive philosophy which we will call: "Doom and BLOOM".

Adherents of the "Doom and Bloom" philosophy view negative current events with an unblinking eye. There is neither denial nor sugarcoating of the factors that might send things south, perhaps in a hurry. This is, if you will, the "Doom" part. Instead of despair and inaction, however, the preparedness community has hope and determination. They see the danger, but also a very special opportunity: The opportunity to become truly self-reliant. This is the "Bloom" part. They see the challenges of today as a wake-up call. It might be an alarm, but it's also a call to action.

Unlike others, the Self-Reliant Nation is positive that there are ways to succeed in the coming hard times. They look to what has worked before there was high technology. They see how their grandparents and great-grandparents succeeded, and they are learning skills that their ancestors had; skills that modern society has lost somewhere along the way.

"Doom and BLOOMERS" see the silver lining in those storm clouds, and are learning how to grow their own food, take care of their own health, and provide for their common defense. There's a learning curve, to be sure, but every bit of knowledge that they can absorb will mean a better future for themselves and their loved ones. They are applying lessons from the past to assure themselves that future.

If the public's perception of the preparedness community is one of "Doom and Bloom" rather than "Doom and Gloom", the association would be one with positivity and "can-do", instead of negativity and inertia. This would allow those who have prepared for tough times to serve as ambassadors of hope. With the acceptance of a positive viewpoint, a rebirth of a collapsed civilization would not only be possible, but would be inevitable. Armed with knowledge and skills to function in a power-down situation, "Doom and Bloomers" would be the vanguard for the establishment of a self-sustainable society.

It is not just wishful thinking. It may be seem daunting to you, but it is well within your potential. It has been said that a 1000 mile journey begins with the first step. Take that first step today, and you'll be ahead of the crowd in terms of assuring your survival and that of your loved ones.

BAD NEWS AND GOOD NEWS

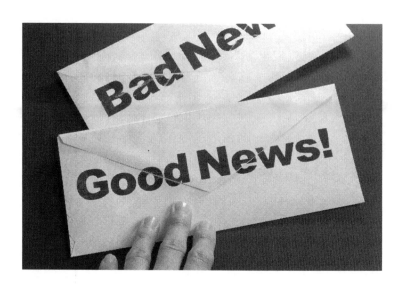

A good percentage of the population has an uneasy feeling about the future. They have heard all the dire predictions of the last 50 years: The Soviet Union and the U.S. will destroy the world in a nuclear war. Y2K will make the entire power grid shut down.

It seems that, every year, there is a Doomsday prediction, and, every year, it fails to come to fruition (whew!). Mayan Apocalypses have come and gone. A new series of predictions, even more dire, for the coming years are also out there. Yet, because we have cried "Wolf" so many times without an actual collapse event happening, the general public has become jaded. Apathy mixed with inertia is their response. This is a dangerous attitude, as the wolf really may show up, eventually, and we are totally unprepared for him.

Have we reached the high water mark as a civilization? There are some signs that we have. One sure sign of the decline of a civilization is the inability to reproduce the technological achievements of its past. Although we are still moving forward technologically in many areas, this sign is now visible. For example, we no longer have the capability or desire to put a man on the moon. The end of the Space Shuttle and International Space Station programs now confines the human race to our own planet. This is not the best course of action for a planet with limited resources and a burgeoning population. Resources that were once earmarked for space travel, however, now are needed simply to keep people fed and the infrastructure in place. This sad state of economic affairs affects many nations that are experiencing difficulties just keeping their heads above water.

Society has faced this issue many times before, with many (now-extinct) cultures. Take Rome, for instance. The Romans were able to develop indoor-plumbing, aqueducts, realistic art, etc. As the civilization went into decline, these advances were unable to be maintained, let alone expanded upon. At one point, collapse of the entire culture occurred. There were still "Romans", but they were at a loss to understand how their ancestors were able to produce such miracles. This period was called a "dark age". We may consider ourselves immune, but we are not; we could, one day, find ourselves on the road to a dark age also.

In many polls, the majority of American citizens feel that the country is in decline. Once the world's undisputed superpower, the prominence of the United States has been in jeopardy for some time from far-away nations such as China and India. What was called the "The American Century" may be slowly grinding to an end. By 2026, the United States is projected to be surpassed by China economically, and by India around 2050. Our leadership in science and technology (especially military) will be challenged between 2020 and 2030, perhaps earlier. This descent has been projected to be gentle and gradual; yet, many of us remember the shocking rapidity of the collapse of the Soviet Union. Why is the United States immune to that fate?

The "end of the world" can be objective, as in a large asteroid striking the planet, or subjective, as in the internet going down for an online business. Why is this subjective? To explain: Not so very long ago, there wasn't an internet at all. We didn't have mobile phones. There were no microwave ovens or televisions and our cars didn't have computers or cruise control. Most of us would consider the loss of these and other items the "end of the world", but life went on without these things just a few decades ago.

Life went on without credit cards, as well. If you didn't have the funds for an item, you went without it. This would be considered cruel and unusual punishment in today's culture. Along with the myriad social services that many governments provide their citizens, we have developed a sense of entitlement; along with it has come a sense of complacency, as well.

Taken together, the possibility of the loss of these modern conveniences and "free" services is heinous to the general population. So heinous, indeed, that they reject the idea of a collapse simply by refusing to even think about the future. Yet, the future is coming, and we are facing uncertain times in a way that is not self-reliant.

What are the issues that could tip a fragile society into dark times? To fully delineate every scenario that can befall us would require a lot more paper and ink than we have, but let's discuss some of them now.

The most likely, in my opinion, is economic collapse. There are at least three major factors in the decline of the United States economically. They are: Trade deficits, the loss of the dollar as the world's currency, and the decline in our status as the world's technological innovator.

Once the world's biggest exporter of goods, the U.S. is now behind China and the European Union. The outsourcing of jobs, especially in manufacturing, has been constant and leaves the nation with less and less products that other countries need. For example, at the time of this writing there are no cellular phones produced in the United States at all. There seems to be no end to this trend, and the unemployment rate attests to it.

China and Russia are no longer using the dollar to transact business with each other, instead using their own currencies. The indiscriminate printing of more and more money to pay our debts has the entire world uneasy. Increasingly, we are seeing calls for an alternative to the current system. If the U.S. dollar ceases to be the world's exchange currency, times will be very tough, indeed, for the country.

A country's technological prowess is dependent on its ability to educate its citizens and to attract the best and brightest that are not yet citizens. Our ranking in math and science education is dropping in every survey. Although we are still attracting students from other countries to our universities (50% of math and science graduate students are from elsewhere), they are no longer planning to live here after they graduate. They see better opportunities in their own countries.

All of the above, combined with an astronomical deficit and near-default, have left the United States as a fading superpower unable to pay its debts. Once the world ceases to use the dollar as its trade currency, no one will want to buy the treasury notes that have served as our way to pay interest on the debt. The costs of imports will rise as a result. To pay for all these rising costs, less money will go to repairing infrastructure, research, and military defense. Do you see where this is headed?

In all likelihood, this will be a gradual downward spiral. The average person will find it more difficult each year to pay his or her bills. Mortgage payments will be behind and more people will find themselves less able to fill up their gas tank or pay for their kids' day care or college tuitions. We will all slowly become poorer than we were. Unemployment or under-employment will further rise, and more adult children will find themselves living at their parent's house. This is already a reality for many folks.

Oil is another major factor where the United States is at a disadvantage. Consumption of foreign oil has risen to 45% in 2011, up from 36% 30 years earlier. The country consumes 18.8 million barrels of oil a day. Even the recent discovery of massive shale oil deposits and new technologies such as hydraulic fracturing (also known as "fracking") will not allow the United States to produce the amount of oil to cover demand. The controversy over environmental impact will make certain of that.

The failure of the U.S. to develop alternative sources of energy leaves the country at the mercy of others. Only 12% of our energy use comes from alternative (solar, hydro, wind, etc.) methods. As other countries, such as China, continue to increase their energy use, the demand for oil rises and so does the price. As the dollar weakens, oil-producing nations may begin to demand payment by other means than U.S. dollars. This will further raise prices.

As low-cost oil becomes a thing of the past, the cost of travel (and export) will skyrocket. Trade will be seriously affected. As winter approaches, the economy stagnates as more and more money is required to simply heat the house. The logical endpoint is bankruptcy, universal poverty and the civil unrest it portends, and eventually, societal collapse.

This scenario is not the only road to perdition. Influenza viruses, with their ability to mutate, are outpacing vaccines. With the ability to travel around the world in a day, outbreaks that would have been localized can become worldwide in a matter of weeks. Widespread use of antibiotics in livestock is producing super-bacteria that can beat drugs that were effective against them previously. In India, strains of tuberculosis, a life-threatening lung disease, are appearing that no antibiotic has so far been able to treat.

Electro-Magnetic Pulses (EMPS), either natural (solar flares) or man-made (terrorism) have the potential to shut down the power grid for decades. If a solar flare approaching the strength of the one that radiated the United States in 1859 occurs, it would take 20 years to manufacture replacements of the transformers that would reinstate the electrical grid. Come to think of it, how would we even power the factories that make them?

Military adventures by various countries might ignite larger conflicts that could destabilize the world. Any number of "acts of God", such as hurricanes, earthquakes, tsunamis, etc., might wreak their havoc. Of course, the likelihood of any one of these situations occurring is small, but what is the likelihood that NONE of these scenarios will occur sometime in your lifetime? Your children's lifetime?

Ok, enough Doom, how about some Bloom? If any of the above actually happens, there will be turmoil. However, after a rocky (perhaps very rocky) period, there will be a transition to a steady state. This transition will probably be gradual with fitful starts and stops. The world may no longer be affluent, but it will be more self-sustainable.

The economy will be an insular one providing the essentials to local communities, using local materials. You won't be able to buy bananas in Montana during the winter. You will, however, be eating organically, and you could be able to grow that food yourself if you're willing to learn how to.

Towards that goal, you'll replace your water-guzzling lawn with vegetable gardens, fruit trees, and berry bushes. Water is just too precious to waste on a putting green. Any remaining grassy areas will become pasture land for goats, cows, and other livestock. By simple necessity, we will all become accomplished homesteaders or have skills that pertain to homesteading.

Self-sufficiency will be the order of the day. If something breaks, you will have learned how to repair it or will barter with someone who does. If you get sick, much of your medicine is already growing in your herb garden. Every family will have someone with the healing touch that will take responsibility for health care in the absence of modern medical facilities.

Is this a lot to swallow in one sitting? Sure it is. It's a major challenge, to be sure, but it's a challenge your great grandparents accepted. You're just as smart as they were. You probably know even more about preventative medicine than they did, or at least have the resources today to learn. All you need is a little motivation and a positive attitude.

What's the end result of all this? Your children will cease wanting to grow up to be runway models and rock stars, and will want to take up truly useful trades that make them an asset to their community. You might wind up living in a larger group; an extended family means more hands to share in the chores. Your children will spend a lot more time interacting with the rest of the family than they do now. Without a computer in front of them, they will actually get to know their loved ones, at last.

Also, there will be a sense of accomplishment. You will have seen that seed that you planted become a plant, and produce something that you can actually eat! Furthermore, it's there because YOU planted and cared for it. Society is so used to specialization today that most people feel like just another cog in a very big machine. The author Robert Heinlein once said: "Specialization is for insects". Humans are much better served being generalists.

In a self-sufficient world, you and your family will likely be the whole ball of wax, from beginning to end. It's a lot of responsibility, but the satisfaction you will have in a job well done will be something you rarely experience today.

So, not so bad, is it? Nobody's anxious for society to start collapsing, but we can be ready for it and have a rewarding life no matter what happens. Keep a quiet determination and a positive outlook with regard to the present, get some skills under your belt, and you will guarantee yourself a productive future.

HISTORY OF PREPAREDNESS

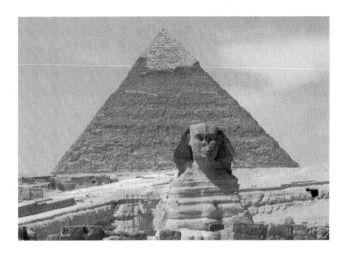

Some say that preparedness has its origin in the animal kingdom. Squirrels, foxes, chipmunks, and various other animals store or bury food which they dig up in the winter to get through lean times. Even though it is instinctual behavior for them, they are assuring their survival in a fashion that we can all learn from. When human beings realize that tough times are on the way, a relatively small percentage will start preparing, and these people are the ones that will be successful in times of trouble.

Preparedness is just the human way to store those nuts for the coming winter. We prepare, as mentioned before, to ensure that there will be food, medical supplies, and all the other things we need to survive. In a true survival situation, most of these necessities will be hard or impossible to obtain. By putting some time, effort and money into accumulating tangible items, we will be able to ensure our well-being if the worst happens. We certainly don't want disasters to occur, but we want to be ready to withstand hard times.

It's not just a sign of intelligence; it signifies a sense of self-preservation and social responsibility to be prepared. It's an achievable goal, and you don't have to be an accomplished outdoorsman to succeed. Anyone, regardless of their station in life, can be successful if they dedicate themselves to their objective.

We all, in the back of our minds, are concerned about the massive calamity: The perfect storm, solar flares, terrorist attacks, economic collapse or any of a number of events that could turn our fragile civilization into a nightmare. We call it "the end of the world as we know it" or "when the **** hits the fan".

These events are horrific, to be sure, but "the end of the world" doesn't have to be nationwide or worldwide; it can just as easily be personal. The loss of a family member or one's employment can easily throw a family into disarray. By storing food and other essential items, the "personal apocalypse" can be a bump in the road instead of the end of the road.

The preparedness community has a long history; as far back as biblical times, in fact. When the Hebrew Joseph was in the Egyptian Pharaoh's jail, he was known for his ability to interpret dreams. After hearing about this ability, Pharaoh sent for the young man, and asked him about a recurring dream that the Egyptian leader was having. In the dream, there were 7 fat, healthy cattle. There then came along 7 thin, diseased cattle and they devoured the healthy ones.

Joseph took this to mean that Egypt would experience 7 years of plenty followed by 7 years of famine. So he recommended that the Pharaoh spend the next 7 bountiful years accumulating grain; in that way, the people would be fed during the subsequent lean years. This was done, and Egypt was prosperous during a famine that left all of its neighbors destitute and starving. This was the very first recorded instance of "prepping"! By following Joseph's recommendation to prepare, we can be a prosperous Egypt instead of its unfortunate neighbors.

In the millennia since the time of Joseph, there have been many instances in which disaster has been averted in times of trouble by the concept of preparedness. Farmers stored grain by erecting silos and "cribs". Every army crossing into enemy territory stockpiled supplies in advance; if they didn't, they would find themselves starving and out of ammunition in a hostile land. In every instance, those who prepared for times of crisis had a head start on everyone around them.

The modern survival community has people with varied skills but of like minds. These people are in the minority, but you will find them scattered everywhere: In cities, suburbs and rural areas. They are diverse: Progressives concerned about global warming prepare and so do conservatives concerned about excessive government. They cross racial, ethnic, and even national boundaries. They might disagree on some issues and they may not always be on the same page at the same time, but they are committed to the same goal. That goal is the continuation of the species, and a life for everyone in the group that is worth living. These are the people that will rebuild a viable society after a catastrophe.

MEDICAL PREPAREDNESS

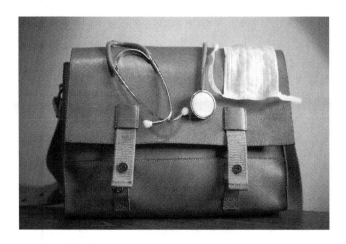

The focus of this book is medical preparedness: That is, the ability to deal with sickness and injuries in tough times. Of course, anyone wishing to survive must first have food, water, and a shelter of some sort. A full stomach and protection from the elements will be the top priority. What, then, is next on the list?

After gathering food and building a shelter, many prepared individuals consider personal and home defense to be the most important priority in the event of a societal collapse. Certainly, defending oneself is important, but have you thought about defending your health?

In a situation where power might be down and normal methods of filtering water and cleaning food don't exist, your health is as much under attack as the survivors in the latest zombie apocalypse movie. Infectious diseases will be rampant in a situation where it will be a challenge to maintain sanitary conditions. Simple activities of daily survival, such as chopping wood, commonly lead to cuts that could get infected. These minor issues, so easily treated by modern medical science, can easily become life-threatening if left untreated in a collapse scenario.

Don't you owe it to yourself and your family to devote some time and effort to obtain medical knowledge and supplies? You may be an accomplished outdoorsman and have plenty of food and your share of defensive weaponry. Yet, what would you say to a member of your family who becomes ill or injured in a remote and austere setting? Take two bullets and call me in the morning? The difficulties involved in a grid-down situation will surely put the health of your entire family or group at risk. It's important to seek education so that you can treat infectious disease and the other ailments that you'll see.

There will likely be a lot more diarrheal disease, for example, than gunfights at the OK corral. History teaches us that, in the Civil War, there were more deaths from dysentery than there were from bullet wounds. Some say "Beans, Bullets and Band-Aids", but I say "Beans and Band-Aids, then Bullets". I suppose, coming from a physician, that's not too surprising. It makes perfect sense that you will, at one point, be responsible for healing the sick and treating wounds.

If you make the commitment to learn how to treat medical issues and to store medical supplies, you're taking a genuine first step towards assuring your family's survival in dark times. The medical supplies will always be there if the unforeseen happens, and the knowledge you gain will be there for the rest of your life. Many medical supplies have long shelf lives; their longevity will be one of the factors that will give you confidence when moving forward. Also, let's not ignore their value as barter items in times of trouble.

When I say to obtain medical knowledge, I am also encouraging you to learn about natural remedies and alternative therapies that may have some benefit for your particular medical problem. I cannot vouch for the effectiveness of every claim that one thing or another will cure what ails you. Suffice it to say that our family has an extensive medicinal garden and that it might be a good idea for your family to have one, also. Many herbs that have medicinal properties grow like weeds, so a green thumb is not required to cultivate them. Many of them do not even require full sun to thrive.

It's important to understand that some illnesses will be difficult to treat if modern medical facilities aren't available. It will be hard to do much about those clogged coronary arteries; there won't be many cardiac bypasses performed. However, by eating healthily and getting good nutrition, you will give yourself the best chance to minimize some major medical issues. In a survival situation, an ounce of prevention is worth, not a pound, but a ton of cure. Start off healthy and you'll have the best chance to stay healthy.

I'm not asking you to do anything that your great-grandparents didn't do as part of their strategy to succeed in life. In a collapse, we'll be thrown back, in a way, to that era. We should learn some lessons from the methods they used to stay healthy. I won't dwell too much on natural remedies in this chapter, as there are chapters devoted to the subject in other parts of this manual.

Some members of my family wonder why I spend all my time trying to prepare people medically for a major disaster. Despite history teaching us otherwise, they are totally certain that there is no scenario that would take away, even for a while, the wonders of high technology. They see the hospital on their way to work and they have health insurance, what could happen? As such, my family is truly puzzled when they read my books and articles. They tell me that I can't turn everyone into doctors, so why I should try?

So I asked myself: Am I trying to turn you all into doctors? No, there's too much to learn in one lifetime; even as a physician, I often come across things I'm not sure about. That's what medical books are for, so make sure that you put together a survival library. You can refer to them when you need to, just as I do.

I AM trying to turn you into something, however: I'm trying to make you a better medical asset to your family and/or survival community than you were before. I firmly believe that, even if you have not undergone a formal medical education, you can learn how to treat the majority of problems you will encounter in a grid-down situation. You can, if you absolutely have to, be the end of the line with regards to the medical well-being of your people.

My efforts are not a fool's quest. If you can absorb the information I'll provide in this handbook, you will be in a position to help when the worst happens. Maybe, one day, you might even save a life; if that happens just once, my mission will have been a success.

THE CONCEPT OF INTEGRATED MEDICINE

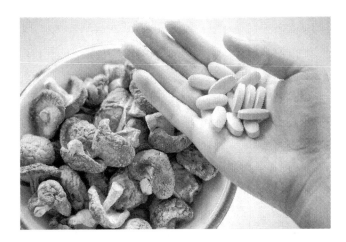

Most of us have a relationship with a conventional healthcare provider. Many regularly see alternative healers as well. Both of these professionals have much to offer in terms of maintaining our medical well-being. Yet, these two disciplines are often at odds with each other. This makes little sense to me, and certainly would be detrimental in a survival situation.

Having an inflexible attitude towards one branch of medicine or another is harmful to your family or survival group. As such, this book is not just geared towards standard medical treatment, but includes other natural healing options. It is not, however, a book solely on alternative medicine either. Those of you that are wholly against one or the other will probably be unhappy with it. If so, I ask you to examine why you are so dead set against one or the other.

I once had a conventional (otherwise known as "allopathic") doctor challenge me to find ANY illness that natural remedies will cure or prevent. I have also heard an herbalist challenge the benefits of the vaccine that eliminated Smallpox from the world. In each case, no amount of evidence would budge either practitioner from their notion that any discipline but their own had any place in the treatment of patients.

This intransigence is akin to entering a fistfight with one hand tied behind your back. We must integrate the practice of medicine to include all methods if we are serious about maintaining the health of our people.

The tools are there, so why not take advantage of all of them and not just some?

Besides having more options, you have more flexibility. Your approach to a patient can change, based upon what the problem is how serious it is. If you break your arm, for example, you will first turn to traditional medicine to set the bone and splint it. Afterwards, however, you might add other approaches to strengthen your immune system to speed the healing process. This method of treating the whole patient is termed "Holistic Medicine". In holistic medicine, we emphasize the need to look at multiple aspects of health, including the physical, nutritional, emotional, lifestyle and social. This practice helps you recover from the mental stress associated with your injury as well as the physical.

Don't forget the part that spirituality plays in the recovery from an injury or illness. For many, it is an important component to the support necessary to foster the healing process. Studies show that those cancer patients with a positive attitude obtained through spiritual means survive longer and have a better quality of life.

Never underestimate the power of positive thinking and spiritual peace when considering the health of your loved ones. Remember that you, as the medical caregiver, will be in charge of their emotional well-being as well as their physical health.

I say this not to endorse a specific religion, philosophy or ritual, but to encourage you to reach inside yourself. There is an inner strength there that many folks don't know they have. If you have what it takes to be an effective medic, it will be most apparent in a crisis. If you're medical prepared, you'll already be halfway there. Consider it just another weapon you'll want in your medical arsenal.

If we ever enter truly bad times, we will have to do a lot of improvising. If the bad times last long enough, our stockpiled drugs will eventually run out. Unless we have the skill and equipment to distill essential oils from plants, they will run out also. Only by applying ourselves to the practice of integrated medicine, incorporating all of the various healing options available to us, will we be likely to weather the aftermath of a societal storm.

What, then, is my message to my colleagues in every medicial discipline? Simply that both alternative and traditional medical professionals should have respect for and encourage cooperation with each other. Both have much to contribute. Each should be willing to learn about the other and incorporate all that is useful from every possible avenue. Together, they can work to ensure a healthy society in good times or bad.

WILDERNESS MEDICINE VS. LONG TERM SURVIVAL MEDICINE

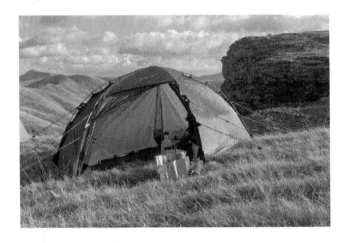

Wilderness Medicine

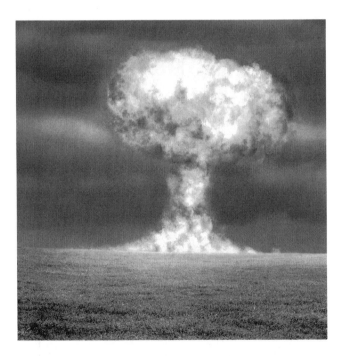

Long Term Survival Medicine

What is wilderness (sometimes called outdoor) medicine? I define it as medical care rendered in a situation where modern care, training and facilities are not readily available. Wilderness medicine would involve medical care rendered during wilderness hikes, maritime expeditions, and sojourns in underdeveloped countries. There is no shortage of excellent books on this subject, some of which I mention in the reference section towards the end of this book.

The basic assumption in emergency medicine is that trained doctors and modern hospitals exist, but are unavailable at the time that medical care is required (perhaps for a significant period of time). You, as temporary caregiver, will be responsible for stabilizing the patient. That means not allowing the injury or illness to get worse.

Your primary goal will be the evacuation of the patient to modern medical facilities, even though they might be hundreds of miles away from the location of the patient. Once you have transferred your patient to the next highest medical resource, your responsibility to the sick or injured individual is over, and you can go on your way. Emergency Medical Technicians or former military corpsman will recognize this strategy as "Stabilize and Transport".

Although principles of wilderness medicine have saved many lives, this approach is different from what I would call "long-term survival" or "collapse" medicine". In a societal collapse, there is no access to modern medical care, and there is no potential for such access in the foreseeable future. As President Harry Truman used to say, "The buck stops here".

As a result of this turn of events, you go from being a temporary first-aid provider to being the caregiver at the end of the line. You are now the highest medical resource left, regardless of whether you have a medical diploma or not.

This fact will lead you to make adjustments to your medical strategy. You are now responsible for the care of the patient from beginning to end. As such, if you want to be successful in your new position, you will have to obtain more knowledge and training than you have now. You will also need more supplies, if you intend to maintain the well-being of your family or survival community, you will have to plan in depth to deal with their potential medical needs.

Medical training and education for non-physicians can include wilderness medical classes, Emergency Medical Technician and even Military Medical Corps training. These courses presuppose that you are rendering care in the hope of later transporting your patient to a working clinic, emergency room or field hospital. As I said previously, "Stabilize and Transport". If you can make the commitment, this training is very useful to have; it's much more likely that you'll experience a short term deficit of medical assistance than a long term one.

Despite this, you must plan for the possibility that you will be completely on your own one day. That includes medically, so the way you think must be modified for a day when intensive care units and emergency rooms are going to be inaccessible. You won't have the luxury of passing the sick or injured individual to a formally trained provider, so you must learn how to diagnose and treat medical problems and you must expect to be there from start to finish.

You will also have to understand how to treat certain chronic medical conditions. Even a paramedic, for example, is unlikely to know how to deal with an abscessed tooth or a thyroid condition. Many of these conditions are treated with drugs and high technology that may no longer be available.

Therefore, you must learn methods that will work in a power-down scenario; you may even have to reach back to older strategies that modern medicine might consider obsolete. Using a combination of prevention, improvisation, and prudent utilization of supplies, you should be able to treat the grand majority of problems you will face in a power-down scenario.

Although all of this might seem daunting, I'm not trying to scare you. In fact, I hope to impart enough information in this handbook to make you more confident. That confidence will come as a result of having planned for both short term disasters and long term ones. When you know what to do in any scenario, you will feel that quiet resolve that comes with the knowledge that you can do the job. You'll be up to the challenge before you, and you'll know it.

THE IMPORTANCE OF COMMUNITY

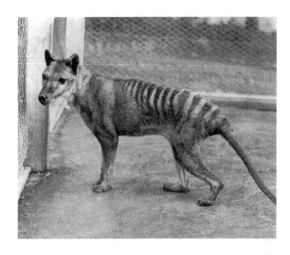

Let's suppose that a calamity has occurred, and you have survived. The power grid is down, and is unlikely to be up again for years. You, however, have prudently stored food, medical supplies, farming and hunting equipment, and are safe in your shelter. You are a fine, young, strapping individual with no medical issues and are reasonably intelligent. Unfortunately, you haven't the slightest idea what the first thing is that you should do to ensure your future health and survival.

The very first way to help assure your medical well-being is very basic. Don't be a lone wolf! The forlorn creature in the above photograph is a Thylacine, sometimes called a Tasmanian wolf. Why did I choose this animal instead of a majestic red or gray wolf? I chose it because the Tasmanian wolf is extinct; if you try to go it alone in a long-term disaster situation, you will be too.

The support of a survival group, even if it's just your extended family, is essential if you are to have any hope of keeping it together when things fall apart.

There will be activities that you would find hard to imagine in an austere setting. You will have to stand watch over your property. You will have to lug gallons of water from the nearest water source. You will, eventually, have to chop wood for fuel. Fill up a 5 gallon bucket with water and walk 100 yards with it (after staying up from midnight to four a.m. standing outside your house) and you'll get the feel of what you might have to go through on a daily basis.

Being the sole bearer of this burden will negatively impact your health and decrease your chances of long-term survival. Exhausted and sleep-deprived, you will find yourself an easy target not only for marauding gangs, but marauding bacteria. Your immune system weakens when exposed to long-term stress; you will be at risk for illnesses that a well-rested individual could easily weather, but you can't. Division of labor and responsibility will make a difficult situation more manageable.

You can imagine how much more possible this will be if you have a group of like-minded individuals helping each other. You can't possibly have all the skills needed to do well by yourself, even if you're Daniel Boone.

For example, we are a physician and nurse who are Master Gardeners for our state, ham radio techs, and raise tilapia as a food fish. Sounds like we have some skills, but neither of us have done any carpentry or raised livestock. Neither have we ever been in charge of the security of others. There are those, however, who have done these things, but could use some of the skills we possess.

Put enough people together with differing skills, and you have put together, even in the middle of a city, a village. A village filled with people that will help each other in a crisis. A rugged individualist might be able to eke out a miserable existence in the wilderness alone, but a society can only be rebuilt by a community.

There's no time like the present to communicate, network and put together a group of like-minded people. The right number of able individuals to assemble for a mutual assistance group will depend on your retreat and your resources. The ideal group will have people with diverse skills but similar philosophies. Unless you are already in such a community, you may feel that it is impossible to find and put together a group of people that could help you in times of trouble. Luckily, that isn't the case. There are many online forums that pertain to preparedness, Many, such as the American Preppers Network and the International Preppers

Network have forums that are specific to (U.S.) states or other countries. Start there and I guarantee you will find others like you.

It's not enough to just be in a group, however. The people in that group must have regular meetings, decide on priorities, and set things in motion. Put together Plan A, Plan B, and Plan C and work together to make their implementation successful. Preparedness means having a plan; have several plans in place for different turns of events. Keep lines of communication open so that all your group members are kept informed.

Practice What You Preach

We mentioned the importance of community in a grid-down environment, but there is another essential part of preparedness. This part is rarely part of the planning process, even for the most self-reliant individual: To optimize your health PRIOR to any catastrophe occurring. If you, as medical caregiver, do not set the example of good health and fitness, how can you expect anyone else to? It's time to practice what you preach.

To do this, you must accomplish the following goals:

- Maintaining a normal weight for your height and age
- Eating a healthy diet
- Maintain good hygiene
- Keeping physically fit
- Eliminating unhealthy habits (smoking, etc.)
- Managing chronic medical issues in a timely fashion

It's important to "tune up" any chronic medical problems that you might currently have. You'll want to have that blood pressure under control, for example. If you have a bum knee, you might consider getting it repaired surgically so that you can function at maximum efficiency if times get tough. Those with poor eyesight might consider having corrective procedures such as LASIK performed to obtain the perfect vision that would be so useful in a survival situation. Use modern technology while it is available. Improve your chances of doing well if, God forbid, it ever becomes inaccessible.

Dental problems should also be managed before bad times make modern dentistry unavailable. Remember how your last toothache affected your work efficiency? If you don't work to achieve all of the above goals, your preparations will be useless.

In a collapse situation, you will be building shelters, walking long distances to find food, tending fires, and many other activities that will test you physically. Getting fit now will prepare you to accept those challenges. Also, doctors say to eat well and exercise for a reason; make sure you get good nutrition and watch those calories. This doesn't mean that you have to run marathons. Even just a daily walk around the block is going to help keep you active and mobile.

This philosophy is pertinent for your mental health and acuity as well. You can't go for long without food and water, but many people will go without a new thought for years on end. Just doing crossword puzzles or reading a newspaper will help keep your mind sharp. Remember that a mind is a terrible thing to waste. Don't waste yours.

If you have bad habits, work to eliminate them. If you damage your heart and lungs by smoking, for example, how will you be able to function in a situation where your fitness and stamina will be continually tested? If you drink alcohol in excess, how can you expect anyone to trust your judgment in critical situations? The same goes for recreational drugs.

Paying careful attention to hygiene is also an important factor for your success in times of trouble. Those who fail to maintain sanitary conditions in their retreat will have a difficult time staying healthy. Infections that are usually seen only in underdeveloped countries will become commonplace. As such, an essential part of your supply storage will be simple items such as soap and bleach.

These two basic strategies, fostering community and practicing preventive medicine/fitness, will take you a long way in your journey to preparedness. They don't cost anything to speak of, and will give you the best chance of succeeding if everything else fails.

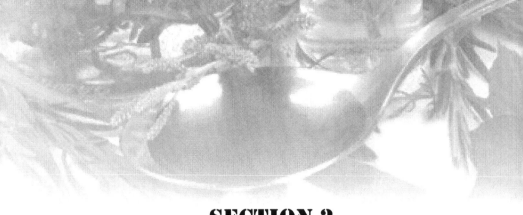

SECTION 2

✚ ✚ ✚

BECOMING A MEDICAL RESOURCE

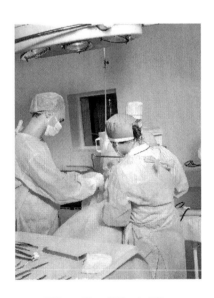

What You Won't Have

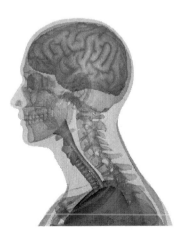

What You Will Have

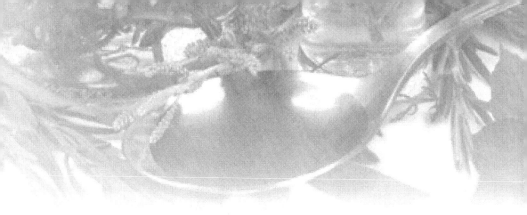

THE SURVIVAL MEDIC

I n a long-term survival situation, it will be an extremely fortunate family or group that has a physician or other formally trained medical professional among its members. When there is no doctor, someone in your group should be assigned the responsibilities of group medic. That person will make the difference between success and failure for a community under duress.

Some people feel that becoming a healthcare provider is a daunting task, and it certainly will be a challenge to accumulate adequate medical stores and obtain the medical knowledge necessary to be effective. Those who will step up and take responsibility for the medical well-being of their loved ones will be special individuals, with a special mission.

If you have been chosen to pick up the flag, your first assignment is to get some training. Some of it will be book learning, and some will be hands-on; the more you learn, the more comfortable you will be in your new role.

Start by studying basic first aid and have a good book on family medicine in your library. A good approach would be to learn as much anatomy and physiology as possible. Anatomy is the blueprint of the body, and physiology is the operating manual. With a working knowledge of these two subjects, you're in a better position to understand disease and injury. This is essential for you to become a successful medic for your group.

Don't forget alternative disciplines such as herbalism. When the commercial medicines run out, you will need a good base of knowledge about plants in your backyard that may have medicinal benefits. Many times, the medic will cultivate favorite herbs specifically for the purpose of having them available in times of trouble.

The most important asset needed to become a competent healthcare provider for your group is just having common sense. A sensible person with good medical supplies, a few medical books and a willingness to learn will be an effective medical resource.

It helps to have a calm demeanor, as sick or injured people take comfort from a focused and level-headed caregiver. Another useful attribute of a good medic is the dedication to teach other members of his/her group some of the skills that he/she learned. One person can't be everywhere at once, and the basics aren't that hard to teach. Cross-training is extremely important, as the medic may, one day, need a medic!

Confidentiality is another important factor to success as a medical resource. You will have to interview your group members so that you'll have all the information you need to keep them healthy. Sometimes that information includes things that your patient doesn't want to be made public. You must never disclose anything that would make others see you as untrustworthy. If you don't have the trust of the community you serve, your effectiveness drops significantly.

There is one last essential characteristic of the successful medic: Self-preservation! This may sound strange to you, but you are an indispensable resource to your entire group. If you place yourself frequently in harm's way, you will eventually find yourself as the patient more often than you or anyone else would like.

Always assess the scene of an injury to determine if you can care for the victim without placing yourself in undue danger. You must abolish all threats; if someone has a gunshot wound, it stands to reason that there's a guy with a gun out there! Always remember that you do a disservice to your survival community by becoming the next casualty.

THE STATUS ASSESSMENT

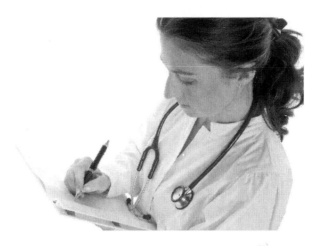

The first thing that the survival medic should perform in preparation for a collapse situation is a status assessment. A number of questions must be asked and answered:

What Will Your Responsibilities Be?

It goes without saying that, as group medic, you will be responsible for the medical well-being of your survival community. But what does that mean? It means that, as well as being the Chief Medical Officer, that you will be:

Chief sanitation officer: It will be your duty to make sure that sanitary conditions at your camp or retreat don't cause the spread of disease among the members. This will be a major issue in an austere setting, and will cause the most medical issues in any survival group.

Some of your responsibilities will relate to latrine placement and construction, others will relate to the supervision of appropriate filtering and sterilization of water. Assurance of proper cleaning of food preparation surfaces will also be very important, as will be the maintenance of good personal and group hygiene.

In areas of extreme climate, it is important to ensure that all members have adequate shelter. Careful attention to these details will be part of a preventative program that will keep your family or community healthy.

Chief dental officer: Medical personnel in wartime or in remote locations report that patients arriving at Sick Call complained of dental problems as much as medical problems. Anyone who has had a bad toothache knows that it affects concentration and, certainly, work efficiency. You will need to know how to deal with dental issues (toothaches, broken teeth, lost fillings) if you are going to be an effective medic. Part of your planning will be the accumulation of appropriate dental supplies.

Chief counselor: It goes without saying that any societal collapse would wreak havoc with peoples' mindsets. You will have to know how to deal with depression and anxiety as well as cuts and broken bones. You will have to sharpen your communication skills as much as your medical skills. A good healthcare provider also understands, as mentioned earlier, the importance of confidentiality in all their patient contacts.

Medical quartermaster: You've done your job and accumulated medical and dental supplies, but when do you break them out and use them? When will you dispense your limited supply of antibiotics, for example? In a collapse situation, these items will no longer be produced, due to the complexity of their manufacture. Careful monitoring of precious supply stock and usage will give you an idea of your readiness to handle medical emergencies for the long term.

Medical Archivist: You are in charge of writing down the medical histories of the people in your group. This record will be useful to remember all the medical conditions that your people have, their allergies, and medications that they might be taking. If your community is large, it would be almost impossible to memorize all of this information.

Also, your histories of the treatments you have performed on each patient are important to put into writing. One day, you might not be there to render care; your archives will be a valuable resource to the person that is in charge when you're not available. Until that day, however, these histories must remain confidential.

Medical education resource: You can't be in two places at once, and you will have to make sure that those in your group have some basic medical knowledge. It's important that they can take care of injuries or illness while you're away. Also, providing all members an education in preventing injuries and infectious disease will give you a head start towards having a healthy survival community.

These responsibilities are many, but may be modified somewhat by the makeup of your group. If you have a pastor or other clergy in your group, they can take some of the burden of psychological counseling away from you. If you have someone skilled in engineering, water treatment, or waste disposal, they might be able to use their knowledge to help maintain sanitary conditions at the retreat, or assure healthy filtered water. Be sure to take whatever help you can get.

What Scenario Are You Preparing For?

It's important to accumulate medical supplies and knowledge that will work in any collapse situation, but what are you actually expecting to happen? Your preparations should be modified to fit the particular situation that you believe will cause modern medical care to be unavailable. There are many possible scenarios that could cause times of trouble, and each of them requires some specialized planning. Your readiness to deal with the most likely illnesses or injuries will increase your effectiveness exponentially.

If you feel that we are on the verge of an economic collapse, you probably believe that the reliable transport of food from farms to the public will no longer exist (nobody is paying the truckers). In that case, malnutrition will be rampant. Your responsibility as medic would be to make sure that your group's food storage includes everything required to give good nutrition. Stockpiling vitamin supplements, commercial or natural, would be a good strategy in this situation. Even if not taken daily, vitamin supplements may be helpful in preventing **diseases caused by** deficiencies.

Knowledge of what nutrients are present in local plant life will be useful. Take the following historical example: In the 1500s, a Spanish exploration party was dying of scurvy (Vitamin C deficiency) in the middle of a pine forest. Native Americans came upon them and took pity on their situation. They walked to the nearest pine tree and picked some green pine needles. They made a tea out of them and nursed the Spaniards back to health. They knew that pine needles were rich in Vitamin C. That knowledge will be useful for you, as well.

Are you concerned about civil unrest? In that case, tailor your supplies and training to equip you to deal with possible traumatic injuries. Stock up on bandages and antiseptics. Other specialized equipment such as splints and blood clotting agents would be necessary in this circumstance.

Many people are concerned about the possibility of a pandemic. If you're worried about a "super flu" descending on your area, stock up on masks and gloves as well as antiviral drugs. Figure out a quarantine strategy and how to put together a sick room that will decrease exposure to healthy family members.

How about a nuclear reactor meltdown? To take this to extremes, perhaps you live near an army base, a large city or a nuclear plant and you're concerned about a terrorist group setting off a nuclear bomb. In that scenario, you'll have to know how to protect your group from radiation, and how to build an effective shelter. You'll want medications like Potassium Iodide to counteract some of the long-term effects of radiation on the thyroid gland.

So, you can see that your supplies and training change somewhat, depending on the course of events. Discuss these scenarios with your family or community, and plan accordingly.

How Many People Will You Be Responsible For?

Your store of medical supplies should correlate well with the number of persons that you will be responsible for. If you have stockpiled 5 treatment courses of antibiotics, it might be enough for a couple or a sole individual, but it will go fast if you are taking care of 20 people.

Remember that most of those people will be out performing tasks that they aren't used to doing. They will be making campfires, chopping wood and toting gallons and gallons of water. You'll see more injuries like sprains and strains, fractures, lacerations, and burns among those people if they are forced to perform activities of daily survival.

It only makes sense to accumulate as many supplies as you possibly can. You might wind up dealing with more survivors than you expected; in reality, you almost certainly will, so you can never have too many medical supplies. The biggest mistake that the survival medic will make is the underestimation of the number of people that will appear on their doorstep in times of trouble. Make allowances for more people than you currently expect.

Don't be concerned that you have too much stored away. Any "excess" items will always be highly sought after for barter purposes. You might spend your money on buying physical silver and gold, but you won't be able to set a broken bone or wrap a sprained ankle with "precious" metals. Food and medical items will be more valuable than mining stocks in hard times. Don't become complacent just because you have a closet full of bandages; they will be used more quickly than you think.

The bottom line is simple: Always have more medical items on hand than you think are sufficient for the number of people in your group.

What Special Needs Will You Have To Care For?

The special issues you will deal with depend on who is in your group. The medical needs of children or the elderly are different from an average adult. Women have different health problems than men. You will have to know if group members have a chronic condition, such as asthma or diabetes. Failure to take things like this into account could be catastrophic. For example, would you be prepared if you found out a group member required adult diapers AFTER a calamity occurs?

Be certain to interview all of your group members, so that you won't be surprised that this person has thyroid problems, or that person has high blood pressure. All of these variables will modify the supplies and medical knowledge you must obtain. Encourage those with special needs to stockpile materials that will help keep them well. Encourage them to have a frank discussion with their physician and obtain extra drug prescriptions in case of emergency (and have them filled in advance).

What Physical Environment Will You Live In?

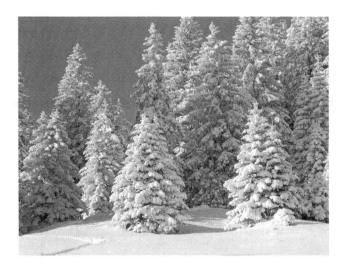

Is your retreat is a cold climate? If so, you will need to know how to keep people warm and how to treat hypothermia. If you're located in a hot climate, you will need to know how to treat heat stroke. Is your environment wet and humid? People who are chronically wet generally don't stay healthy, so you will have to have a strategy to keep your group members dry. Are you in a dry, desert-like environment? If you are, you will have to provide strategies for providing lots of clean water.

Some people live in areas where all of the above conditions exist at one point or another during the year. These considerations might even be a factor in where you would choose to live if a collapse situation is imminent.

How Long Do You Expect To Be The Sole Medical Resource?

Some catastrophes, such as major damage from tornadoes or hurricanes, may limit access to medical care for a relatively short period of time. A societal breakdown, however, could mean that there is no availability of advanced medical care for the foreseeable future.

The longer you will be the healthcare resource for your group, the more supplies you will have to stockpile and the more varied those supplies should be. If the catastrophe means a few weeks without medical care, you probably can get away without, for example, equipment to extract a diseased tooth. If it's a true long-term collapse, however, that equipment will be quite important. Spend some time thinking about all the possible medical issues you might face as the end of the line caregiver for your family. Prepare a plan of action to handle each one. Remember to plan for issues that may occur further down the road, such as birth control issues for a daughter who has not yet reached puberty.

How Do You Obtain The Information You Will Need To Be An Effective Healthcare Provider?

A good library of medical, dental, survival and nutritional books will give you the tools to be an effective medic. Even if you were already a doctor, let's say a general practitioner, you would need various references to learn how to perform surgical procedures that you ordinarily would send to the local surgeon. If you're a surgeon, you would need references to refresh your knowledge of the treatment of diabetes. Even the most resourceful homesteader can't know everything!

Luckily, medical reference books are widely available, with tens of thousands on sale at online auction sites like EBay or retail sites like Amazon.com on any given day. Often, they are deeply discounted. If money is tight, many libraries have a medical section and many local colleges have their own medical library.

Don't ignore online sources of information. Take advantage of websites with quality medical information; there are thousands of them. By printing out information you believe will be helpful to your specific situation, you will have a unique store of knowledge that fits your particular needs. I recommend printing this information out because you never know; one day, the internet may not be as accessible as it is today.

The viral video phenomenon, at sites like YouTube, has thousands of medically oriented films on just about every topic. They range from suturing wounds to setting a fractured bone to extracting a damaged tooth. You will have the benefit of seeing things done in real time. To me, this is always better than just looking at pictures.

The number of medical resources is almost endless; take advantage of them. I have compiled a list of reference books and useful videos at the back of this book. Review them and consider adding them to your library.

How Do You Obtain Medical Training?

There are various ways to get practical training. Almost every municipality gives you access to various courses that would help you function as an effective healthcare provider.

EMT (Emergency Medical Technician) Basic: This is the standard for providing emergency care. The courses are set out by the U.S. Department of Transportation, and are offered by many community colleges. The course length is usually several hundred hours.

I know that this represents a significant commitment of time and effort, but it is the complete package short of going to medical or nursing school for four years. You will receive an overview of anatomy and physiology, and an introduction to the basics of looking after sick or injured patients.

These programs are based around delivering the patient to a hospital as an end result. As medical facilities may not be accessible in the aftermath of a disaster, these classes may not be perfect for a long-term survival situation; nevertheless. you will still learn a lot of useful information and I highly recommend them.

It should be noted that there are different levels of Emergency Medical Technician. EMT-Basic is the primary course of study, but you can continue your studies and become a Paramedic. Paramedics are taught more advanced procedures, such as placing airways, using defibrillators, and placing intravenous lines. In remote areas, they might even take on the roles of physicians and nurses to give injections, place casts or stitch up wounds. These skills are highly pertinent during a disaster.

Most of us will not have the time and resources to commit to such an intensive course of training. For most of us, a Red Cross First Responder or CERT (Community Emergency Response Team) course is the ticket. These programs cover a lot of the same subjects (albeit in much less detail) and would certainly represent a good start on your way to getting trained. The usual course length is 40-80 hours. A number of community outreach groups also offer the course.

Of course, the American Heart Association and others provide standard CPR (cardio-pulmonary resuscitation) courses and everyone should take these, whether or not they will have medical responsibility in times of trouble.

There are a number of "specialty" courses provided by private enterprises which might be helpful. Wilderness EMT/Tactical EMT courses are programs meant to teach medical care in a potentially hostile environment. Sometimes, they have a prerequisite of at least EMT-Basic.

There are many wilderness "schools" out there, however, that will offer some practical training to non-medical professionals that might be useful in difficult times. At the very least, they are cognizant that such a scenario could exist and that your goal of transporting the patient to modern medical facilities might not be a valid option. It pays to research the schools that provide this training, as the quality of the learning experience probably varies.

LIKELY MEDICAL ISSUES YOU WILL FACE

It is important to tailor your education and training to the probable medical issues you will have to treat. In an austere or post-collapse setting, it might be difficult to predict what these might be. Therefore, it's helpful to examine the statistics of those who provide medical care in underdeveloped areas. With this information, you will be able to determine what medical supplies will be needed and prepare yourself for the probable emergencies you'll face.

Looking at one healthcare provider's experience over an extended time in a remote area is a good way to identify likely medical issues for the collapse medic. It wouldn't be unusual to see the following:

Trauma

- Minor Musculoskeletal injuries (sprains and strains)
- Minor trauma (cuts, scrapes)
- Major traumatic injury (fractures, occasional knife and/or gunshot wounds)
- Burn injuries (all degrees)

Infection

- Respiratory infections (pneumonia, bronchitis, influenza, common colds)
- Diarrheal disease (sometimes in epidemic proportions)
- Infected wounds
- Minor infections (for example, urinary infections, "pinkeye")
- Sexually transmitted diseases
- Lice, Ticks, Mosquitos and the diseases they carry

Allergic reactions

- Minor (bees, bed bugs or other insect bites and stings)
- Major (anaphylactic shock)

Dental

- Toothaches
- Broken or knocked-out teeth
- Loss fillings
- Loose crowns or other dental work

Womens' Issues

- Pregnancy
- Miscarriage
- Birth control

A short aside here: If you have purchased this volume, you probably have done some research into collapse scenarios which could lead to society unraveling. You have probably been given a great deal of advice as to what to do in this situation or that, but you have never been given this advice:

If you want to be fruitful, don't multiply; at least in the early going of a major collapse.

It should be clear that you are going to need all of your personnel at 110% efficiency. Anyone who has been pregnant knows that there may be a "glow" associated with it, but you sure aren't at peak performance. Even those who are well-prepared for just about any disaster often forget that pregnancies happen, and don't plan ahead for them. When a member of your family or group is unexpectedly with child, you may find it difficult to be mobile when you need to be. As well, your manpower supply, especially in a small family, has taken a big hit.

Pregnancy is relatively safe these days, but there was a time in the not too distant past where the announcement of a pregnancy was met as much with concern as joy. Complications such as miscarriage, postpartum bleeding and infection took their toll on women, and you must seriously plan to prevent pregnancy, at least until things stabilize. Condoms are fine, but will become brittle after two or three years.

Consider taking the time to learn about natural methods of birth control, such as the Natural Family Planning method. This is a simple method that predicts ovulation by taking body temperatures, and is relatively effective. A discussion of this method and other options will take place later in this book.

Don't misunderstand me: I am not saying that you should not rebuild our society and follow your personal or religious beliefs. I just want you to understand that your burden, in a collapse, will be heavier if you don't plan for every possibility.

MEDICAL SKILLS YOU WILL WANT TO LEARN

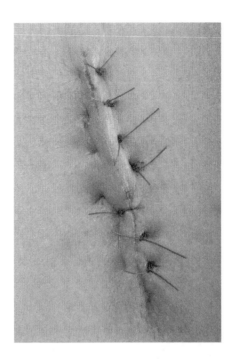

A very reasonable question for an aspiring medic to ask is "What exactly will I be expected to know?" The answer is: As much as you're willing to learn! Using the previous list of likely medical issues will give you a good idea what skills you'll need. You can expect to deal with lots of ankle sprains, colds, cuts, rashes, and other common medical issues that affect you today. The difference will be that you will need to know how to deal with more significant problems, such as a leg fracture or other traumatic injury. You'll also need to know what medical supplies will be required and how to follow your patient's status until they are fully recovered. Here are the skills that an effective medic will have learned in advance of a long-term survival situation:

- Learned how to take vital signs, such as pulses, respiration rates and blood pressures.
- Learned how to place wraps and bandages on injuries

- Learned how to clean an open wound
- Learned how to treat varying degrees of burns
- Learned the indications for use of different medications, essential oils and alternative therapies. As well, know the dosages, frequency of administration, and side effects of those substances. You can't do this on your own; you'll need resources such as the Physician's Desk Reference. This is a weighty volume that comes out yearly and has all the information you'll need to use both prescription and non-prescription drugs. Also consider purchasing a good book on home remedies and alternative therapies as well.
- Learned how to perform a normal delivery of a baby and placenta.
- Learned how to splint, pad and wrap a sprain, dislocation, or fracture.
- Learned how to identify bacterial infectious diseases (such as Strep throat, etc.)
- Learned how to identify viral infectious diseases (such as influenza, etc.)
- Learned how to identify parasitic/protozoal infectious diseases (such as Giardia, etc.)
- Learned how to identify and treat head, pubic, body lice, and ticks
- Learned how to identify venomous snakes and treat the effects of their bites
- Learned how to identify and treat various causes of abdominal, pelvic and chest pain
- Learned how to treat allergic reactions and anaphylactic shock
- Learned how to identify and treat sexually transmitted diseases
- Learned how to evaluate and treat dental disease (replace fillings, treat abscesses and perform extractions)
- Learned how to identify and treat skin disease and rashes
- Learned how to care for the bedridden patient (treating bedsores, transport considerations)
- Learned basic hygiene, nutrition and sanitary practices (this couldn't be more important)
- Learned how to counsel the depressed or anxious patient (you will see a lot of this in times of trouble)
- Learned how to insert an IV (EMT classes teach this),
- Learned how to place sutures in a wound.

Actually, more important that knowing how to suture is knowing WHEN to suture. Most wounds that will occur in a power down situation will be dirty wounds, and closing such an injury will lead to bacteria being locked into the tissues, causing infection. See our discussion on this topic later in this book.

Perhaps the most important skill to obtain is how to prevent injuries and illnesses. You will spend much of your time observing simple things, such as whether your people are appropriately dressed for the weather. You will be required to enforce the use of hand and eye protection during work sessions. Learn to recognize situations that place your family at risk, and you will avoid many of the problems that can crop up.

I know, this is a lot to absorb, but don't feel that learning this information is impossible, or that you can't be of benefit if you only learn some of the above. The important thing to do is to learn at least enough to treat some of the more common medical issues. Once you've learned the basics, you'll be able to take care of 90% of the problems that are brought before you in times of trouble. After that, any additional information you learn will just make you even more effective as a medical resource. Knowledge gives you power: The power to keep everyone as healthy as possible.

MEDICAL SUPPLIES

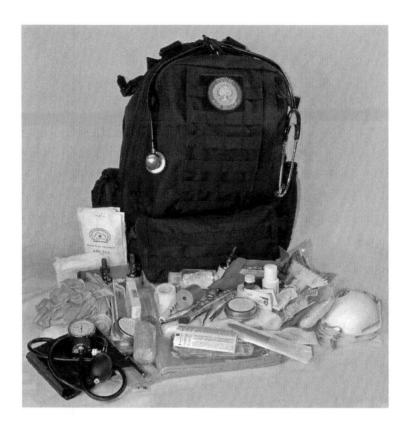

For anyone to do their job properly, they'll need the right equipment. Imagine a carpenter having to use a steak knife as a saw, or a hunter using a pea shooter instead of a rifle. The same goes for the medic. The successful healthcare provider has spent a lot of time and energy (and some money) on accumulating a good amount and variety of medical supplies. The more the better, since you don't know how long you might have to function without access to modern medical care.

It's important to note that the value of many medical supplies depends largely on the knowledge and skill that the user has obtained through study and practice.

A blood pressure cuff isn't very useful to someone who doesn't know how to take a blood pressure. Concentrate on first obtaining items that you can use effectively, and then purchase more advanced equipment as your skills multiply.

Don't forget that many items can be improvised; a bandanna may serve as a triangular bandage, an ironing board as a stretcher or thin fishing line and a sewing needle might be useful as suturing equipment. A careful inspection of your own home would probably turn up things that can be adapted to medical use. Look with a creative eye and you'll be surprised at the medical issues you are already equipped to deal with.

Sterile Vs. Clean

A significant factor in the quality of medical care given in a survival situation is the level of cleanliness of the equipment used. You may have heard of the terms "sterile" and "clean", but do you have more than a vague idea of what they mean?

When it comes to medical protection, "sterility" means the complete absence of microbes. Sterile technique involves hand washing with special solutions and the use of sterile instruments, towels, and dressings. When used on a patient, the area immediately around these items is referred to as a "sterile field". The sterile field is isolated and closely guarded to prevent contact with anything that could allow micro-organisms to invade it.

To guarantee the elimination of all organisms, a type of pressure cooker called an "autoclave" is used for instruments, towels, and other items that could come in contact with the patient. All hospitals, clinics, and medical offices clean their equipment with this device. Having a pressure cooker as part of your supplies will allow your instruments to approach the level of sterility required for, say, minor surgical procedures.

Of course, it may be very difficult to achieve a sterile field if you are in an extremely austere environment. In this case, we may only be able to keep things "clean". Clean techniques concentrate on prevention by reducing the number of microorganisms that could be transferred from one person to another by medical instruments or other supplies. Meticulous hand washing with soap and hot water is the cornerstone of a clean field.

In most survival settings, this may be as good as it gets, but is that so bad? With regards to wound care, there is very little research that compares clean vs. sterile technique. In one study, an experiment was conducted in which one group of patients had their wounds was cleaned with sterile saline solution, the other group with tap water. Amazingly, the infection rate was 5.4% in the tap water group as opposed to 10.3% in the sterile saline group. Another study revealed no difference in infection rates in wounds treated in a sterile fashion as opposed to clean technique. Therefore, I usually recommend clean, drinkable water to treat most wounds.

To maintain a clean area, certain chemicals are used called "disinfectants". Disinfectants are substances that are applied to non-living objects to destroy microbes. This would include surfaces where you would treat patients or prepare food. Disinfection does not necessarily kill all bugs and, as such, is not as effective as sterilization, which goes through a more extreme process to reach its goal. An example of a disinfectant would be bleach.

Disinfection removes bacteria, viruses, and other bugs and is sometimes considered the same as "decontamination". Decontamination, however, may also include the removal of noxious toxins and could pertain to the elimination of chemicals or radiation. The removal of non-living toxins like radiation from a surface would, therefore, be decontamination but not disinfection.

It's useful to know the difference between a disinfectant, an "antibiotic", and an "antiseptic". While disinfectants kill bacteria and viruses on the surface of non-living tissue, antiseptics kill microbes on living tissue surfaces. Examples of antiseptics include Betadine, Chlorhexidine (Hibiclens), Iodine, and Benzalkonium Chloride (BZK).

Antibiotics are able to destroy microorganisms that live inside the human body. These include drugs such as Amoxicillin, Doxycycline, Metronidazole, and many others. We'll discuss these in detail later in the book.

Medical Kits

Most commercial first aid kits are fine for the family picnic or a day at the beach, but we will talk about serious medical stockpiles here.

There are four levels of medical kits that we will identify. The first kit is a personal carry or individual first aid kit, sometimes called an IFAK. Every member of a group can carry this lightweight kit; it allows, in most cases, treatment of some common medical problems encountered in the wilderness or when traveling.

In some military services, the IFAK or personal carry kit is useful to the medic as a source of supply. If a squad member is injured, the medic will first use items, as needed, from the wounded soldier's kit. This is a resource multiplier and allows the corpsman to carry more advanced medical equipment in their pack.

The second kit listed below is the "nuclear family bag": This kit is mobile, with the items fitting in a standard large backpack, and will suffice as a medical "bug-out" bag for a couple and their children. It is, in my opinion, the minimum amount of equipment that a head of household would need to handle common emergencies in a long-term survival situation.

The third kit is a "medic at camp" kit, one that the person responsible as medical resource for the group would be expected to maintain in an expedition camp. The fourth kit is the "community clinic", or everything that a skillful medic will have stockpiled for long term care of his/her survival family or group.

Don't feel intimidated by the sheer volume of supplies in the clinic version; it would be enough to serve as a reasonably well-equipped field hospital. Few of us have the resources or skills to purchase and effectively use every single item. If you can put together a good nuclear family bag, you will have accomplished quite a bit.

IFAK or Personal Carry Kit

1   Cold pack/Hot pack
1   4" Ace wrap
1   6" Israeli bandage or other compression bandage
1   2g Celox or Quikclot hemostatic agent
1   Tourniquet
2   Eye pads

1   Pack (2 sheets) steri-strips
1   Nail scissors
1   Straight hemostat clamp 5"
1   2-0 Nylon suture
1   Super glue or Medical glue packet
1   Tweezers
1   LED penlight
1   Stainless steel bandage scissors 7.25"
20 1" x 3" Adhesive bandages
10 2" x 3" Adhesive bandages
2   Sterile ABD dressings 5" x 9"
5   Pairs Large Nitrile Gloves
20 Non-sterile 4" x 4" gauzes
10 Sterile 4" x 4" gauze
5   Non-Stick sterile dressing 3" x 4"
1   Roller gauze sterile dressing
1   Mylar solar blanket
1   Cloth Medical Tape 1" x 10 yds.
1   Duct tape 2" x 5 yds.
1   Triangular Bandage with safety pins
1   Tube of triple antibiotic ointment
10 Alcohol wipes
10 Povidone-iodine (Betadine) wipes
6   BZK anti-microbial wipes
2   Packets burn gel
6   Sting Relief Towelettes
1   Hand sanitizer

For all of the following, quantities will be dependent on the number of people you are medical responsible for.

Nuclear Family Kit

First aid reference book
Antibacterial Soap/Hand Sanitizers
Antiseptic/Alcohol Wipes
Gauze pads-(4" x 4" – sterile and non-sterile)
Gauze rolls-(Kerlix, etc.)

MEDICAL SUPPLIES

Non-Stick pads (Telfa brand)
Triangular bandages or bandannas
Safety Pins (large)
Israeli Battle Dressings or other Compression bandage
Adhesive Band-Aids (various sizes/shapes)
Large absorbent pads (ABD or other brand)
Medical Tape – (Elastoplast, Silk, Paper varieties), 1 inch, 2 inch
Duct Tape
Tourniquet
Moleskin or Spenco Second Skin Blister kit
Cold Packs/Heat Packs (reusable if possible)
Cotton Eye Pads, Patches
Cotton Swabs (Q-tips), Cotton Balls
Disposable Nitrile Gloves (hypoallergenic)
Face Masks (surgical and N95)
Tongue Depressors
Bandage Scissors (all metal is best)
Tweezers
Magnifying Glass
Headlamp or Penlight
Kelly Clamp (straight and curved)
Needle Holder
2-0, 4-0 Nylon Sutures
Scalpel or field knife
Styptic pencil (stops bleeding from superficial cuts)
Hemostatic Agents (Celox or Quikclot powder)
Saline Solution (liter bottle or smaller)
Steri-Strips/butterfly closures - thin and thick sizes
Survival Sheet/Solar Blanket
Thermometer (rectal or ear)
Antiseptic Solutions (Betadine, Hibiclens, etc.)
3% Hydrogen Peroxide
Benzalkonium Chloride wipes
Rubbing Alcohol
Witch Hazel
Antibiotic Ointment
Sunblock

Lip balms
Insect Repellant
1% Hydrocortisone Cream
2.5% Lidocaine cream (local anesthetic)
Acetaminophen/Ibuprofen/Aspirin
Benadryl (Diphenhydramine)/Claritin (Loratadine)
Imodium (Loperamide)
Pepto-Bismol (Bismuth Subsalicylate)
Rid shampoo (for lice)
Oral Rehydration Packs (or make it from scratch)
Water Purification Filter or Tablets
Gold Bond foot powder
Silvadene Cream (burns)
Oral Antibiotics (discussed later)
(or natural equivalents of all the above)
Birth Control Accessories (condoms, birth control pills, cervical caps, etc.)
Herbal Teas, Tinctures, Salves, and Essential Oils
Neti pot (use only with sterile solutions)

Dental Tray:

Cotton pellets and rolls
Dental mirror
Dental pick, toothpicks
Dental floss
Clove bud oil (anesthetic for toothache)
Zinc Oxide (make a paste with oil of cloves and you get temporary dental cement), or...
Commercial dental kits (Den-Temp, Cavit)
Hank's Solution (used to preserve viability in knocked-out teeth)
4-0 Chromic suture
Needle holder
Actcel oral hemostatic agent (stops dental bleeding)
Extraction equipment (forceps and elevators)
Gloves, masks, and eye protection

The "Medic Bag at Away Camp" List

(medical supplies for an expedition)

All of the above in larger quantities, plus:

Medical reference book(s)
Combat Dressings (Israeli bandages aka The Emergency Bandage)
"Bloodstopper" dressing (inexpensive multipurpose dressing)
Tourniquet
Quik-Clot or Celox dressings (these are impregnated with substances that help stop bleeding) or larger powder packs
Extra-Large gauze dressings
Neck Collar
Eye cups, eye wash
Ammonia inhalants
Head Lamp
Slings
Splints
Irrigation Syringes (60-100 ml is good)
Needle Syringes (various sizes- 20 gauge, 6 ml is common)
Surgical scissors (Mayo or Metzenbaum)
Needle holders and clamps, (enough to do basic minor surgery)
Scalpel and disposable blades (lots)
Emergency Obstetric Kit (comes as a pack)
Vicryl or Silk 0, 2-0, 3-0, 4-0, 5-0 suture material (very fine nylon fishing line will work if necessary)
Suture removal tray
Fels-Naptha/Zanfel Soap (poison ivy, oak and sumac)
Saline solution- for irrigation of open wounds (sterilized water will also be acceptable for this purpose)
Cidex solution-for cleaning instruments
1% or 2% (Lidocaine) (local anesthetic in injectable form-prescription medication)
More varied supply of antibiotics (prescription)
Zofran (for nausea and vomiting-prescription)
Tramadol (stronger pain medicine- prescription)

Oral Rehydration powder (this can be made using home ingredients as well)
Epinephrine (Epi-pen, prescription injection for severe allergic reactions)
Rid lotion/Nix Shampoo (lice/scabies treatment)
Terconazole cream (antifungal)
Fluconazole 100 or 150mg tablets (prescription antifungal)
Wart removal cream/ointment/solution
Hemorrhoid cream/ointment
Tincture of Benzoin ("glue" for bandages)

The Community Clinic Supply List

(long-term care center)

All of the above in larger quantities, plus:

Extensive medical library
Treatment Table
Plaster of Paris cast kits (to make casts for fractures) (4in/6in)
Naso-oropharyngeal airway tubes (to keep airways open)
Nasal airways (keeps airways open)
Resuscitation facemask with one-way valve
Resuscitation bag (Ambu-bag)
Endotracheal tube/ Laryngoscope (allows you to breathe for patient)
Portable Defibrillator (expensive)
Blood Pressure cuff (sphygmomanometer)
Stethoscopes
CPR Shield
Otoscope and Ophthalmoscope – (instruments to look into ears and eyes)
Urine test strips
Pregnancy test kits
Sterile Drapes (lots)
Air splints (arm/long-leg/short-leg)
SAM splints
Scrub Suits
IV equipment, such as:
Normal Saline solution
Dextrose and 50% Normal Saline IV solution

IV tubing sets - maxi-sets + standard sets
Blood collection bags + filter transfusion sets
Syringes 2/5/10/20 mL
Needles 20/22/24 gauge
IV kits 16/20/24 gauge
Paper tape (1/2 in/1in) for IV lines
IV stands (to hang fluid bottles)
Saline Solution for irrigation (can be made at home as well)
Foldable stretchers
Paracord (various uses)
Triage tags (for mass casualty incidents)

Surgery Tray items (extremely ambitious):

Sterile Towels
Sterile Gloves
Mayo scissors
Metzenbaum scissors
Small and medium needle holders
Bulb syringes (for irrigating wounds during procedures)
Assorted clamps (curved and straight, small and large)
Scalpel handle and blades (sizes 10, 11, 15) or disposable scalpels
Emergency Obstetric Kit (includes cord clamps, bulb suction, etc.)
Obstetric forceps (for difficult deliveries)
Uterine Curettes (for miscarriages, various sizes), Uterine "Sound" (checks depth of uterine canal)
Uterine Dilators (to open cervix; allows removal of dead tissue)
Bone saw (for amputations)
Sutures, such as:
Vicryl; 0, 2-0, 4-0 (absorbable)
Chromic 0, 2-0 (absorbable)
Silk, Nylon or Prolene 0, 2-0, 4-0(non-absorbable)
Surgical staplers and staple removers
Chest decompression kits and drains – various sizes for collapsed lungs
Penrose drains (to allow blood and pus to drain from wounds)
Foley Catheters – Sizes 18, 20 for urinary blockage
Urine Bags

Nasogastric tubes (to pump a stomach)
Pressure Cooker (to sterilize instruments, etc.)

Additional Prescription Medications

Medrol dose packs, oral steroids
Salbutamol inhalers for asthma/severe allergic reactions
Antibiotic/anesthetic eye and ear drops
Oral Contraceptive Pills
Metronidazole, oral antibiotic and anti-protozoal
Amoxicillin, oral antibiotic
Cephalexin, oral antibiotic
Ciprofloxacin, oral antibiotic
Doxycycline, oral antibiotic
Clindamycin, oral antibiotic
Trimethoprin/Sulfamethoxazole, oral antibiotic
Ceftriaxone, IV antibiotic
Diazepam IV sedative to treat seizures
Diazepam in oral form, sedative
Alprazolam, oral anti-anxiety agent
Oxytocin (Pitocin) IV for post-delivery hemorrhage
Percocet, (oxycodone with paracetamol/acetaminophen),
strong oral pain medicine
Morphine Sulfate or Demerol, strong injectable analgesic

I'm sure there is something that I might have missed, but the important thing is to accumulate supplies and equipment that you will feel competent using in the event of an illness or an injury. Some of the above supplies, such as stretchers and tourniquets, can be improvised using common household items.

It should be noted that many of the advanced items are probably useful only in the hands of an experienced surgeon, and could be very dangerous otherwise. Also, some of the supplies would be more successful in their purpose with an intact power grid. These items just represent a wish list of what I would want if I were taking care of an entire community.

MEDICAL SUPPLIES

You should not feel that the more advanced supply lists are your responsibility to accumulate alone. Your entire group should contribute to stockpiling medical stores, under the medic's coordination. The same goes for all the medical skills that I've listed. To learn everything would be a lifetime of study; truthfully, more than even most formally-trained physicians can accomplish. Concentrate on the items that you are most likely to use regularly and be grateful of assistance from others in your group.

NATURAL REMEDIES

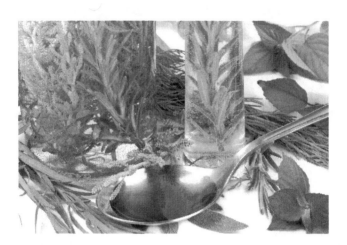

There are many issues that are best handled with the support of the latest technology and modern equipment and facilities. Sure enough, I've just spent the last chapter telling you to stock up on all sorts of high-tech items (even defibrillators!) and, indeed, many of these things are indispensable when it comes to dealing with certain medical conditions.

Unfortunately, you probably will not have the resources needed to stockpile a massive medical arsenal. Even if you are able to do so, there are concerns. Your supplies will last only a certain amount of time. Depending on the number of people you are medically responsible for, you can expect to be shocked at the rapidity with which precious medications and other items are used up. Tough decisions may have to be made when you're down to that last box of gauze.

One solution is to grossly overstock on commonly used medical supplies, but this, too, is costly and doesn't really solve your problem; even large stockpiles will eventually dry up when dealing with the common injuries and illnesses you'll encounter.

Therefore, you must devise a strategy that will allow you to provide medical care for the long run. You will need a way to produce substances that will have a medical benefit without having a pharmaceutical factory at your disposal.

Well, there is another option: The plants in your own backyard or nearby woods. You might ask yourself, "I thought I was reading a book by a medical doctor. What's all this plant stuff?"

To answer this, we have to look at the history of medicine. Physicians have occupied different niches in society over the ages, from priests during the time of the pharaohs, to slaves and barbers in imperial Rome and the dark ages, and artists during the Renaissance.

All of these ancient healers used different methods but there was one thing they had in common: They knew the use of natural products for medicinal purposes. If they needed more of a particular plant than occurred in their native environment, they cultivated it. They learned to make teas, tinctures and salves containing these products and how best to use them to treat illness. If modern medical care is no longer available one day, we will have to take advantage of their experience.

A little more history: Salicin is a natural pain reliever found in the under bark of Willows, Poplar and Aspen trees. In the 19th century, we first developed a process to commercially produce Aspirin (Salicylic acid) from these trees commonly found in our environment. Today, most artificially produced drugs involve many different chemicals in their manufacture. To make Insulin or Penicillin, for example, so many chemicals are used that it would be impossible to reproduce the process in any type of collapse scenario. Do we even know what effect all of these ingredients have on our health? Despite this, we have gone so far in our ability to synthesize medications that we use them far too often in our treatment of patients.

Even organized medicine is realizing that we are too fast and loose in our utilization of pharmaceuticals. Medical journals now call for physicians to focus on prevention instead of reflexively reaching for the prescription pad. Additionally, doctors are now being asked to prescribe only one drug at a time, due to the interactions that multiple medications have with each other. There's a new skepticism regarding the conventional medical wisdom that might just be good for your health.

Having said this, not all pharmaceuticals are bad. Indeed, some of them can save your life. Natural remedies, however, should be integrated into the medical toolbox of anyone willing to take responsibility for the well-being of others. Why not use all the tools that are available to you? At one point or another, the medicinal herbs and plants you grow in your garden may be all you have.

Natural substances can be used in "home remedies" via several methods, including:

Teas: A hot drink made by infusing the dried, crushed leaves of a plant in boiling water.

Tinctures: Plant extracts made by soaking herbs in a liquid (such as water, grain alcohol, or vinegar) for a specified length of time, then straining and discarding the plant material. (also known as a "decoction").

Essential Oils: Liquids comprised of highly concentrated aromatic mixtures of natural compounds obtained from plants. These are typically made by a process called "distillation"; most have long shelf lives.

Salves: Highly viscous or semisolid substances used on the skin (also known as an ointment, unguent, or balm).

Some of these products may also be ingested directly or diluted in solutions. A major benefit of home remedies is that they usually have fewer side effects than commercially produced drugs.

It is the obligation of the group medic to obtain a working knowledge of how to use and, yes, grow these plants. Consider learning the process of distillation to obtain concentrated versions for stronger effect. A number of reference books are available on the subject of natural remedies, and are listed in the appendix of this book.

Another alternative therapy thought by some to boost immune systems and treat illness is colloidal silver. Colloidal silver products are made of tiny silver particles, silver ions or silver combined with protein, all suspended in a liquid — the same type of precious metal used in jewelry and other consumer goods. Silver compounds were used in the past to treat infection before the development of antibiotics.

Recently, laboratory studies at the department of Biochemistry at Jiaxing College, China, have shown that "silver-containing alginate fibers" provide a sustained release of silver ions when in contact with samples of wound drainage, and are "highly effective against bacteria".

Colloidal silver products are usually marketed as dietary supplements that are taken by mouth. Colloidal silver products also come in forms that can be applied to the skin, where they are thought to improve healing by preventing infection. Silver use is only rarely associated with ill effects. Continuous use of silver, especially internally, may result in a condition known as Argyria. This rare condition causes your skin to turn blue; this is mostly a cosmetic concern.

Ionic silver (Ag^+) and silver particles in concentration has been shown to have an antimicrobial effect in certain laboratory studies. Physicians use wound dressings containing silver sulfadiazine (Silvadene) to help prevent infection. Wound dressings containing silver are being used more and more often due to the increase in bacterial resistance to antibiotics. A study under the aegis of the Hull York Medical School found that a dressing containing silver was "a highly effective and reliable barrier to the spread of MRSA into the wider hospital." As a topical agent, Silvadene has been used on burn injuries for many years.

Less evidence is available from traditional medical sources regarding ionic silver solutions for internal use. Silver ions are like members of the lonely hearts club; they are a positively charged particle desperately looking to bond with another, negatively charged, ion. Once inside our body, they have a willing partner in the form of the Chloride from the salt in our cells. Once bonded as Silver Chloride, the compound is essentially inert. As such, it is uncertain how much benefit that internal use of silver will give you.

Despite this, there are many prominent naturopaths who strongly support its use. Home ionic silver generators are available for sale at a multitude of online sites.

Silver proteins bind organic materials to silver, so they are a different product than ionic silver. Unless suspended in a gelatin base, they have a tendency to drop to the bottom of the bottle (this is called "precipitation") and lose their antimicrobial effect. The larger the Silver particle, the more likely this will occur. In rare circumstances, the presence of organic matter in the compound could lead to contamination.

It is important to understand that colloidal effectiveness is determined by particle surface area. Large silver particles tend to precipitate, so smaller is better. Since the smallest silver particles do not require a protein to be suspended in the solution, more surface area will be available for anti-microbial effects. If you pursue this option, seek out products that will produce the smallest silver particles in their solutions.

I have to mention that the FDA has banned colloidal silver sellers from claiming any therapeutic or preventive value. As a result, the product is a dietary supplement by status, and cannot be marketed as preventing or treating any illness. More evidence is warranted before silver becomes a standard part of the medical arsenal.

ESSENTIAL OILS

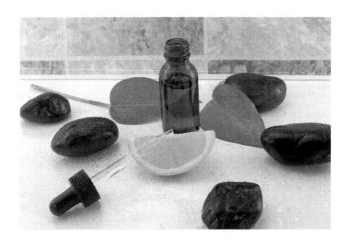

As a medical doctor/registered nurse practitioner team, we received conventional medical training at university hospitals while getting our degrees. Since that time, however, we have explored various alternative methods of healing; this is not to replace our education, but as a supplement and as an additional tool in the medical woodshed.

Nature may, one day, be our pharmacy. The knowledge of herbal remedies had been passed down generation after generation. In a situation where regular medications are no longer produced, it is imperative to learn the medicinal benefits of plants that you can grow in your own garden.

One class of alternative remedies that are commonly used is Essential Oils. These substances are called "essential" because they capture the "essence" of the plant. Unlike cooking oils, such as olive or corn, these oils are less fixed and more volatile. That means that they tend to evaporate easily, unlike the "fixed" oils, which don't evaporate even in high temperatures. As such, essential oils are popular in aromatherapy. Essential oils are distilled from whole plant material, not a single ingredient; therefore, every oil has multiple uses.

Although you might not realize it, you've been using essential oils all your life. You've no doubt used them in soaps, furniture polishes, perfumes and ointments. Previous generations of conventional physicians commonly included them in their medical bags. Indeed, many standard medical texts of the past were, essentially, treatises on how to use these products.

Although it only takes a few leaves of peppermint to make a tea, it takes 5 pounds of leaves to make 1 ounce of essential oil. One source states that it takes an entire acre of peppermint to produce just 12 pounds. The same source says that 12,000 rose blossoms are required to produce a tablespoon of rose oil! These concentrated versions are the ones you see marketed in small, dark bottles. As such, they should be used sparingly. A reference book or two about essential oils would be a great addition to your medical library; see the medical reference section in the back of this book.

You might be surprised to learn that the Food and Drug Administration only requires 10% essential oil in the bottle to be considered "Pure Essential Oil". Beware of claims of FDA certification; the FDA has no certification or approval process for these products.

Essential oils are produced by plants to serve as either an attractant to pollinator insects (hence their strong fragrance) or as a repellant against invading organisms, from bacteria to animal predators. These substances usually contain multiple chemical compounds, making each plant's essential oil unique. Oils may be produced by leaves, bark, flowers, resin, fruit or roots. For example, Lemon oil comes from the peel, Lavender oil from flowers, and Cinnamon oil from bark.

Some plants are sources of more than one essential oil, dependent on the part processed. Some plant materials produce a great deal of oil; others produce very little. The strength or quality of the oil is dependent on multiple factors, including soil conditions, time of year, sub-species of plant, and even the time of day the plant is harvested.

The manufacture of essential oils, known as "extraction", can be achieved by various methods:

- **Distillation Method**: Using a "still" like old-time moonshiners, water is boiled through an amount of plant material to produce a steam that travels through cooled coils. This steam condenses into a "mixture" of oil and water (which doesn't really mix) from which the oil can be extracted.

- **Pressing Method:** The oils of citrus fruit can be isolated by a technique which involves putting the peels through a "press". This works best only with the oiliest of plant materials, such as orange skins.
- **Maceration Method**: a fixed oil (sometimes called a "carrier" oil) or lard may be combined with the plant part and exposed to the sun over time, causing the fixed oil to become infused with the plant "essence". Oftentimes, a heat source is used to move the process along. The plant material may be added several times during the process to manufacture a stronger oil. This is the method by which you obtain products such as "garlic-infused olive oil". A similar process using flowers is referred to as "Enfleurage".
- **Solvent Method:** Alcohol and other solvents may be used on some plant parts, usually flowers, to release the essential oil in a multi-step process.

As each essential oil has different chemical compounds in it, it stands to reason that the medicinal benefits of each are also different. As such, an entire alternative medical discipline has developed to find the appropriate oil for the condition that needs treatment. The method of administration may differ, as well. Common methods are:

1. **Inhalation Therapy:** This method is also known as "aromatherapy". Add a few drops of the essential oil in a bowl of steaming water (distilled or sterilized), and inhale. This method is most effective when placing a towel over your head to catch the vapors. Many people will place essential oils in potpourri or use a "diffuser" to spread the aroma throughout the room; this technique probably dilutes any medicinal effects, however.
2. **Topical Application:** The skin is an amazing absorbent surface, and using essential oils by direct application is a popular method of administration. The oil may be used as part of a massage, or directly placed on the skin to achieve a therapeutic effect on a rash or muscle. Before considering using an essential oil in this manner, always test for allergic reactions beforehand. Even though

the chemical compounds in the oil are natural, that doesn't mean that they couldn't have an adverse effect on you (case in point: poison ivy).

A simple test involves placing a couple of drops on the inside of your forearm with a cotton applicator. Within 12-24 hours, you'll notice a rash developing if you're allergic. Mixing some of the essential oil with a fixed or "carrier" oil such as olive oil before use is a safer option for topical use. Another concern, mostly with topically-applied citrus oils, is "phototoxicity" (an exaggerated burn response to sun exposure).

I have some reservations about whether applying an essential oil on the skin over a deep organ, such as the pancreas, will really have any specific effect on that organ. It is much more likely to work, however, on the skin itself or underlying muscle tissue.

3. **Ingestion:** Direct ingestion is unwise for many essential oils, and this method should be used with caution. Most internal uses of an essential oil should be of a very small amount diluted in at least a tablespoon of a fixed oil such as olive oil. Professional guidance is imperative when considering this method. You can always consider a tea made with the herb as an alternative. This is a safer mode of internal use, although the effect may not be as strong.

Essential oils have been used as medical treatment for a very long time, but it's difficult to provide definitive evidence of their effectiveness for several reasons. Essential oils are difficult to standardize, due to variance in the quality of the product based on soil conditions, time of year, and other factors that we mentioned above. An essential oil of Eucalyptus, for example, may be obtained from Eucalyptus Globulus or Eucalyptus Radiata and have differing properties as a result. These factors combine to make scientific study problematic.

In most university experiments, a major effort is made to be certain that the substance tested caused the results obtained. As essential oils have a number of different chemicals and are often marketed as blends, which ingredient was the cause of the effect? If the oil is applied with massage, was the effect related to the oil itself or the therapeutic benefit of the physical therapy?

The majority of studies on essential oils have been conducted by the cosmetics and food industries; some have been conducted by individuals or small companies. Standard studies for medicinal benefit are usually performed by the pharmaceutical industry, but they generally have little interest in herbal products. This is because they have few options in patenting these products.

Therefore, serious funding is hard to find because of the limited profit potential. Despite this, essential oils have various reported beneficial effects, mainly based on their historical use on many thousands of patients by alternative healers. Although there are many essential oils, a number of them are considered mainstays of any herbal medicine cabinet. Here are just some:

Lavender Oil: An analgesic (pain reliever), antiseptic, and immune stimulant. It is thought to be good for skin care and to promote healing, especially in burns, bruises, scrapes, acne, rashes and bug bites. Lavender has a calming effect, and is used for insomnia, stress and depression. It has been reported effective as a decongestant through steam inhalation. Lavender oil may have use as an antifungal agent, and may be used for Athlete's foot or other related conditions.

Eucalyptus Oil: An antiseptic, antiviral, and decongestant (also an excellent insect repellent), Eucalyptus oil has a "cooling" effect on skin. It also aids with respiratory issues and is thought to boost the immune system. Consider its use for flus, colds, sore throats, coughs, sinusitis, bronchitis, and hay fever. When exposure is expected, it has been reported to have a preventative effect. Eucalyptus may be used in massages, steam inhalation, and as a bath additive. Although eucalyptus oil has been used in cough medicine, it is likely greatly diluted and should not be otherwise ingested in pure form.

Melaleuca (Tea Tree) Oil: Diluted in a carrier oil such as coconut, Tea Tree oil may be good for athlete's foot, acne, skin wounds, and even insect bites. In the garden, Tea Tree oil is a reasonable organic method of pest control. In inhalation therapy, it is reported to help relieve respiratory congestion. Studies have been performed which find it effective against both Staphylococcus and fungal infections. Some even recommend a few drops in a pint of water for use as a vaginal douche to treat yeast. Tea Tree oil may be toxic if used in high concentrations, around sensitive areas like the eyes, or ingested.

Peppermint Oil: This oil is said to have various therapeutic effects: antiseptic, antibacterial, decongestant, and anti-emetic (stops vomiting). Peppermint oil is applied directly to the abdomen when used for digestive disorders such as irritable bowel syndrome, heartburn, and abdominal cramping. Some herbalists prescribe Peppermint for headache; massage a drop or two to the temples as needed. For sudden abdominal conditions, achy muscles or painful joints, massage the diluted oil externally onto the affected area. As mentioned previously, definitive proof of topical application effects on deep organs is difficult to find.

Lemon Oil: Used for many years as a surface disinfectant, it is often found in furniture cleaners. Many seem to think that this disinfecting action makes it good for sterilizing water, but there is no evidence that it is as effective as any of the standard methods of doing so, such as boiling. Lemon oil is thought to have a calming effect; some businesses claim to have better results from their employees when they use it as aromatherapy. Don't apply this oil on the skin if you will be exposed to the sun that day, due to increased likelihood of burns.

Clove Oil: Although thought to have multiple uses as an anti-fungal, antiseptic, antiviral, analgesic, and sedative, Clove oil particularly shines as an anesthetic and antimicrobial. It is marketed as "Eugenol" to dentists throughout the world as a natural pain killer for toothaches. A toothpaste can be made by combining clove oil and baking soda; when mixed with zinc oxide powder, it makes an excellent temporary cement for lost fillings and loose crowns. Use Clove oil with caution, as it may have an irritant effect on the gums if too much is applied.

Arnica Oil: Arnica oil is used as a topical agent for muscle injuries and aches. Thought to be analgesic and anti-inflammatory, it is found in a number of sports ointments. As a personal aside, I have tested this oil on myself, and found it to be effective though not very long lasting. Frequent application would be needed for long term relief. Although some essential oils are excellent as aromatherapy, Arnica oil is toxic if inhaled.

Chamomile Oil: There are at least two versions of Chamomile oil, Roman and German. Roman Chamomile is a watery oil, while German

Chamomile seems more viscous. Both are used to treat skin conditions such as eczema as well as irritations due to allergies. Chamomile oil is thought to decrease gastrointestinal inflammation and irritation, and is thought have a calming effect as aromatherapy, especially in children.

Geranium Oil: Although variable in its effects based on the species of plant used, Geranium oil is reported to inhibit the production of sebum in the skin, and may be helpful in controlling acne. Some believe that it also may have hemostatic (blood-clotting) properties, and is often recommended for bleeding from small cuts and bruising. When a small amount of oil is diluted in shampoo, it may be considered a treatment for head lice.

Helichrysum Oil: Thought to be a strong analgesic and anti-inflammatory, Helichrysum is used to treat arthritis, tendonitis, carpal tunnel syndrome, and fibromyalgia as part of massage therapy. It has also been offered as a treatment for chronic skin irritation.

Rosemary Oil: Represented as having multiple uses as an antibacterial, anti-fungal, and anti-parasitic, Rosemary oil is proven to control spider mites in gardens. Use a few drops with water for a disinfectant mouthwash. Inhalation, either cold or steamed, may relieve congested or constricted respiration. Mixed with a carrier oil, it is used to treat tension headaches and muscle aches.

Clary Sage Oil: One of the various chemical constituents of Clary Sage has a composition similar to estrogen, and has been used to treat menstrual irregularities, premenstrual syndrome, and other hormonal issues. It is also believed to have a mild anticoagulant effect, and may have some use as a blood thinner. Clary Sage also is thought to have some sedative effect, and has been used as a calming agent.

Neem Oil: With over 150 chemical ingredients, the Neem tree is referred as "the village pharmacy" in its native India. The majority of Ayurvedic alternative remedies have some form of Neem oil in them. Proven as a natural organic pesticide, we personally use Neem Oil in our vegetable garden. Reported medicinal benefits are too numerous to list here and seem to cover just about every organ system. It should be noted, however, that it may be toxic when the oil is taken internally.

Wintergreen Oil: A source of natural salicylates, Wintergreen oil is a proven anticoagulant and analgesic. About 1 fluid ounce of Wintergreen Oil is the equivalent of 171 aspirin tablets if ingested, so use very small amounts. It may also have beneficial effects on intestinal spasms and might reduce elevated blood pressures.

Frankincense Oil: One of the earliest documented essential oils, evidence of its use goes back 5000 years to ancient Egypt. Catholics will recognize it as the incense used during religious ceremonies. Studies from Johns Hopkins and Hebrew Universities state that Frankincense relieves anxiety and depression in mice (how, exactly, was this determined?). Direct application of the oil may have antibacterial and antifungal properties, and is thought to be helpful for wound healing. As a cold or steam inhalant, it is sometimes used for lung and nasal congestion.

Blue Tansy Oil: Helpful as a companion plant for organic pest control, Blue Tansy is sometimes planted along with potatoes and other vegetables. The oil has been used for years to treat intestinal worms and other parasites. One of its constituents, Camphor, is used in medicinal chest rubs and ointments. In the past, it has been used in certain dental procedures as an antibacterial.

Oregano Oil: An antiseptic, oregano oil has been used in the past as an antibacterial agent. It should be noted that Oregano oil is derived from a different species of the plant than the Oregano used in cooking. One of the minority of essential oils that are safe to ingest, it is thought to be helpful in calming stomach upset, and may help relieve sore throats. Its antibacterial action leads some to use the oil in topical applications on skin infections when diluted with a carrier oil. Oregano Oil may reduce the body's ability to absorb iron, so consider an iron supplement if you use this regularly.

Thyme Oil: Reported to have significant antimicrobial action, diluted Thyme oil is used to cure skin infections, and may be helpful for ringworm and athlete's foot. Thyme is sometimes used to reduce intestinal cramps in massage therapy. As inhalation therapy, it may loosen congestion from upper respiratory infections.

"Thieves' Oil": Many essential oils are marketed as blends, such as "Thieves' Oil". This is a combination of clove, lemon, cinnamon bark, eucalyptus and rosemary essential oils. Touted to treat a broad variety of ailments, studies at Weber State University indicate a good success rate in killing airborne viruses and bacteria. Of course, the more elements in the mixture, the higher chance for adverse reactions, such as phototoxicity.

Some important caveats to the above list should be stated here. Most of the essential oils listed are unsafe to use in pregnancy, and may even cause miscarriage. Also, allergic reactions to essential oils, especially on the skin, are not uncommon; use the allergy test I described earlier before starting regular topical applications.

Even though essential oils are natural substances, they may interact with medicines that you may regularly take or have adverse effects on chronic illness such as liver disease, epilepsy or high blood pressure. Thorough research is required to determine whether a particular essential oil is safe for you.

Having said that, essential oils are a viable option for many conditions. Anyone interested in maintaining their family's well-being should regard them as just another weapon in the medical arsenal. Learn about them with an open mind, but maintain a healthy skepticism about "cure-all" claims.

THE MEDICINAL GARDEN

Planting your own medicinal garden is a prudent way to provide alternatives to modern medicine. Until pharmaceuticals were produced in factories, communities and homesteads had to grow their own "medicine". This common practice was a natural part of the landscape and provided needed remedies for many medical issues. Oftentimes, a community would have a person that served as an herbalist and supervised the cultivation and processing for proper administration.

Growing your own medicinal garden is both rewarding and beneficial; in times of trouble, you will likely have limited access to pharmaceuticals. The learning curve when gardening can be steep, so don't delay planting those medicinal seeds until the situation is critical.

Select a well-drained, sunny area with healthy soil. Although some herbs grow well in shade, most plants need at least 6-8 hours of full sun for proper growth and development. Potting is appropriate for medicinal plants that will need to be transported inside during a cold winter. Water should be provided on a regular basis to allow the soil to stay moist, but not muddy or waterlogged. A small amount of natural mulch is perfect for maintaining an even moisture level in very dry conditions.

Learn about permaculture if you are planting in the ground. This method has many benefits and will reduce your maintenance schedule. Use only organic pest and disease control. A soapy spray of 1 tablespoon of neem oil, 1 teaspoon of Dr. Bronner's lavender, tea tree or peppermint castile soap and, optional, a few drops of tea tree essential oil to 4-8 cups of water makes a great disease and natural pest control. Spray foliage in the late afternoon every 5-7 days or after a heavy rain.

The medicinal plants you select should match your climate as best as possible. However, with certain plants, you may be able to grow warmer climate plants by protecting them from the cold with greenhouses or using row covers. This will expand the range of medicinal plants you may choose to grow either in pots or around your homestead.

Here is a short list of medicinal plants you may consider growing, with the most common part of the plant used and some of the conditions it might help:

Aloe Vera (Aloe Vera)- the slimy gel from the leaf is used to heal and soothe rashes, burns, and cuts.

Angelica (Angelica archangelica)- rhizomes (similar to a root but actually an underground stem) are used to make a tinctures and infusions to treat menstrual cramps.

Arnica (Arnica montana)- flowers and rhizomes are utilized to produce very dilute concentrations of an ointment or salve. Used only externally on unbroken skin for bruises or joint/muscle pain.

Calendula (Calendula officinalis)- the flowers are used fresh or dried and made into teas, tinctures, creams and salves. Drinking a calendula tea or tincture may relieve menstrual cramps, intestinal cramps and decrease the severity of a viral infection. Rich in antioxidants, it can be applied externally as a cream, salve, infused oil or as a compress. Calendula reduces pain and heals minor burns, cuts, rashes, ringworm and athlete's foot. Cool, weak tea compresses may heal an eye infection; apply to the affected eye three times daily.

Cayenne (Capsicum frutescens)- the pepper (fruit) is used dried and powdered, infused in oil, as a tincture or mixed in a salve or cream. Good externally for arthritic pain as a salve, cream or infused oil, and may be useful to stop mild to moderate bleeding in a wound if direct pressure is not working. Cayenne can be taken internally as a tincture or as a pinch of powder in a tea for to treat intestinal infections, sore throat pain or gas. Some consider it a broad spectrum antibacterial.

Chamomile, German (Matricaria recutita)- the flowers are used in teas, salves and creams. Internally taken, the tea is known to be relaxing and is used as an antispasmodic (relaxes muscle tension and cramps). It also helps with insomnia, calms an upset stomach, and may also reduce the inflammation of joints. Externally used, cooled tea compresses or eye-wash may treat eye infections. Applied to painful rashes, itchy skin, or sore nipples, a poultice (a mass of warmed crushed flowers), cream or salve may relieve and heal skin conditions.

Comfrey (Symphytum officinale)- the leaves, aerial parts, and root are used in creams, salves, infused oils, ointments, poultices and tinctures. Use is limited to external use on unbroken skin only. Common uses for comfrey externally are to help heal broken bones, sprains, strains and bruises. Comfrey may help with acne and reduce scarring.

Echinachea (Echinacea purpurea, augustifolia or pallida)- the flowers and roots are used to produce tinctures, teas, capsules, and pills. It is known to be a strong antibacterial and antiviral due to its immune stimulating effects. Some use it to help reduce allergies, such as hay fever.

Elder (Sambucus nigra)- this tree produces two parts used medicinally: the fresh or dried flowering tops and the berries. A tea, tincture or syrup made of the flowering tops are good for coughs, colds, flu and reducing allergies. Cooking is needed to prevent poisoning from elderberries, which can be used for the same ailments as the flowering tops but are not considered as effective. Wine is commonly made from elderberries.

Witch Hazel (Hamamelis virginiana)- tincture of the bark is used as an astringent to reduce hemorrhoids, stop itching from insect stings.

Feverfew (Tanacetum parthenium)- the fresh or dried aerial parts (stems, leaves and flowers) are used to produce a tea, tincture, capsules or pills. Use the leaves to produce a tea or tincture for the treatment or prevention of migraine headaches and also to reduce fevers. This herb may also help with arthritic conditions. Do not use in combination with blood-thinning medications.

Garlic (Allium sativum)- the fresh cloves are used (crushed) to make a tea, tincture, syrup, or capsules. Garlic may help lower blood pressure, reduce cholesterol, thin the blood to help protect against blood clots, and lower blood sugar levels. It has antibacterial and antiviral properties, which makes it effective for treating both digestive and respiratory infections. It can be applied externally to dress wounds for reduced infection rates. Use with caution if taking blood thinners or antihypertensive medications.

Ginger (Zingiber officinale)- the rhizomes are used to make a tea, essential oil, capsule or tincture. Ginger is excellent for use in digestive disorders. It can help relieve both morning sickness and motion sickness. Some types of food poisoning may be treated effectively with ginger. Ginger may lower blood pressure. It increases sweating, which is beneficial to reduce a fever.

Ginkgo (Ginkgo biloba)- the leaves are the most commonly used part in Western medicine; the dehusked seed, however, is occasionally used in Chinese medicine. The fresh or dried leaves are used to make a tea, tincture or fluid extract. It is typically utilized to help improve memory and circulation. Gingko also has anti-allergenic properties, which makes it helpful to relieve wheezing in asthmatics.

Ginseng, Siberian (Eleutherococcus seticosus)- the roots are used to make a tea, tincture or incorporated into capsules. It is used to reduce the effects of physical stress and mental stress. It stimulates the immune system to help the body fight viruses and bacterial infections.

Goldenseal (Hydrastis canadensis)- the rhizomes are used to produce a tincture, tea, powder or infusion. It is said to be a mild laxative; it also reduces heavy menstrual bleeding. A dilute infusion can be used as eyewash for infections, as a mouthwash for swollen or infected gums, or as an external treatment for psoriasis. Goldenseal is not appropriate for use in pregnancy.

Lavender (Lavendula officinalis)- the fresh or dried flowers are used to produce a tea, tincture, infusion or essential oil. It enhances relaxation and calms nervous conditions, including muscle or intestinal cramps, and loosens tight airways in asthmatics. Applied externally, it is an antiseptic for open wounds and mild burns. It relieves itching and inflammation, and can be used to relieve bug bites and rashes.

Lemon Balm (Melissa officinalis)- the fresh or dried aerial parts are used to produce a juice, tea, tincture, infusion, lotion and salve/cream. It can reduce nervous conditions and cramping, and is useful for anxiety, intestinal cramps, and muscle aches. Lemon balm can relieve cold sores and reduce future outbreaks.

Licorice (Glycyrrhiza glabra)-the dried or fresh root is used to create a tea, fluid extract, tincture, dried juice stick or powder. It is a gentle laxative. It is considered to have anti-inflammatory effects. It helps with canker sores, upset stomach, and acid reflux. This same action also helps it reduce arthritic pain and inflamed joints. Do not take if anemic, have high blood pressure or during a pregnancy.

Peppermint (Mentha piperita)-the fresh or dried aerial parts are used to make a tea, tincture, lotion, capsules and essential oil. The tea or tincture is helpful for digestive problems and may reduce gas, cramps, and diarrhea. As a lotion or diluted essential oil, it helps relieve headaches and migraines when a small amount is applied to the temples in a gentle massage.

Rosemary (Rosmarinus officinalis)-the fresh or dried leaves are used to produce a tea, tincture or essential oil. The tea or tincture can help reduce stress and relieve headaches. Applied as a diluted essential oil or lotion it may relieve sore muscles or joint pain. Do not take the essential oil internally.

Sage (Salvia officinalis)-the fresh or dried leaves are used to make a tea, tincture or fresh leaves are crushed and applied directly to the skin. The fresh crushed leaves are helpful to relieve stings and bug bite irritation. The tea is good to relieve a sore throat, canker sores or sore gums when used as a gargle. Drinking the tea can help reduce menopausal symptoms.

Skullcap (Scutellaria lateriflora)-the fresh or dried aerial parts are used to create an infusion, tincture or capsules. It is said to calm and relax nervous conditions, including insomnia and menstrual pain. The tincture may help relieve headaches.

Senna (Cassia senna or Senna alexandrina)-the fresh or dried pods are used commonly to make a tea. It is a laxative and over-the-counter preparations are available to treat constipation. Senna should be used only in dilute, small dosages. Do not take for more than 10 days.

St. John's Wort (Hypericum perforatum)- the fresh or dried flowering tops are used to make a tea, tincture, cream or infused oil.. Most commonly said to be a relaxant and helpful to treat depression, PMS and menopausal symptoms. The infused oil is useful when applied externally to help with stimulating tissue repair on wounds and burns; it may also may reduce joint and muscle pains. This herb may cause sensitivity to sunlight.

Thyme (Thymus vulgaris)- the fresh or dried aerial parts including leaves are used to produce a tea, tincture, syrup and essential oil. A tea may be helpful for use in treating colds and flu. Syrup made from thyme is a traditional cough remedy. A tincture applied externally may help with vaginal fungal infections. Thyme has been used as a treatment for intestinal worms. Do not use the essential oil during pregnancy

Turmeric (Curcuma longa)-the fresh or dried rhizome is used in a tea, tincture, poultice or powder. It is said to have a strong anti-inflammatory action, and may help with asthma, arthritis and eczema. A beneficial effect on stomach and intestinal cramps is also attributed to this herb. Turmeric has blood thinning properties and should be avoided if taking anti-coagulants. Externally it is useful in treating fungal infections, psoriasis and other itchy rashes and could be utilized as a replacement for hydrocortisone if modern medicines are unavailable. Turmeric may cause stomach upset or heartburn if taken regularly. It may cause sensitivity to sunlight if taken regularly.

Valerian (Valerian officinalis)- the roots and rhizome are used to produce a tea, tincture or powder.. Commonly used to reduce stress, induce relaxation and treat insomnia. It can help relax muscle tension, intestinal cramps and menstrual pain. Do not take with alcohol or if using sleep-inducing medications.

Yarrow (Achillea millefolium)-fresh or dried aerial parts are used to make a tea, tincture, essential oil or a poultice. Yarrow is used externally to heal wounds as a poultice. Traditionally mixed with other herbs in a tea, it may help with colds and flus. Some claim that it reduces menstrual bleeding. There are reports of allergic reactions to Yarrow by some, and it should not be used during pregnancy.

The same issues regarding proof of effectiveness and uncertainty of dosage that we related in the essential oil chapter are relevant for the herbs on this list. Perform your own research into these alternatives and come to your own conclusions. For useful books on herbalism and other medical subjects, go to the reference section at the end of this book.

THE PHYSICAL EXAM

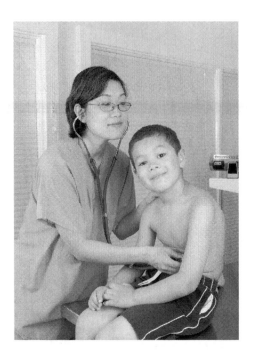

By reading this book, you have made the decision to take responsibility for the medical well-being of your family in the aftermath of a disaster. Therefore, you will have to build a store of knowledge of how to evaluate a patient and make a diagnosis.

You will have to put your (gloved) hands on them and be able to look for physical signs of illness or check out a wound in a systematic manner. Sometimes the problem is obvious in seconds; other times, you will have to examine the entire body to determine the problem. During an exam, always communicate to your patient who you are, what you are doing and why. Remain calm and be very careful about forcing them to move or perform an action that is beyond their capability.

The most basic information is obtained by checking the vital signs. This includes the following;

- **Pulse rate** – this can be taken by using 2 fingers to press on the side of the neck or the inside of the wrist (by the base of the thumb). A normal pulse rate at rest is 60-100 beats per minute. You may choose to feel the pulse for, say, 15 seconds and multiply the number you get by 4 to get beats per minute. A full minute would be more accurate, however. You will find that most people who are agitated from having suffered an injury will have a high pulse rate. This is called "**tachycardia**".

- **Respiration rate** – this is best evaluated for an entire minute to get an accurate reading. The normal adult rate at rest is 12-18 breaths per minute, somewhat more for children. Note any unusual aspects, such as wheezing or gurgling noises. A respiration rate over 20 per minute is a sign of a person in distress, and is known as "**tachypnea**".

- **Blood pressure** – blood pressure is a measure of the work the heart has to do to pump blood throughout the body. You're looking for a pressure less than 140/90 at rest. Blood pressure may be high after extreme physical exertion but goes back down after a short while. Of course, some people have high blood pressure as a medical condition. A very low blood pressure may be seen in a person who has hemorrhaged or is in shock. Instructions on how to take a blood pressure can be found in the chapter on high blood pressure, also called "**hypertension**".

- **Mental status** – You want to know that your patient is alert and, therefore, can respond to questions and commands. Ask your patient what happened. If they seem disoriented, ask simple questions like their name, where they are, or what year it is. Note whether the patient appears lethargic or agitated. Some patients may appear unconscious, but may respond to a spoken command. For example: "Hey! Open your eyes!" If no result, determine if they respond to a stimulus, such as gentle pressure on their breastbone. If they don't, they are termed "unresponsive" and something very serious is going on.

- **Body Temperature** - Take the person's temperature to verify that they don't have a fever. A normal temperature will range from 97.5 to 99.0 degrees Fahrenheit. A significant fever is defined as a temperature above 100.4 degrees Fahrenheit

(38 degrees Celsius). Very low temperatures (less than 95 degrees Fahrenheit (35 degrees Celsius) may indicate cold-related illness, also known as hypothermia. On the opposite hand is heat stroke (hyperthermia), where the temperature may rise above 105 degrees Fahrenheit (40.5 degrees Celsius).

Once you've taken the vital signs and determined that there is no obvious injury, perform a general exam from head to toe in an organized fashion. Touch the patient's skin; is it hot or cold, moist or dry? Is there redness, or is the patient pale? Examine the head area and work your way down. Are there any bumps on their head, are they bleeding from the nose, mouth, or ears? Evaluate the eyes and see if they are reddened and if the pupils respond equally to light.

Have the patient open their mouth and check for redness, sores, or dental issues with a light source and a tongue depressor. Check the neck for evidence of injury and feel the back of the head and neck, especially the neck bones (vertebrae).

Take your stethoscope and listen to the chest. This is called "**auscultation**". Do you hear the patient breathing as you place the instrument over different areas of each lung? Are there noises that shouldn't be there? Practice listening on healthy people to get a good idea of what clear lungs should sound like. Abnormal sounds would include wheezing, gurgles, and crackles. I have included some references to videos that allow you to hear these sounds at the end of this book.

Listen to the heart and see if the heartbeat is regular or irregular in rhythm. Check along the ribs for rough areas that might signify a fracture. Check the armpits (also known as the axilla) for masses. Perform a breast exam by moving your fingers in a circular motion over the breast tissue, starting from the periphery near the axilla and ending at the nipple.

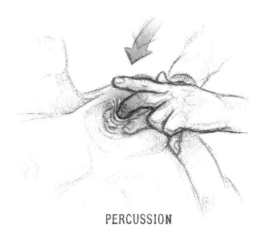

PERCUSSION

Press on the abdomen with your open hand. This is referred to as "**palpation**". Is there pain? Is the belly soft or is it rigid and swollen? Do you feel any masses? Use your stethoscope to listen to the gurgling of bowel sounds. Lack of bowel sounds may indicate lack of intestinal motility; excessive bowel sounds may be seen in some diarrheal disease. Place your open hand on the different quadrants of the abdomen and tap on your middle finger. This is called "**percussion**". The abdomen will sound "hollow" normally, but dull where there might be a mass. Press down on the right side below the rib cage to determine if the liver is enlarged (you won't feel it if it isn't). An enlarged spleen will appear as a mass on the left side under the bottom of the rib cage.

Check along the patient's spine for evidence of pain or injury. Pound lightly with a closed hand on each side of the back below the last rib; this is where the kidneys are, and injury or infection would cause this action to be very painful to the patient.

Check each extremity by feeling the muscle groups for pain or decreased range of motion. Make sure that there is good circulation by checking the color on the tips of the fingers and toes. Poor circulation will make these areas white or blue in color. Check for sensation by lightly tapping with a safety pin. Place your hands on their thighs and ask them to lift up, to check for normal strength and tone. Ask them to grasp your fingers with each hand; then, try to pull your hand away. If you can't, that's good. The strength on each side should be about equal.

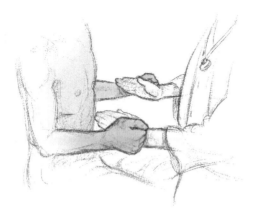

STRENGTH TESTING

Human beings are what we call "bilaterally symmetrical". If you draw a line vertically down the length of their body, each side is essentially the same. This means that, if you are uncertain whether a limb is injured or deformed, you can compare it to the other side.

These are just some basics. Certainly, there's a lot more to a physical exam than what you've just read, but practicing exams on others will give you experience. As time goes by, you'll get the feel of what is normal and what isn't. Once you get the hang of it, your efforts will prepare you for making a diagnosis if we find ourselves without access to modern medical care.

THE MASS CASUALTY INCIDENT

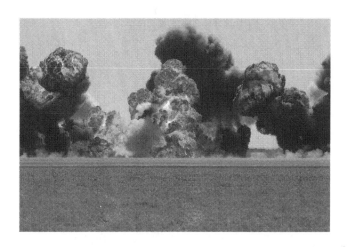

The last section discussed performing a general physical exam. Most of these exams will be unhurried and routine, but, occasionally, you will have to make some quick decisions. For major trauma, it is important to take note of the "golden hour". A victim's chance of survival decreases significantly if not treated within 1 hour of the injury. It gets even worse with every 30 minutes that pass without care.

The responsibilities of a medic in times of trouble will usually be one-to-one; that is, the healthcare provider will be dealing with one ill or injured individual at a time. If you have dedicated yourself to medical preparedness, you will have accumulated significant stores of supplies and some knowledge. Therefore, your encounter with any one person should be, with any luck, within your expertise and resources. There may be a day, however, when you find yourself confronted with a scenario in which multiple people are injured. This is referred to as a **Mass Casualty Incident** (MCI).

A mass casualty incident is any event in which your medical resources are inadequate for the number and severity of injuries incurred. Mass Casualty Incidents (we'll call them "MCIs") can be quite variable in their presentation. They might be:

- Doomsday scenario events, such as nuclear weapon detonations
- Terrorist acts, such as occurred on 9/11 or in Oklahoma City

- Consequences of a storm, such as a tornado or hurricane
- Consequences of civil unrest
- Mass transit mishap (train derailment, plane crash, etc.)
- A car accident with, say, three people significantly injured (and only one ambulance)
- Many others

The effective medical management of any of the above events requires rapid and accurate triage. **Triage** comes from the French word "to sort" ("Trier") and is the process by which medical personnel (like you, survival medic) can rapidly assess and prioritize a number of injured individuals, thereby doing the most good for the most people. Note that I didn't say: "Do the best possible care for EACH individual victim".

Let's assume that you are in a marketplace somewhere in the Middle East or perhaps in your survival village near the border with another (hostile) group. You hear an explosion. You are the first one to arrive at the scene, and you are alone. There are twenty people on the ground, some moaning in pain. There were probably more, but only twenty are, for the most part, in one piece. The scene is horrific.

S.T.A.R.T.

As the first to respond to the scene, medic, you are Incident Commander until someone with more medical expertise arrives on the scene. What do you do? Your initial actions may determine the outcome of the emergency response in this situation. This will involve what we refer to as the 5 S's of evaluating a MCI scene:

- Safety
- Sizing up
- Sending for help
- Set-up of areas
- **START** – Simple Triage And Rapid Treatment

1. **Safety Assessment**: In the Middle East, an insidious strategy on the part of terrorists is the use of primary and secondary bombs. The main bomb causes the most casualties, and the second bomb

is timed to go off or is triggered just as the medical/security personnel arrive.

Many medical professionals wince when I talk about not approaching the injured in a hostile setting. Why am I suggesting that you do NOT immediately go to the nearest victim? Because your primary goal as medic is your own self-preservation; keeping the medical personnel alive is likely to save more lives down the road. Therefore, you do your family and community a disservice by becoming the next casualty.

In the immediate aftermath of the Oklahoma City bombing, various medical personnel rushed in to aid the many victims. One of them was a heroic 37 year old Licensed Practical Nurse who, as she entered the area, was struck by a falling piece of concrete. She sustained a head injury and died five 5 days later.

As you arrive, be as certain as you can that there is no ongoing threat. Do not rush in there until it is certain that you and your helpers are safe entering the area.

2. **Sizing up the Scene:** Ask yourself the following questions:
    *   What's the situation? Is this a mass transit crash? Did a building on fire collapse? Was there a car bomb?
    *   How many injuries and how severe? Are there a few victims or dozens? Are most victims dead or are there any uninjured that could assist you?
    *   Are they all together or spread out over a wide area?
    *   What are possible nearby areas for treatment/transport purposes?
    *   Are there areas open enough for vehicles to come through to help transport victims?

3. **Sending for Help:** If modern medical care is available, call 911 and say (for example): "I am calling to report a mass casualty incident involving a multi-vehicle auto accident at the intersection of Hollywood and Vine (location). At least 7 people are injured and will require medical attention. There may be people trapped in their cars and one vehicle is on fire."

In three sentences, you have informed the authorities that a mass casualty event has occurred, what type of event it was, where it occurred, an approximate numbers of patients that may need care, and the types of care or equipment that may be needed. I'm sure you could do even better than I did above, but you want to inform the emergency medical services without much delay.

If you are the current Incident Commander, get your walkie-talkie or handie-talkie and notify base camp of the situation and what you'll need in terms of personnel and supplies. If you are not medically trained, contact the person who is the group medic. The most experienced medical person who arrives then becomes the new Incident Commander.

4. **Set-Up:** Determine likely areas for various triage levels (see below) to be further evaluated and treated. Also, determine the appropriate entry and exit points for victims that need immediate transport to medical facilities, if they exist. If you are blessed with lots of help at the scene, determine triage, treatment, and transport team leaders.

5. **S.T.A.R.T.:** Triage uses the acronym S.T.A.R.T., which stands for Simple Triage And Rapid Treatment. The first round of triage, known as "primary triage", should be fast (30 seconds per patient if possible) and does not involve extensive treatment of injuries. It should be focused on identifying the triage level of each patient. Evaluation in primary triage consists mostly of quick evaluation of respirations (or the lack thereof), perfusion (adequacy of circulation), and mental status. Other than controlling massive bleeding and clearing airways, very little treatment is performed in primary triage.

Although there is no international standard for this, triage levels are usually determined by color:

Immediate (Red tag): The victim needs immediate medical care and will not survive if not treated quickly (for example, a major hemorrhagic wound/internal bleeding). This person has top priority for treatment.

Delayed (Yellow tag): The victim needs medical care within 2-4 hours. Injuries may become life-threatening if ignored, but can wait until Red tags are treated (for example, open fracture of femur without major hemorrhage).

Minimal (Green tag): Generally stable and ambulatory ("walking wounded") but may need some medical care (for example, broken fingers, sprained wrist).

Expectant (Black tag): The victim is either deceased or is not expected to live (for example, open fracture of cranium with brain damage, multiple penetrating chest wounds).

Knowledge of this system allows a patient marking system that easily allows a caregiver to understand the urgency of a patient's situation. It should go without saying that, in a power-down situation without modern medical care, a lot of red tags and even some yellow tags will become black tags. It will be difficult to save someone with major internal bleeding without surgical intervention.

The above is good to know, but let's go through an example of a mass casualty incident; we'll discuss how you would perform your triage duties.

Primary Triage: MCI scenario

Here's our hypothetical scenario: you are in your village near the border with another (hostile) group. You hear an explosion. You are the first one to arrive at the scene, and you are alone. There are about twenty people down, and there is blood everywhere. What do you do?

Referring back to the 5 S's, let's say that you have already determined the SAFETY of the current situation and SIZED UP the scene. There appears to have been a bomb that exploded. There are no hostiles nearby, as far as you can tell, and there is no evidence of incoming ordinance. Therefore, you believe that you and other responders are not in danger. The injuries are significant (there are body parts) and the victims are all in an area no more than, say, 30 yards.

The incident occurred on a main thoroughfare in the village, so there are ways in and ways out. You have SENT a call for help on your handie-talkie and described the scene, and have received replies from several group members, including a former ICU nurse who is contacting everyone else with medical experience. The area is relatively open, so you can SET UP different areas for various triage categories. Now you can START (Simple Triage And Rapid Treatment).

You will call out as loudly as possible: "I'm here to help, everyone who can get up and walk and needs medical attention, get up and move to the sound of my voice. If you are uninjured and can help, follow me."

You're lucky, 13 of the 20, mostly from the periphery of the blast, sit up, or at least try to. 10 can stand, and 8 go to the area you designated for walking wounded. These people have cuts and scrapes, and a couple of them are limping; one has obviously broken an arm. 2 beaten-up but sturdy individuals join you. By communicating, you have made your job as temporary Incident Commander easier by identifying the walking wounded (Green Tags) and getting some immediate help. You still have 10 victims down.

You then go to the closest victim on the ground. Start right where you are and go to the next nearest victim in turn. In this way, you will triage faster and more effectively than trying to figure out who needs help the most from a distance or going in a haphazard pattern.

Let's cheat just a little and say that you happen to have SMART tags in your pack. SMART tags are handy tickets which allow you to mark a particular triage level on a patient. Once you identify a victim's triage level, you remove a portion of the end of the tag until you reach the appropriate color and place it around the patient's wrist.

You could, instead, use colored adhesive tape, colored markers, or numbers placed on the forehead. If you use numbers:

- Priority 1 is immediate/red (top priority)
- Priority 2 is delayed/yellow
- Priority 3 is minimal/green
- Priority 4 is dead/expectant/black

The number method is used in some other countries; it is useful if you're color blind).

It is important to remember that you are triaging, not treating. The only treatments in START will be stopping massive bleeding, opening airways, and elevating the legs in case of shock. As you go from patient to patient, stay calm, identify who you are and that you're here to help. Your goal is to find out who will need help most urgently (red tags). You will be assessing **RPMs** (Respirations, Perfusion, and Mental Status):

Respirations: Is your patient breathing? If not, tilt the head back or, if you have them, insert an oral airway (Note: in a MCI triage situation, the rule against moving the neck of an injured person before ruling out cervical spine injury is, for the time being, suspended) If you have an open airway and no breathing, that victim is tagged black. If the victim breathes once an airway is restored or is breathing more than 30 times a minute, tag red. If the victim is breathing normally, move to perfusion.

Perfusion: Perfusion is an evaluation of how normal the blood flow or circulation is. Check for a (wrist or neck) pulse and/or press on the nail bed (I sometimes use the pad of a finger) firmly and quickly remove. It will go from white to pink in less than 2 seconds in a normal individual. This is referred to as the **Capillary Refill Time (CRT)**. If there is no pulse or it takes longer than 2 seconds for nail bed color to return to pink, tag red. If a pulse is present and CRT is normal, move to mental status.

Mental Status: Can the victim follow simple commands ("open your eyes", "what's your name")? If the patient is breathing and has normal perfusion but is unconscious or disoriented: Tag red. If they can understand you and follow commands, tag yellow if they can't get up or green if they can. Remember that, as a consequence of the explosion, some victims may not be able to hear you well.

It might be easier to remember all this by just thinking 30 -2- Can Do:

30 (respirations)
2 (CRT)
Can Do (Commands)

If there is any doubt as to the category, always tag the highest priority triage level. Not sure between yellow and red? Tag red. Once you have identified someone as triage level red, tag them and move immediately to the next patient unless you have major bleeding to stop. Any one RPM check that results in a red result tags the victim as red. For example, if someone wasn't breathing but began breathing once you repositioned the airway, tag red, stop further evaluation if not hemorrhaging and move to the next patient. Elevate the legs if you suspect shock.

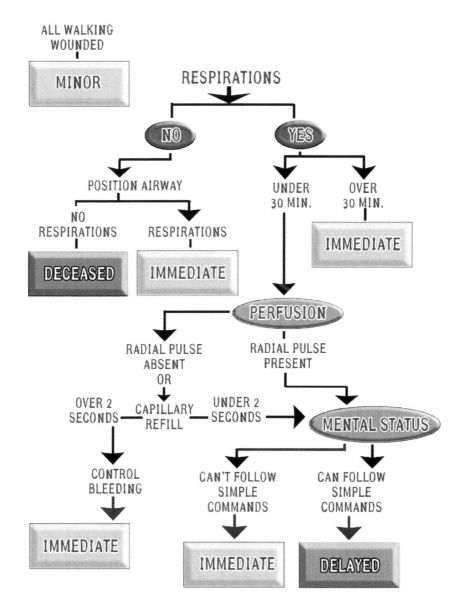

TRIAGE CASCADE

Now, let's return to our mass casualty event. You have identified 8 walking wounded and moved them to a designated area. You have 2 relatively unhurt victims who will assist your triage efforts. Finally, the list below contains your 10 patients on the ground, in order. Read the descriptions and decide the primary triage level; utilize your helpers wisely. We'll discuss how we triaged them in detail in the next section:

1. Male in his 30s, complains of pain in his left leg (obviously fractured), Respirations 24, pulse strong, CRT 1 second, no excessive bleeding.
2. Female in her 50s, bleeding from nose, ears, and mouth. Trying to sit up but can't, respirations 20, pulse present, CRT 1 second, not responding to your commands.
3. Teenage girl bleeding heavily from her right thigh, respirations 32, pulse thready, CRT 2.5 seconds, follows commands.
4. Another teenage girl, small laceration on forehead, says she can't move her legs. Respirations 20, pulse strong, CRT 1 second.
5. Male in his 20s, head wound, respirations absent. Airway repositioned, still no breathing.
6. Male in his 40s, burns on face, chest, and arms. Respirations 22, pulse 100, CRT 1.5 seconds, follows commands.
7. Teenage boy, multiple cuts and abrasions but not hemorrhaging, says he can't breathe, respirations 34, radial pulse present, CRT 2.5 seconds.
8. Female in her 20s, burns on neck and face, respirations 22, pulse present, CRT 1 second, asks to get up and can walk, although with a limp.
9. Elderly woman, bleeding profusely from an amputated right arm (level of forearm), respirations 36, pulse on other wrist absent, CRT 3 seconds, unresponsive.
10. Male child, multiple penetrating injuries, respirations absent. Airway repositioned, starts breathing. Radial pulse absent, CRT 2 seconds, unresponsive.

MCI Scenario Results

On the previous pages, we described a mass casualty incident scene with 20 victims and told you about initial considerations before beginning

START (Simple Triage and Rapid Treatment). You ended up with 10 victims on the ground, 8 walking wounded, and 2 uninjured but unskilled helpers. You moved the walking wounded to a separate area and are now ready to quickly triage the remaining 10 victims.

To review the primary triage categories:

Immediate (Red tag): The victim needs immediate medical care and will not survive if not treated quickly. (for example, a major hemorrhagic wound/internal bleeding) Top priority for treatment.

Delayed (Yellow tag): The victim needs medical care within 2-4 hours. Injuries may become life-threatening if ignored, but can wait until Red tags are treated. (for example, open fracture of femur without major hemorrhage)

Minimal (Green tag): Generally stable and ambulatory ("walking wounded") but may need some medical care. (for example, 2 broken fingers, sprained wrist)

Expectant (Black tag): The victim is either deceased or is not expected to live. (for example, open fracture of cranium with brain damage, multiple penetrating chest wounds)

And here are your triage evaluation parameters (**RPMs**):

Respirations: Is your patient breathing? If not, tilt the head back or, if you have them, insert an oral airway (Note: in a MCI triage situation, the rule against moving the neck of an injured person before ruling out cervical spine injury is, for the time being, suspended) If you have an open airway and no breathing, that victim is tagged black. If the victim breathes once an airway is restored or is breathing more than 30 times a minute, tag red. If the victim is breathing normally, move to perfusion.

Perfusion: Perfusion is an evaluation of how normal the blood flow or circulation is. Check for a radial pulse and/or press on the nail bed (I sometimes use the pad of a finger) firmly and quickly remove. It will go from white to pink in less than 2 seconds in a normal individual. This is referred to as the **Capillary Refill Time (CRT)**. If no radial pulse or it takes longer than 2 seconds for nail bed color to return to pink, tag red. If a pulse is present and CRT is normal, move to mental status.

Mental Status: Can the victim follow simple commands ("open your eyes", "what's your name")? If the patient is breathing and has normal perfusion, but is unconscious or can't follow your commands, tag red. If they can follow commands, tag yellow if they can't get up or green if they can. Remember that, as a consequence of the explosion, some victims may not be able to hear you well.

Remember this: **30** (respirations) – **2** (CRT) – **Can Do** (follows commands)

Your 2 uninjured helpers are an able-bodied man and woman. The woman knows how to take a pulse. You have no medical equipment with you other than some oral airways and triage tags to work with.

Begin with the nearest victim (#1 on the list in the previous section:

1. Male in his 30s, complains of pain in his left leg (obviously fractured), Respirations 24, pulse strong, CRT 1 second, no excessive bleeding.
    Respirations are within acceptable range (less than 30), pulse and CRT normal. Complains of pain, and is communicating where it hurts, so mental status probably normal. This patient is tagged YELLOW: needs care but will not die if there is a reasonable (2-4 hour) delay. Move on.

2. Female in her 50s, bleeding from nose, ears, and mouth. Trying to sit up but can't, respirations 20, pulse present, CRT 1 second, not responding to your commands.
    This victim has a significant head injury, but is stable from the standpoint of respirations and perfusion. As her mental status is impaired, tag RED (immediate). Move on.

3. Teenage girl bleeding heavily from her right thigh, respirations 32, pulse thready, CRT 2.5 seconds, follows commands.
    This victim is seriously hemorrhaging, one of the reasons to treat during triage. Respirations elevated and perfusion impaired. You use your unskilled male helper to apply pressure by placing his hands on the bleeding and applying pressure, preferably using his shirt or bandanna as a "dressing". Tag RED. As the patient is

already RED, you don't really have to assess mental status. You and your female helper move on.

4. Another teenage girl, small laceration on forehead, says she can't move her legs. Respirations 20, pulse strong, CRT 1 second.

   Probable spinal injury but otherwise stable and can communicate. Tag YELLOW. Move on.

5. Male in his 20s, head wound, respirations absent. Airway repositioned, still no breathing.

   If not breathing, you will reposition his head and place an airway. This fails to restart breathing. This patient is deceased for all intents and purposes. Tag BLACK, move on.

6. Male in his 40s, burns on face, chest, and arms. Respirations 100, CRT 1.5 seconds, follows commands.

   This victim has significant burns on large areas, but is breathing well and has normal perfusion. Mental status is unimpaired, so you tag YELLOW and move on.

7. Teenage boy, multiple cuts and abrasions but not hemorrhaging, says he can't breathe, respirations 34, radial pulse present, CRT 2.5 seconds.

   This victim doesn't look so bad but is having trouble breathing and has questionable perfusion. Mental status is unimpaired, but he likely has other issues, perhaps internal bleeding. You tag RED (respirations over 30, impaired perfusion) and move on.

8. Female in her 20s, burns on neck and face, respirations 22, pulse present, CRT 1 second, asks to get up and can walk, although with a limp.

   Obviously injured, this young woman is otherwise stable and communicating. With assistance, she is able to stand up, and can walk by herself. She becomes another of the walking wounded, tag GREEN. Point her to the other GREEN victims and move on.

9. Elderly woman, bleeding profusely from an amputated right arm (level of forearm), respirations 36, pulse on other wrist absent, CRT 3 seconds, unresponsive.

Obviously in dire straits, you use your shirt as a tourniquet and sacrifice your remaining helper to apply pressure on the bleeding area. Tag RED, move on.

10. Male child, multiple penetrating injuries, respirations absent. Airway repositioned, starts breathing. Radial pulse absent, CRT 2 seconds, unresponsive.

You initially think this child is deceased, but you follow protocol and reposition his airway by tilting his head back. In normal circumstances you would be very reluctant to do this because of the possibility of a neck injury. A Mass Casualty Incident is one of the few circumstances where you don't worry about cervical spine injuries in making your assessment. He starts breathing even without an oral airway, to your surprise, so you tag him RED. If he is bleeding heavily from his injuries, you apply pressure and wait for the additional help you originally requested to arrive.

You have just performed triage on 20 victims, including the walking wounded, in 10 minutes or less. Help begins to arrive, including the ICU nurse that you contacted initially. You are no longer the most experienced medical resource at the scene, and you are relieved of Incident Command. The nurse begins the process of assigning areas for yellow, red and black tags where secondary triage and treatment can occur.

There is still much to do, but you have performed your duty to identify those victims who need the most urgent care. In a normal situation, your modern medical facilities will already have ambulances and trained personnel with lots of equipment on the scene. In a collapse situation, however, the prognosis for many of your victims is grave. Go over our list of victims and see who you think would survive if modern medical care is not available. Many of the RED tags and even some of the YELLOW tags would be in serious danger of dying from their wounds.

PATIENT TRANSPORT

As we mentioned earlier, the main goal of a medic in a survival situation is to transfer the injured or ill person to a modern medical facility. These facilities will be non-existent in the scenarios that this book deals with. As such, you will have to make a decision as to whether your patient can be treated for their medical problem at their present location or not. If they cannot, you must consider how to move your patient to where the bulk of your medical supplies are.

Before deciding whether to move a patient, stabilize them as much as possible. This means stopping all bleeding, splinting orthopedic injuries, and verifying that the person is breathing normally. If you cannot assure this, consider having a group member get the supplies needed to support the patient before you move them. Have as many helpers available to assist you as you can. The most important thing to remember is that you want to carry out the evacuation with the least trauma to your patient and yourself.

An important medical supply to have in this circumstance is a stretcher. Many good commercially-produced stretchers are available, but improvised stretchers can be put together without too much effort. Even an ironing board can become an effective transport device. A person with a spinal injury should be rolled onto the stretcher without bending their neck or back if at all possible.

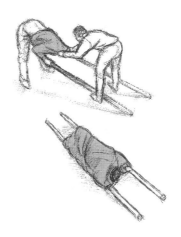

SHIRT STRETCHER

Other options include taking two long sticks or poles and inserting coats or shirts through them to handle the weight of the victim. If the rescuer grasps both poles, a helper could pull their coat off. This automatically moves the coat onto the poles. Lengths of Paracord or rope can also be crisscrossed to form an effective stretcher.

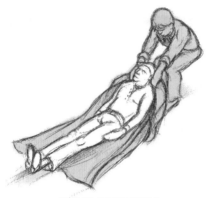

THE BLANKET PULL

If you must pull a person to safety, grasp their coat or shirt at the shoulders with both hands, allowing their head to rest on your forearms. You could also place a blanket under the patient, and grasp the end of the blanket near their head and pull. Again, if you are uncertain about the extent of any spinal injuries, do your best to not allow much bending of the body or neck during transport.

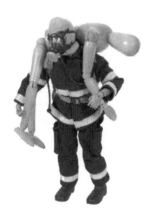

Fireman's Carry

If your patient can be carried, there are various methods available. The "Fireman's Carry" is effective and keep's the victim's torso relatively level and stable. In a squatting or kneeling position, you would grasp the person's right wrist with your left hand and place it over your right shoulder. Keeping your back straight, place your right hand between their legs and around the right thigh. Using your leg muscles to lift, rise up; you should end up with their torso over your back and the right thigh resting over your right shoulder. Their left arm and leg will hang behind your back if you have done it correctly. Adjust their weight so as to cause the least strain.

Another option is the "Pack-Strap Carry". With your patient behind you, grasp both arms and cross them across your chest. If squatting, keep your back straight and use your legs and back muscles to lift the victim. Bend slightly so that the person's weight is on your hips and lift them off the ground.

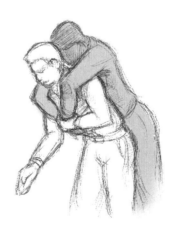

PACK STRAP CARRY

If you have the luxury of an assistant, you might consider placing your patient on a chair and carry using the front legs and back of the chair. This constitutes a sitting "stretcher". Another two person carry involves one rescuer wrapping their arms around the victim's chest from behind while the second rescuer (facing away from the patient) grabs the legs behind each knee. This is done in a squatting position, using the leg muscles to lift the patient.

It's important to remember this simple acronym when pulling or carrying a person: **B.A.C.K**.

- **B**ack Straight – muscles and discs can handle more load safely when the back is straight.
- **A**void Twisting – joints can be damaged when twisting.
- **C**lose to body – avoid reaching to pick up a load; it causes more strain on muscles and joints.
- **K**eep Stable – the more rotation and jerking, the more pressure on the discs and muscles.

Be sure to check the Video Resources section at the back of this book to see some of these methods being used in real time.

THE IMPORTANCE OF PATIENT ADVOCATES

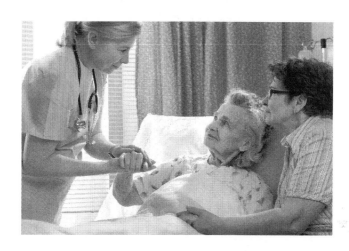

Before we move on, let's talk about an important aspect of holistic patient care. We spend a lot of time in this book talking about medical issues in times of trouble, from storms to a complete societal breakdown. However, times of trouble can be very personal, such as when you find yourself or a loved one battling a debilitating medical condition.

In certain instances, it is easy for the patient to "fall through the cracks" of a huge medical establishment. This has happened to one of my sons, Daniel. Daniel is a 30 year old who has had severe diabetes since he was nine years old. Due to his disease, he has developed kidney failure and partial blindness, and has been on dialysis for the last year. He has been on a kidney and pancreas transplant list since that time.

After a number of false alarms, a kidney and pancreas became available as a result of a drunk driver taking the life of a young father of two as he was riding his bicycle. He underwent the surgery at a large hospital, one of the few in the state that performed this type of procedure. The good news is that the new organs functioned well from the very start, producing urine and lowering his blood sugars to almost normal levels within 24 hours.

Several days after the operation, he was deemed fit enough to leave the Intensive Care Unit and go to a regular floor. This means that, instead of having a nurse specifically for him, he shared a nurse with several other patients. This is standard operating procedure, and usually has no ominous implications.

However, when I went to see him that day, he wasn't looking well. He seemed pale to me, and his abdomen seemed more distended that it did before. There was a drain coming out of his belly, and it was full of, what seemed to me, frank blood. He was getting vital signs (blood pressure, pulse, etc.) taken every 4 hours, and the chart appeared to show that he was stable and doing fine.

Seeing the blood draining out of his abdomen concerned me. I took his vitals myself earlier than scheduled; he was tachycardic (pulse very fast) and his blood pressure had dropped. As I was unable to find medical staff, I emptied the bloody drain and it filled up again (and again) within 2-3 minutes. It was clear to me that he was bleeding internally, and it was a significant amount. He was heavily sedated and wasn't complaining; I doubt , since he is nearly blind, he could find the button to push to notify the nurse even if he was awake.

This was late at night, and most visitors had left. Staffing was light, also, and it took some time to find his nurse, who was attending to another patient. My surgeon's hackles were raised, and I (not ashamed to say) raised a ruckus which led to an overworked resident to take a look at him. To her credit, it was clear that something was wrong, and he returned to surgery. They wound up removing 3000-4000cc of free blood from his abdomen and stopping the hemorrhage.

He recovered from this ordeal and, thankfully, his transplanted kidney and pancreas are still functioning. However, thinking about this episode, it was clear to me that it could have ended very badly. If not identified in time, it's very likely that I would have received a call in the morning notifying me that he passed away during the night.

I'm telling you this story not to gain sympathy or a pat on the back, but to convince you of the importance of being a patient advocate. If, like many of our readers, you are working to become a better medical asset to your people in hard times, then you must take patient advocacy as serious as learning first aid. As a healthcare provider in tough times, you must put yourself in the shoes of your patient and walk a mile in them.

You may already see yourself as an advocate for your patient as a survival medic. Indeed, most doctors today feel they know what's best for their patients. You may, however, also find yourself limited by a major workload in times of trouble, and this may make it difficult for you to see things from another person's perspective. This is no reflection on you as a person; it's just the way things might be. Your patient may "fall through the cracks" if you're not careful, simply due to the amount of pressure on you to care for a large survival community.

Consider appointing a family member or other individual to follow a sick patient with you, not necessarily to provide care but to provide support. Allow your patient to participate in medical decisions regarding their health and never resent their questions. If they are too week to do so, communicate with their appointed advocate; let them know what your plan of action is.

Here are my **Three A's of Advocacy**:

1. **Accept** the importance of a patient's rights.
2. **Advise** the patient so that they can be a full partner in the therapeutic process.
3. **Allow** an advocate to be an intermediary if the patient is too weak to actively participate in his or her care.

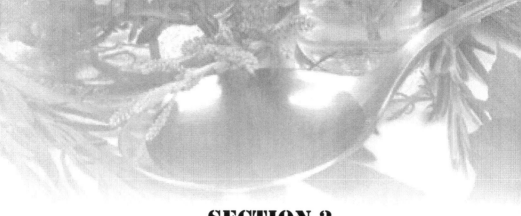

SECTION 3

✚ ✚ ✚

HYGIENE AND SANITATION

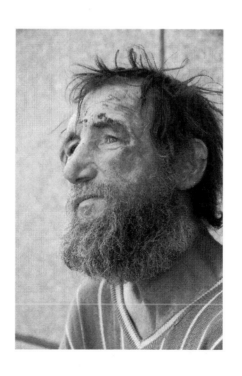

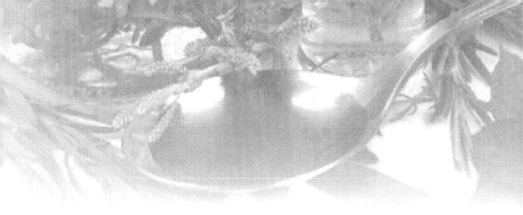

HYGEINE-RELATED MEDICAL PROBLEMS

In nature, many animals make specific efforts to preen and groom themselves. Their instinctual tendency to remain clean keeps them healthy. The human urge to be clean, although not related to instinct, has done its job as well. Time and effort spent in remaining clean translates into resistance to disease. When humans are under stress, attention to hygiene suffers because all available energy has to be directed to activities of daily survival.

As survival medic, you will have some control over the likelihood that your family or group will be exposed to unsanitary conditions. Indeed, your diligence in this matter is one of the major factors that will determine your success as a caregiver.

When we consider a person with hygiene issues, we generally expect them to have a foul smell. Body odors occur when sweat mixes with bacteria, and we all know that certain bacteria can lead to disease. It is up to the medic to ensure that hygiene issues do not put the survival group at risk. Strict enforcement of good sanitation and hygiene policies will do more to keep your family healthy than anything that any medic, nurse or medical doctor can do.

In a situation where there is no longer access to common cleansing items such as soap or laundry detergent, the goal of staying clean is difficult to achieve even with the best of intentions. Therefore, accumulation of these items in quantity is in your best interest.

Cleanliness issues extend to various important areas, such as dental care and foot care. With the increase of physical labor that we will be required to perform, we will get sweaty and dirty. The dirtier and wetter we get, the more prone we will be to problems such as infections or infestations. With careful attention, we can decrease our chances of dealing with these illnesses.

LICE, TICKS, AND WORMS

Lice

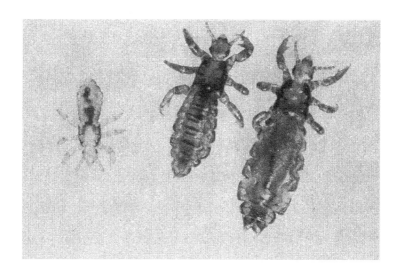

Typical head lice.

A common health problem pertaining to poor hygiene is the presence of lice, also known as "**Pediculosis**". Lice (singular: louse) are wingless insects that are found on many species. On humans, there are three types: Head, Body and Pubic. Some diseases use lice as vectors, causing major implications for entire survival groups. Sometimes, itching caused by lice causes breaks in the skin which allows other infections to develop.

Although it is thought that human lice evolved from organisms on gorillas and chimpanzees, they are, generally speaking, species-specific. That means that you cannot get lice from your dog, like you could get fleas. You get them only from other humans. It is interesting to note that human lice and chimpanzee lice diverged from each other, evolutionarily, about 6 million years ago; this is almost exactly when their hosts went their separate ways.

Lice spread rapidly in crowded, unsanitary conditions or where close personal contact is unavoidable. These conditions occur, for example, in many schools where children come into contact with each other during the course of the day (head lice, mostly). The sharing of personal items can also lead to louse infestations; combs, articles of clothing, pillows, and towels that are used by multiple individuals are common ways that lice are spread.

Adult **head lice** (Pediculus humanus capitis) are greyish-white and can reach the size of a small sesame seed. Infestation with head lice can cause itching and, sometimes, a rash. However, this type of lice is not a carrier of any other disease. Even in developed countries, head lice are relatively common, with 6-12 million cases a year in the United States, mostly among young children.

With their less developed immune systems, kids sometimes don't even know they have them; adults are usually kept scratching and irritated unless treated. An interesting fact is that African-Americans are somewhat resistant to head lice, probably due to the shape and width of the hair shaft.

The diagnosis is made by identifying the presence of the louse or its "nits" (eggs). Nits look like small bits of dandruff that are stuck to hairs. They are more easily seen when examined using a "black light". This causes them to fluoresce as light blue "dots" attached to the hair shafts near the scalp. As "black lights" will be rare in a collapse, a fine-tooth comb run through the hair will also demonstrate adult lice and nits. Special combs are used to remove as many lice as possible before treatment and to check for them afterwards. Many prefer the metal nit combs sold at pet stores to plastic ones sold at pharmacies.

You will find that the nits are firmly attached to the hair shaft about ¼ inch from the scalp. Nits will generally appear as yellow or white and oval-shaped. Olive oil may be applied to the comb; this may make the nits easier to remove.

Body lice (Pediculus humanus corporis) are latecomers compared to head lice, probably appearing with the advent of humans wearing clothes 110,000-170,000 years ago. As the concept of cleaning clothes occurred quite later, the constant contact with dirty garb caused frequent infestations.

This may be a common issue with the homeless today, but will likely be an epidemic in a collapse situation when regular bathing and clothes washing becomes problematic. Body lice are slightly larger than head lice; they also differ in that they live on dirty clothes (especially the seams), not on the body. They go to the human body only to feed. They are, also, sturdier than their cousins, and can live without human contact for 30 days or so.

Removal and, preferably, destruction of the infested clothing is the appropriate strategy here. Sometimes, using medication is unnecessary as the lice have left with the clothes (don't bet on it, however). Body lice, unlike head lice, ARE associated with infectious diseases such as typhus, trench fever and epidemic relapsing fever. Continuous exposure to body lice may lead to areas on the skin that are hardened and deeply pigmented.

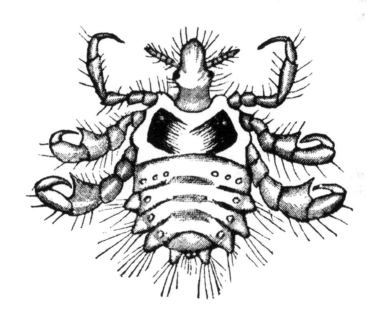

Crab Louse

Pubic infestations may be either caused by lice or mites. **Pubic lice** (Pthirus pubis), also known as "**crabs**", usually start in the pubic region but may eventually extend anywhere there is hair, even the eyelashes. They are most commonly passed by sexual contact. Severe itching is the main symptom and can involve the axillary (armpit) hair or even the eyelashes.

Although they are sometimes seen in a patient that has other sexually transmitted diseases, pubic lice do not actually transmit other illnesses. It should be noted that pubic lice is one of the few sexually transmitted diseases that is NOT prevented by the use of a condom.

Scabies is different from "crabs" and is caused by tiny eight-legged organisms called mites (Sarcoptes scabiei), not lice. The mites burrow through the skin forming small raised red bumps. Itching is noted and is most intense at night. Scabies can affect skin folds, even those with little hair such as the folds of the wrists, elbows, or between the fingers or toes.

These types of infestation are killed by medications called "Pediculocides". They include:

- Nix Lotion (1% Permethrin)
- Rid Shampoo (pyrethrin)
- Kwell Shampoo (Lindane)
- Malathion 5% in isopropanol

Nix lotion (permethrin) will kill both the lice and their eggs. Rid shampoo will kill the lice, but not their eggs; be certain to repeat the shampoo treatment 7 days later. This may not be a bad strategy with the lotion, as well. Ask your physician for a prescription for Kwell (lindane) shampoo to stockpile. It is a much stronger treatment for resistant cases. It may cause neurological side-effects in children, so avoid using this medicine on them. To use these products:

- Start with dry hair. If you use hair conditioners, stop for a few days before using the medicine. This will allow the medicine to have the most effect on the hair shaft.
- Apply the medicine to the hair and scalp.
- Rinse off after 10 minutes or so.
- Check for lice and nits in 8 to 12 hours.
- Repeat the process in 7 days

Wash all linens that you don't throw away in hot water (at least 120 degrees). Unwashable items, such as stuffed animals, that you cannot bring yourself to throw out should be placed in plastic bags for 2 weeks (for head lice) to 5 weeks (for body lice), then opened to air outside. Combs and brushes should be placed in alcohol or very hot water. Your patients should change clothes daily, although this may be difficult in a survival situation.

Natural remedies for lice have existed for thousands of years. Even commercial medications like Rid Shampoo use pyrethrin, which is extracted from the chrysanthemum flower. Another favorite anti-lice product is Clearlice, a natural product containing peppermint, among other things, and is thought by many to be superior to standard treatments.

Another good combination utilizes tea tree and neem oils. For external use only, mix a blend of salt, vinegar, tea tree oil and neem oil and apply daily for 21 days. Alternatively, Witch Hazel and tea tree oil applied daily after showering for 21 days has been reported as effective against hair lice.

A triple blend of tea tree, lavender, and Neem oil applied to the public region for 21 days may be effective in eliminating Scabies. Witch Hazel and tea tree oil, again, may be helpful for lice in this region as well. Some have advocated bathing with ½ cup of Borax and ½ cup of hydrogen peroxide daily for 21 days.

Although I have seen recommendations to "suffocate" lice with margarine, lard, butter, or coconut/olive oil, there isn't enough evidence to be certain that this method will work.

Ticks

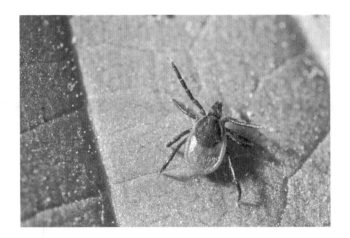

Common Deer Tick

Ticks are not as clearly associated with poor hygiene as lice. Although they are commonly thought of as insects, they are actually arachnids like scorpions and spiders. The American dog tick carries pathogens for Rocky Mountain spotted fever, and the blacklegged tick, also known as the deer tick, carries the microscopic parasite that's responsible for Lyme disease. Some tick-borne illness is similar to influenza with regards to symptoms; it is often missed by the physician. Lyme disease sometimes has a tell-tale rash, but other tick-related diseases may not.

Most Lyme disease is caused by the larval or juvenile stages of the deer tick. These are sometimes tough to spot because they're not much bigger than a pinhead. Each larval stage feeds only once and very slowly, usually over several days. This gives the tick parasites plenty of time to get into your bloodstream. The larval ticks are most active in summer. Although most common in the Northeastern U.S., they seem to be making their way further West every year.

Ticks don't jump like fleas do; they don't fly like, well, flies, and they don't drop from trees like your average spider. The larvae like to live in leaf litter, and they latch onto your lower leg as you pass by. Adults live in shrubs along game trails (hence the name Deer Tick) and seem to transmit disease less often. In inhabited areas, you might find them in woodpiles (especially in shade).

Many people don't think to protect themselves outdoors from exposure to ticks and other things like poison ivy, and many wind up being sorry they didn't. If you're going to spend the day in the fresh air, you should be taking some precautions:

- Don't leave skin exposed below the knee.
- Wear thick socks (tuck your pants into them).
- Wear high-top boots
- Use insect repellant

A good bug repellant is going to improve your chances of avoiding bites. Citronella can be found naturally in some areas and is related to plants like lemon grass; just rub the leaves on your skin. Soybean oil and oil of eucalyptus will also work. Consider including these in your medicinal garden if your climate allows it.

It is important to know that your risk of Lyme disease or other tick-spread illness increases the longer it feeds on you. The good news is that there is generally no transmission of disease in the first 24 hours. After 48 hours, though, you have the highest chance of infection, so it pays to remove that tick as soon as possible. Ticks sometimes don't latch onto your skin for a few hours, so showering or bathing after a wilderness outing may simply wash them off. This is where good hygiene pays off, as far as tick-related diseases go.

If you find a tick feeding on you, remove it as soon as possible. To remove a tick, take the finest set of tweezers you have and try to grab the tick as close to your skin as you can. Pull the tick straight up; this will give you the best chance of removing it intact. If removed at an angle, the mouthparts sometimes remain in the skin, which might cause an inflammation at the site of the bite. Fortunately, it won't increase your chances of getting Lyme disease.

Afterwards, disinfect the area with Betadine or triple antibiotic ointment. I'm sure you've heard about other methods of tick removal, such as smothering it with petroleum jelly or lighting it on fire. No method, however, is more effective that pulling it out with tweezers.

Luckily, only about 20% of deer ticks carry the Lyme disease or other parasite. A rash that appears like a bulls-eye occurs in about half of patients. If you get a rash along with flu-like symptoms that are resistant to medicines, you'll need further treatment.

Oral antibiotics will be useful to treat early stages. Amoxicillin (500 mg 3x/day for 14 days) or Doxycycline (100mg 2x/day for 14 days) should work to treat the illness. These can be obtained without a prescription in certain veterinary medications. See the chapter in this book on antibiotics and their uses. Don't be surprised if your patient still experiences muscle aches and fatigues for a time after treatment.

Parasitic Worms

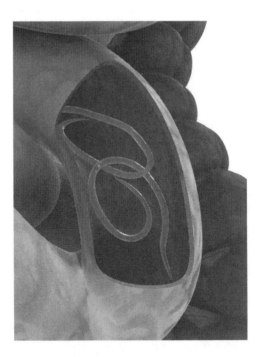

In a long-term survival situation, you can bet that you will be exposed to some pretty strange diseases and infestations. Simply being outside more often will expose you to mosquitos that carry illness. As well, your food and water may be contaminated or poorly cooked; this is yet another vector to allow infection to enter your body.

The organisms involved might be bacteria, viruses, or even parasites. Just walking barefoot in your garden can cause you to pick up one of these organisms. You gardeners know that nematodes (a type of roundworm) live in and on the soil.

Parasitic worms (also known as helminthes) are what we call internal parasites, because they live and feed inside your body. This differentiates them from external parasites such as lice or ticks, which live and feed on the outside of your body. When infected or infested, you are called a "host".

There are three types of parasitic worms: tapeworms, roundworms, and flukes. They range in size from microscopic to almost a foot long, depending on the species. The most common infection we'll see in the U.S. is the tiny Pinworm, which affects 40 million Americans.

Underdeveloped countries in Africa and Asia have the highest incidence of parasitic worms, but it is thought that over a quarter of the world's population has one type or another in their system. Children are especially vulnerable, with harmful consequences; parasites may account for stunted growth and poor development.

Worms attach themselves mostly to the intestinal tract, although some flukes infect the liver and lungs as well. Worm eggs or larvae enter through the mouth, nose, anus or breaks in the skin. Many helminthes are dependent on the acid in the stomach to dissolve the egg shell, and cannot hatch without it. The worm itself, however, is immune to the effects of stomach acid.

Many infections are asymptomatic or just involve some itching in the anal area (especially Pinworms). With some species, however, a large concentration of organisms can cause serious problems. Symptoms include stomach pains, nausea and vomiting, diarrhea, fatigue, and even intestinal obstruction. In rare cases, an obstruction can cause so much damage to the bowel that the patient may die. Organisms that invade the liver or lungs can even cause respiratory distress or a weakened metabolism.

Your body knows when it has been invaded, and sets up an immune response against the worm. It is unlikely to kill it, however, and all the energy put into defending the body may weaken the ability to fight other infections. As such, people with worms are more prone to secondary infections. The more issues the body has to deal with, the less effective it is in fighting them.

Some worms actually compete with your body for the food that you take in. Ascaris, for example, will attach to the wall of your intestine and eat partially digested food that comes its way. This competition prevents you from absorbing the nutrients effectively. Anemia and malnutrition may result. This may not matter much now, when you have access to as much food as you want. In a collapse, however, you will not have this luxury. Combined with diarrhea, you could be at a significant nutritional deficit.

There are various drugs such as Vermox, which are called "vermicides" (worm-killers). These are effective in destroying the worms inside your body, and might be a good choice to stockpile if you're in an area that has seen parasitic worm infections before. It is thought that overuse or multiple uses of these drugs may eventually cause the organism to become resistant. This is especially becoming an issue with livestock. Natural anti-helminthic plants also exist. Wormwood, Clove, and Plumeria have been reported as effective. Interestingly, tobacco will also help eliminate worms.

Parasitic worm infections are contagious in that they can be passed through contact with the infected individual. Careful attention to hygiene and, among medical providers, strict glove use will decrease this likelihood. Hand washing is considered important in preventing a community-wide epidemic, especially before preparing food.

Scratching during sleep may transmit eggs to fingernails, so be certain to wear clothing that will prevent direct hand contact with the anus. Known worm patients should wash every morning to remove any eggs deposited overnight in that area.

It's important to realize that unusual illnesses and infections will be problems that the survival medic may have to deal with. Obtaining knowledge of which organisms exist in your area, even if they are not major problems today, will be key in keeping your loved ones healthy.

DENTAL ISSUES

Many of our readers are often surprised that a book on survival medicine devotes a portion of its pages to dental issues. Few who are otherwise medically prepared seem to devote much time to dental health. History, however, tells us that problems with teeth take up a significant portion of the medic's patient load. In the Vietnam War, medical personnel noted that fully half of those who reported to daily sick call came with dental complaints. In a long-term survival situation, you might find yourself as dentist as well as nurse or doctor.

Anyone who has had to perform a task while simultaneously dealing with a bad toothache can attest to the decrease in work efficiency caused by the problem. If it's bad enough, it's unlikely that your mind can concentrate on anything at all, other than the pain that you're experiencing. Therefore, it only makes sense that you must learn basic dental care and procedures to keep your people at full work efficiency; it may be the difference between success and failure in a collapse.

A survival medic's philosophy should be that an ounce of prevention is worth a pound of cure. This thinking is especially apt when it comes to your teeth. By enforcing a regimen of good dental hygiene, you will save your loved ones from a lot of pain (and yourself a lot of headache).

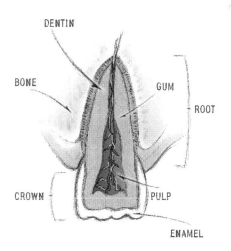

TOOTH ANATOMY

The anatomy of the tooth is relatively simple for such an important part of our body, and is worth reviewing. The part of the tooth that you see above the gum line is called the "crown". Below it, you have the "root". The bony socket that the tooth resides in is called the "alveolus". Teeth are anchored to the alveolar bone with ligaments, just like you have ligaments holding together your ankle or shoulder.

The tooth is composed of different materials:

- Enamel: The hard white external covering of the tooth crown.
- Dentin: Bony yellowish material under the enamel, and surrounding the pulp.
- Pulp: Connective tissue with blood vessels and nerves endings in the central portion of the tooth.

Most dental disease is caused by bacteria. Your mouth is chock full of them, so anything that decreases the amount of bacteria there will reduce the chances of developing dental disease. By keeping up their oral hygiene, a person will decrease their risk of an appointment at the survival dental office.

A daily brushing routine is essential, but at one point or another you will run out of toothbrushes. As an alternative, you can use your finger with a little toothpaste in a circular motion; this method will work long-term, or at least as long as you have fingers. A piece of cloth can also be utilized for this purpose.

Another option is to chew on the end of a twig until it gets fibrous and use that to clean your teeth. Any bendable twig (that is, live wood) will serve the purpose. Dead wood will just fall apart in your mouth, and cause more problems than give benefits. Native Americans prized black birch (also known as "sweet birch") due to its mild minty taste. This twig can serve dual purposes in that you could use the other end as a toothpick.

At one point or another, commercially-made toothpaste will no longer be available. Consider Baking soda as an alternative. Baking soda is inexpensive and less abrasive to dental enamel than manufactured silica-based toothpaste. It is an excellent choice, and it doesn't have fluoride.

Fluoride is sometimes useful as a direct treatment to strengthen teeth in those less than 12 years old, but adults really get very little benefit from it. There is even a school of thought that there are major medical risks associated with long term exposure to it. Significant controversy surrounds the topic.

Every time you eat a meal and, especially, before going to bed, you should be brushing your teeth or at least rinsing your mouth with warm salt water or a good antibacterial rinse. This will decrease inflammation in the gums and the risk of infection.

An effective and inexpensive option would be to use a solution made of ½ water and ½ 3% hydrogen peroxide. Swish it around in your mouth for 1-2 minutes to obtain the full effect. Most don't include mouth rinses as part of their survival storage, but this is a great way to prevent tooth issues. Beware of higher concentrations of hydrogen peroxide, as these could burn the inside of your mouth.

Another method of preventing tooth decay is faithful flossing. It may be inconvenient for some, but a lot of bacteria like to accumulate between your teeth. You can prove this by flossing and then smelling the floss. Unless you're flossing regularly, it will have a foul odor due to the large amounts of bacteria you have just dislodged. Flossing is also useful for removing foreign objects, such as food particles, from between teeth; tie a simple knot in the floss if the object is particularly difficult to remove.

How Teeth Decay

The stages of tooth decay

1. Healthy tooth with plaque
2. Decay in enamel
3. Decay in dentin
4. Decay in pulp

It's important to understand how bacteria causes tooth disease. Bacteria live in your mouth and they colonize your teeth. Usually, they will accumulate in the crevices on your molars and at the level where the teeth and gums meet. These colonies form an irregular thick film on the base of your enamel known as "tartar" or "plaque". The more tartar you have, the less healthy your gums and teeth are.

When you eat, these bacterial colonies also have a meal; they digest the sugars you take in and produce a toxic acid. This acid has the effect of slowly dissolving the enamel of your teeth (the outside of the tooth that's shiny). This commonly happens around areas where you've had dental work already, like the edges of fillings and under crowns or caps.

Once the enamel has broken down, you have what is called a "cavity". This could take just a few months to cause problems or could take 2-3 years. Once the cavity becomes deep enough to invade the soft inner part of the tooth (the pulp), the process speeds up and, because you have living nerves in each tooth, starts to cause pain. If the cavity isn't dealt with, it can lead to infection once the bacteria dig deep enough into the nerve or the surrounding gum tissue.

Inflamed gums have a distinctive appearance: They'll bleed when you brush your teeth and appear red and swollen. This is called "gingivitis", and is very common once you reach adulthood. As the condition worsens, it could easily lead to infection. If it affects the gums, it may spread to the roots of teeth or even the bony socket.

Once the root of the tooth is involved, you could develop a particularly severe infection called an "abscess". This is an accumulation of pus and inflammatory fluid that causes swelling and can be quite painful. Once you have an abscess, you will need antibiotic therapy and/or perhaps a procedure to drain the pus that has accumulated. The tooth will likely be unsalvageable at this point.

Diet plays an important part in the process of cavity formation. A diet that is high in sugar causes bacteria to produce the most acid. The longer your mouth bacteria are in eating mode, the longer your mouth has acid digging into your teeth. The two most important factors that cause cavities are the number of times per day and the duration of time that the teeth are exposed to this acid.

Let's say you have a can of soda in your hand. If you drink the entire thing in 10 minutes, you've had one short episode in which your mouth bacteria are producing high quantities of acid. The acid level drops after about 30 minutes or so. If you nurse that soda, however, and sip from it continuously for hours, you've increased both the number of exposures to sugar and the amount of time it's swishing around in there. The acid level never really gets a chance to drop, and that leads to decay.

Toothache

Treatment of a toothache starts with finding the bad tooth. Have your patient open their mouth so that you can investigate the area. A dental mirror and dental pick are good tools to start with. First, you will carefully look around for any obvious cavity or fracture. If there is nothing that you can see, however, you may still have serious decay between teeth or below the gums.

So how do you tell which tooth is the problem if you don't see anything obvious? Do this: Touch the teeth in the area of the toothache with something cold. The bad tooth will be very sensitive to cold. Now, touch it with something hot. If there is no sensitivity to heat, the tooth is salvageable.

A tooth that is, likely, beyond hope will cause significant pain when you touch it with something hot (only touch the tooth). It will continue to hurt for 10 seconds or so after you remove the heat source. This is because the nerve has been irreversibly damaged. Once the nerve is damaged at the level of the root, you might not feel either hot or cold. It will, however, be painful to even the slightest touch.

The basis of modern dentistry is to save every tooth if at all possible. In the old days (not biblical times, I mean 50 years ago), the main treatment for a diseased tooth was extraction. If we find ourselves in a grid-down situation, that's how it will be in the future.

If you delay extracting a severely decayed tooth, it will likely get worse. Decay could spread to other teeth or cause an infection that could spread to your bloodstream (called "sepsis") and cause major damage.

The important thing to know is this: 90% **of all dental emergencies can be treated by extracting the tooth.**

Besides a dental pick and mirror, what else needs to be in the group medic's dental kit? Gloves are one item that you should have in quantity. Don't ever stick your hands in someone's mouth without gloves; what they say about human bites isn't too far from the truth. Instead of latex, buy nitrile gloves, as they will not irritate someone who is allergic to latex. Other items that are useful to the survival dentist are:

- Dental floss, Toothbrushes.
- Dental or orthodontic wax as used for braces; even a candle will do in a pinch. Wax can be used to splint a loose tooth to its neighbors.
- A Rubber bite block to keep the mouth open. This will help you see the dentition and prevent yourself from getting bitten. One of those large pink erasers would serve the purpose just fine.
- Cotton pellets, Q tips, gauze sponges (cut into small squares).
- Temporary filling material, such as Tempanol, Cavit or Den-temp.
- Oil of cloves (eugenol), a natural anesthetic. Commercial toothache medications that have this include Red Cross Toothache Medicine containing 85% eugenol, Dent's Toothache Drops containing another anesthetic called benzocaine and eugenol in combo, and Orajel or Hurricaine containing benzocaine. This might come in a kit that includes dental tweezers and cotton pellets that you'll need for placement. It's important to know that eugenol burns the tongue, so never touch anything but teeth with it.
- Zinc oxide powder; mixed with 2 drops of clove oil, it will harden into temporary filling cement.
- Oil of oregano, a natural antibacterial.
- Dental tweezers, dental mirrors, and a dental pick.
- Extraction forceps. These are like pliers with curved ends. They come in versions specific to upper and lower teeth. Although there are many types of dental extractors, you should at least have 2: #151 or #79N for lower teeth and #150A or #150 for upper teeth.
- Elevators, one small, one medium. These are thin but solid chisel-like instruments that help with extractions by separating

ligaments that hold teeth in their sockets (some parts of a Swiss army knife might work in a pinch).
- A dental scaler to remove tartar.
- Pain medication and antibiotics.

If a collapse situation lasts long enough, you will come across people who have lost fillings or have loose caps or crowns. Although the commercial filling cements listed above are useful, a more economical way to get temporary filling material is available: Make it yourself.

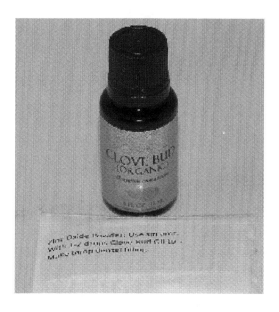

Clove bud oil and Zinc Oxide

Take 2 drops of Oil of Cloves (eugenol) and mix it with zinc oxide powder until you make a paste. Roll this into a ball and apply this to the area and it will harden, relieving pain at the same time.

Use your dental pick to scrape out black decay, especially at the edges of the cavity. Your paste should cover the entire area previously occupied by the original filling. Scrape off excess so that the person can close their teeth normally when they bite. You can use carbon paper or paper that you have rubbed a pencil on to identify areas where you have placed excess cement. Have your patient bite down; the carbon will stain the excess filling material dark.

It should be noted that these methods are temporary measures. Unless modern dentistry becomes available again, you will likely have to repeat the filling process multiple times.

Dental Fractures

Today's dentists have high technology on their side, but this technology will not be available if things go south. Therefore, we look to historical methods of treating these problems. Although some of these methods may not currently be in use, they may suffice to at least temporarily deal with the issue in times of trouble. Of these issues, some will be related to trauma.

Dental trauma may appear in various forms. After an injury to the oral cavity, a person may have:

- **A Dental Fracture**: a portion of a tooth chipped or broken off
- **A Dental Subluxation**: a loose tooth
- **A Dental Avulsion:** a tooth knocked out completely

When a portion of a tooth is broken off, it is categorized based on the number of layers of the tooth that are exposed. Classically, dentists have referred to these as Ellis class 1, 2, and 3 fractures.

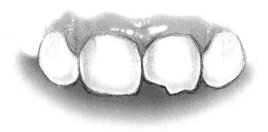

ELLIS no.1

- **Ellis 1 fractures**: In a Ellis 1 fracture, only the enamel has been broken and no dentin or pulp is exposed. This is only a problem if there is a sharp edge to the tooth. You can consider filing the edge smooth or using a mixture of Oil of Cloves, also known as eugenol, and zinc oxide powder as temporary cement.

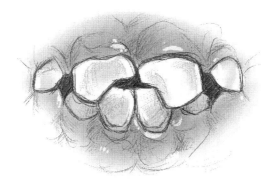

ELLIS no.2

- **Ellis 2 fractures**: Ellis 2 fractures show yellow or beige dentin under the enamel. This area may be sensitive and should be covered if possible. The composition of dentin is different than enamel and bacteria may enter and infect the tooth. This is especially the case with pediatric dental trauma.

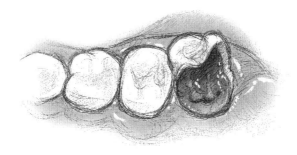

ELLIS no.3

- **Ellis 3 fractures**. Here the pulp and dentin are both exposed, and Ellis 3 fractures can be quite uncomfortable. If the pulp is exposed, it may bleed. Protective coverings will be most necessary here, and the risks of permanent damage most likely, especially in a collapse.

When you identify a fracture of a tooth, you should evaluate the patient for associated damage, such as to the face, inside of the cheek, tongue, and jaw. On occasion, a tooth fragment may be lodged in the soft tissues and must be removed with instruments.

There is likely to be blood due to the trauma, so thoroughly clean out the inside of the mouth so you can fully assess the situation. Then, using your gloved hand or a cotton applicator, lightly touch the injured tooth to see if it is loose. Don't forget your bite block.

For sensitive Ellis II fractures of dentin, cover the exposed surface with a calcium hydroxide composition (commercially sold as "Dycal"), a fluoride varnish (fluoride is rarely beneficial in drinking water, in my opinion, but is acceptable as a direct application to the tooth defect in this situation) or even clear nail polish or a medical adhesive such as Dermabond (medical super glue) to decrease sensitivity. Provide pain medications and instruct the patient to avoid hot and cold food or drink.

- Ellis III fractures into pulp are trouble, due to the risk of infection, among other reasons. Calcium hydroxide on the pulp surface coupled with additional temporary cement can be used as coverings. Provide for analgesics and antibiotics. Penicillin and Doxycycline are acceptable options. Despite all this, the prognosis is not favorable without modern dental intervention.

A particularly difficult dental fracture involves the root. Sometimes, it is not until the gum is peeled back that a fracture in the root is identified. If this is the case, the tooth is likely unsalvageable (especially in vertical fractures) and, in a power-down situation, should be extracted.

Dental Subluxations and Avulsions

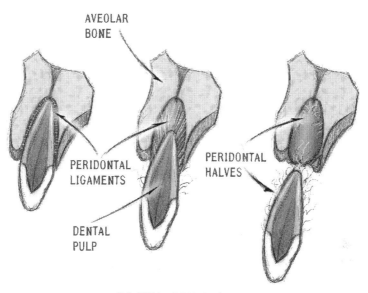

AVEOLAR
BONE

PERIDONTAL
LIGAMENTS

PERIDONTAL
HALVES

DENTAL
PULP

TOOTH AVULSION

A tooth that is knocked loose but not out of its alveolar socket is called a "subluxation". Lightly using your gloved hand or a cotton applicator should identify if it is loose and how much. Minimal trauma may require no major intervention.

If a tooth is loose, it should be pressed back into the alveolus (socket) and "splinted" to neighboring teeth for stability. Dentists use wire or special materials for this purpose, but you might find yourself having to use soft wax if professional help is not at hand. If you can, use enough wax to anchor the loose tooth to neighboring teeth both in front and in back. Prevent further trauma by placing on a liquid diet (juices, gelatin) for a time, until the tooth appears well anchored. Soft diets (things like puddings or soft cereals) are also ok.

The most favorable situation when a tooth is completely knocked out (an "avulsion") is that it came out in one piece, down to its root and ligaments. In this circumstance, time is a very important factor in possible treatment success. If the tooth is not replaced or at least placed in a preservation solution, the success of re-implantation drops 1% every MINUTE the tooth is not in its socket.

A good preservation liquid for teeth that have been knocked out is "Hank's Solution". This is a balanced salt solution that has been used to culture living cells, and it helps protect raw ligament fibers for a time. Hank's Solution is available commercially as "Save-a-Tooth". Although you can make your own Hank's Solution, it is a fairly complex process.

If you are not at your retreat at the time of injury:

- Find the tooth
- Pick it up by the crown, avoid touching the root as it will damage the already damaged ligament fibers.
- Flush the tooth clean of dirt and debris with water or saline solution. Don't scrub it, as it will damage the ligament further.
- If you don't have preservation solution, place the tooth in milk, saline solution, or saliva (put it between your cheek and gum, or under your tongue). This will keep your ligament cells alive longer than plain water will.

If the tooth has been out for less than 15 minutes, you may attempt to re-implant it. Flush the tooth and the empty socket with Hank's solution (Save-a-Tooth), replace the tooth and cover with cotton or gauze. Then, have the patient bite down firmly to keep it in place. Splint it with soft wax to the neighboring teeth and place your patient on a liquid diet. Antibiotics such as Penicillin (veterinary equivalent: Fish-Pen) or doxycycline (Bird-Biotic) will be helpful to prevent infection.

You may have to soak the tooth for a half hour or so in Hank's Solution before you replace it, if it has been out for more than 15 minutes. The longer you wait to replace the tooth, the more painful it will likely be to replace, so make sure you have lots of pain relief meds in your supplies.

After a couple of hours of being out, the ligament fibers dry out and die, and the tooth is for most intents and purposes dead. Replacing it at this point is problematic, as the pulp will decay like all dead soft tissue does. This may cause a chronic inflammation; as such, the rotting pulp is usually removed in a root canal procedure by a dentist. The dead tooth (which may turn dark in color) then scars down into its bony socket, acting like a dental implant. This is called "Ankylosis". This is part of the reason why you should not replace "baby teeth", because the scarring process may prevent the permanent teeth from emerging.

It's important to know that, in mature permanent teeth, the pulp doesn't survive the injury even if the ligament does. As such, without the availability of modern dental care to remove dead tissue, even your best efforts may be unsuccessful. Serious infection in the dead pulp often ensues, and your patient may be in a worse situation than just missing a tooth.

Life with dentists may be unpleasant sometimes (root canals, for example), but life without dentists will leave us with few options in most dental emergencies. In such circumstances, we may have to return to tooth extraction as the treatment of choice.

Dental Extraction

You, as medic, will eventually find yourself in a situation where you have to remove a diseased tooth. The important thing to know is that 90% of all dental emergencies can be treated by extracting the tooth.

Tooth extraction is not an enjoyable experience as it is, and will be less so in a long-term survival situation with no power and limited supplies. Unlike baby teeth, a permanent tooth is unlikely to be removed simply by wiggling it out with your (gloved) hand or tying a string to it and the nearest doorknob and slamming. Knowledge of the procedure, however, will be important for anyone expecting to be the medical caregiver in the aftermath of a major disaster.

Before we go any further, I have to inform you that I am not a dentist, just an old country doctor. It is illegal and punishable by law to practice dentistry without a license. The lack of formal training or experience in dentistry may cause complications that are much worse than a bum tooth. If you have access to modern dental care, seek it out.

Proper positioning will help you perform the procedure more easily. For an upper extraction (also called a "maxillary extraction"), the patient should be tipped at a 60 degree angle to the floor. The patient's mouth should be at the level of the medic's elbow. For a lower extraction, (also called a "mandibular extraction"), the patient should be sitting upright with the level of the mouth lower than the elbow. For right-handed medics, stand to the right of the patient; for left-handers, stand to the left. For uppers and most front lower extractions, it is best to position yourself in front. For lower molars, some prefer to position themselves behind the patient.

To begin with, you will want to wash your hands and put on gloves, a face mask, and some eye protection. You will want to keep the area around the tooth as dry as possible, so that you can see what you're doing. There will be some bleeding, so you might want to place cotton balls or rolled gauze squares around the tooth to be removed. These may have to be changed from time to time.

The teeth are held in place in their sockets by ligaments, which are fibrous connective tissue. These ligaments must be severed to loosen the tooth. This is accomplished with an elevator, which looks like a small flathead screwdiver or small chisel. See the image below for the proper way to hold the instrument.

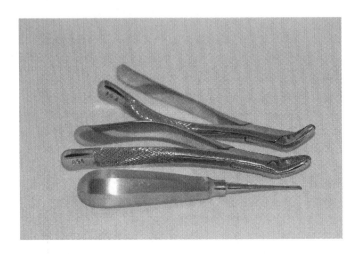

Dental Extractors and Elevator

Go between the tooth in question and the gum on all sides and apply a small amount of pressure to get down to the root area. This should loosen the tooth. Expect some bleeding.

Take your extraction forceps and grasp the tooth as far down the root as possible. This will give you the best chance of removing the tooth in its entirety the first time. For front teeth (which have 1 root), exert pressure straight downward for uppers and straight upward for lowers, after first loosening the tooth with your elevator. For teeth with more than 1 root, such as molars, a rocking motion will help loosen the tooth further as you extract. Once loose, avoid damage to neighboring teeth by extracting towards the cheek (or lip, for front teeth) rather than towards the tongue. This is best for all but the lower molars that are furthest back (wisdom teeth).

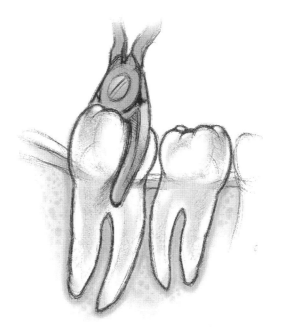

DENTAL EXTRACTOR
GRASPING ROOT

Use your other hand to support the mandible (lower jaw) in the case of lower extractions. If the tooth breaks during extraction (not uncommon), you will have to remove the remaining root. Use your elevator to further loosen the root and help push it outward.

Afterwards, place some gauze on the bleeding socket and have the patient bite down. A product known as Actcel hemostatic gauze is helpful to slow excessive bleeding; cut the gauze into small moistened squares and place directly on the bleeding area. It should form a gel which can be rinsed away with water in 24 hours.

Occasionally, a suture may be required if bleeding is heavy. Use 4-0 chromic catgut absorbable suture material in this case. In a recent Cuban study, veterinary super glue (N-butyl-2-cyanoacrylate) was used in over 100 patients in this circumstance with good success in controlling both bleeding and pain. Dermabond has been used in some cases in U.S. emergency rooms for temporary relief. Hot liquids and hard foods should be avoided for 24-72 hours.

Expect some swelling, bruising, and pain over the next few days. Cold packs will decrease swelling for the first 24-48 hours; afterwards, use warm compresses to help with jaw stiffness. Also, consider antibiotics, as infection is a possible complication. Liquids and a diet of soft foods should be given to decrease trauma to the area.

Use non-steroidal anti-inflammatory medicine such as Ibuprofen for pain. Stay away from aspirin, as it may hinder blood clotting in the socket. The blood clot is your friend, so make sure not to smoke, spit, or even use straws; the pressure effect might dislodge it, which could cause a painful condition called Alveolar Osteitis or "dry socket".

You will notice that the clot is gone and may notice a foul odor in the person's breath. Antibiotics and warm salt water gargles are useful here, and a solution of water with a small amount of Clove oil may serve to decrease the pain. Don't use too much clove oil, as it could burn the mouth.

In a long-term survival situation, difficult decisions will have to be made. If modern dentistry is gone due to a mega-catastrophe, the survival medic will have to take on that role as well as the role of medical caregiver. Performing dental procedures without training and experience, however, is a bad idea in any other scenario. Never perform a dental procedure on someone if you have modern dental care available to you.

RESPIRATORY INFECTIONS

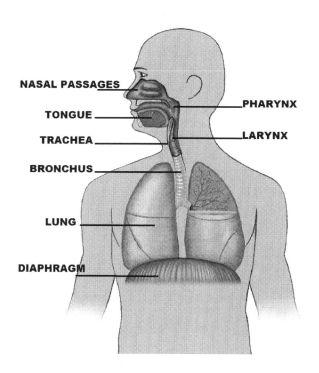

Even with today's modern medical technology, most of us can't avoid the occasional respiratory infection. Without strict adherence to sanitary protocol, it would be very easy in a collapse situation for your entire community to come down with colds, sinusitis, influenza or even pneumonia. Common colds may be caused by any of 200 different viruses. Influenza comes from viruses in the Influenza A, B, and C categories.

The societal risk of influenza is significant, mostly from Influenza A viruses. Over the course of time, influenza outbreaks from this category have included:

- The Russian Flu in 1889-90 (1 million deaths)
- The Spanish Flu in 1918 (50-100 million deaths)
- The Asian Flu in 1957-8 (1-1.5 million deaths)
- The Hong Kong Flu in 1968-9 (750,000 deaths)
- The Swine Flu in 2009-2010 (18,000 deaths)

Most of the above deaths associated with influenza are not caused by the virus, itself. They are due to bacterial pneumonia, a secondary infection which invades the patient through a virus-weakened immune system.

In general, most respiratory infections are spread by viral particles, and the organisms that cause these infections can live for up to 48 hours on common household surfaces, such as kitchen counters, doorknobs, etc. Contagious viral particles can easily travel 4 to 6 feet when a person sneezes.

Respiratory issues are usually divided into upper and lower respiratory infections. The upper respiratory tract is considered to be anything at the level of the vocal cords (larynx) or above. Oftentimes, the diagnosis will be related to the part of the upper respiratory system affected. This includes:

- The nose: Rhinitis
- The throat: Pharyngitis
- The sinuses: Sinusitis
- The voice box: Laryngitis
- The epiglottis: Epiglottitis
- The tonsils: Tonsilitis
- The ear canal: Otitis

(the suffix "-itis" simply means "inflammation of")

The lower respiratory tract includes the lower windpipe, the airways (taken together, called "bronchi") and the lungs themselves. Respiratory infections, such as bronchitis and pneumonia, are the most common cause of infectious disease in developed countries.

Symptoms of the common cold can include fever, cough, sore throat, runny nose, nasal congestion, headaches, and sneezing. Symptoms of lower respiratory infections (pneumonia and some bronchitis) include cough (with phlegm, it is referred to as a "productive" cough), high fever, shortness of breath, and weakness/fatigue. Most respiratory infections start showing symptoms 1 to 3 days after exposure to the causative organism. They can be expected to last for 7 to 10 days if upper and somewhat longer if lower.

Colds vs. Influenza

There are differences between the common cold and influenza that are helpful to make a diagnosis. The symptoms are similar, but are more likely and more severe in one or the other. Consult the list below to identify what you're most likely dealing with:

Symptoms	Cold	Influenza
Fever	Rare, Low	Common, High
Headache	Rare	Common
Nasal Congestion	Common	Occasional
Sore Throat	Common	Occasional
Cough	Mild	Severe
Aches and Pains	Common	Severe
Fatigue	Mild	Severe

For influenza, the administration of antiviral medications such as Tamiflu or Relenza will shorten the course of the infection if taken in the first 48 hours after symptoms appear. After the first 48 hours, antivirals have less medicinal effect.

For colds, concentrate your treatment on the area involved; nasal congestion medication for runny noses or sore throat lozenges for pharyngitis, for example. Ibuprofen or Acetaminophen will alleviate muscle aches and fevers. Steam inhalation and good hydration also give some symptomatic relief. Various natural remedies are also useful to relieve symptoms, which we will discuss in the next section of this book.

Although most upper respiratory infections are caused by viruses, some sore throats may be caused by a bacterium called Beta-Streptococcus (Also known as Strep Throat). These patients will often have small white spots on the back of their throat and/or tonsils, and are candidates for antibiotics. Amoxicillin (veterinary equivalent: Fish-Mox) or Keflex (Fish-Flex) are some of the drugs of choice in those not allergic to Penicillin drugs. Erythromycin (Fish-Mycin) family drugs are helpful in those who are Penicillin-allergic.

In most cases, however, it is not appropriate to use antibacterial agents such as antibiotics for upper respiratory infections. Antibiotics have been overused in treating these problems, and this has led to resistance on the part of some organisms to the more common drugs. Resistance has made some of the older antibiotics almost useless in the treatment of many illnesses.

Lower respiratory infections, such as pneumonia, are the most common cause of death from infectious disease in developed countries. These can be caused by viruses or bacteria. The more serious nature of these infections leads many practitioners to use antibiotics more often to treat the condition. Most bronchitis is caused by viruses, however, and will not be affected by antibiotics. Antibiotics may be appropriate for those with a lower respiratory infection that hasn't improved after several days of treatment with the usual medications for upper respiratory infections.

The patients who are at-risk will appear to have worsening shortness of breath or thicker phlegm over the course of time despite the usual therapy. There is a school of thought that recommends more liberal use of antibiotics in sick persons over the age of 60 or those with other serious medical conditions. This population has a higher risk of death because of decreased resistance to secondary bacterial infections.

Both upper and lower respiratory infections are different than asthma, which is a condition where the airways become constricted in a type of spasm, causing a particularly vocal kind of breathing called a "wheeze". Asthma may occur as an allergic response, or may be associated with some respiratory infections, such as childhood "croup". The treatment of asthma involves different medicines than colds or flus, such as certain antihistamines and epinephrine, than those used in treating respiratory infections.

Good respiratory hygiene is important to prevent patients with respiratory infections from transmitting their infection to others. Practicing good hygiene is not only a good strategy for you and your family, but demonstrates social responsibility and could prevent a pandemic. This is what needs to be done:

- Sick individuals should cover their mouth and nose with tissues and dispose of those tissues safely.

- Use a mask if coughing. Although others caring for the sick individual may wear masks (N95 masks are best for healthcare providers), it is most important for the afflicted person to wear one.
- Have caregivers perform rigorous hand hygiene before and after contact. Wash with soap and warm water for 15 seconds or clean your hands with alcohol-based hand sanitizers if they do not appear soiled.
- Sick persons should keep at least 4 feet away from other persons, if possible, due to droplet spread.
- Wash down all possibly contaminated surfaces such as kitchen counters or doorknobs with an appropriate disinfectant (dilute bleach solution will do).
- Isolate the sick individual in a specific quarantine area, especially if he/she has a high fever.
- Have medical care providers wear gloves at all times when treating the patient.
- Don't self-medicate, especially with antibiotics, unless modern medical care is not accessible for the foreseeable future;

Many of the strategies and treatments described above will deal with respiratory infections quite well, but what is modern pharmaceuticals are not available or are no longer produced due to a major catastrophe? In that circumstance, we must look to our own backyard and, if we planned wisely, our medicinal garden. We will have to consider natural substances that might help alleviate various respiratory symptoms and strengthen the body's immune response.

Historically, Vitamin C, Vitamin E, and other antioxidants taken regularly are supposed to decrease the frequency and severity of respiratory infections. Many studies confirm their usefulness, although the amount of down time due to colds/flus per year was only decreased 1 day in one study. Despite this, antioxidant support of the immune system can be obtained through good nutrition or supplements and should be part of any approach to survival food storage.

Most natural remedies are meant to target individual symptoms, such as nasal congestion or fever. There are, however, a number of alternative treatments for various respiratory infections that are reported to help stimulate the entire immune system. Consider these essential oils:

- Geranium
- Clove Bud
- Tea Tree
- Lavender

To use these oils, you would use a procedure called "direct inhalation therapy". Place 2-3 drops on the palm of your hand. Warm the oil by rubbing your hands together, and then bring your hands to your nose and mouth. Breathe 3-5 times slowly and deeply. Relax and breathe normally for 2 minutes, then repeat the process. Wipe any excess oil onto throat and chest.

Many herbs may be helpful when used internally as a tea. Popular ones for general respiratory support are Elderberry, Echinacea, Licorice root, Goldenseal, Chamomile, Peppermint, and Ginseng. Additionally, anti-bacterial action has been found in Garlic and Onion oil, fresh Cinnamon, and powdered Cayenne Pepper. Other options include raw unprocessed honey, lemon, and apple cider vinegar, which are often added to one of the above herbal teas.

Other than general treatments, there are several good remedies to treat specific symptoms associated with colds and flu. To treat **fever**, for example, consider teas made from the following herbs:

- Echinacea
- Licorice Root
- Yarrow
- Fennel
- Catnip
- Lemon Balm

The underbark of willow, poplar, and aspen trees are known to be a source of Salicin, the essential ingredient in aspirin. Strip off the outer bark, take several strips of the green underbark and make a tea out of it. It should work as aspirin does to decrease fever.

Other strategies to combat fever include sponge baths with water and vinegar. It has also been reported that slices of raw onion on the bottom of the feet are effective in some cases (wear socks to hold them in place). I haven't tested this last method myself, so I would appreciate input from people who have tried it. Although I can't tell you if it is effective, I can tell you that it probably isn't very practical.

Others have used herbal aerosol "spritzers". Combine several drops of Chamomile, Lavender or Thyme essential oil with water and spray on the chest, back, arms, and legs (avoid spraying the face). The cooling effect alone will be beneficial in those with fevers.

To deal with the **congestion** that goes along with most respiratory infections, consider using direct inhalation therapy (described above) or salves with these essential oils:

- Eucalyptus
- Rosemary
- Anise
- Peppermint
- Tea Tree
- Pine
- Thyme

Another inhalation method of delivering the above herbs or even traditional medications involves the use of steam. Steam inhalation is beneficial for many respiratory ailments and is easy to implement. Just place a few drops of essential oil into steaming water and lower your face to inhale the vapors. Cover the back of your head with a towel to concentrate the steam.

Herbal teas that relieve congestion include: Stinging Nettles, Licorice Root, Peppermint, Anise, Cayenne Pepper, Sage and Dandelion. Mix with honey and drink 3-4 times per day as needed. Fresh horseradish is used to open airways by taking ¼ teaspoon orally 3 times a day. Plain sterile saline solution (via nasal spray or in a "neti pot") is also used by both traditional and alternative healers.

For **aches and pains** due to colds, try using salves consisting of essential oils of:

- St. John's Wort
- Eucalyptus
- Camphor
- Lavender
- Peppermint
- Rosemary
- Arnica (dilute)

Helpful teas to relieve muscle ache include: Passionflower, Chamomile, Valerian Root, Willow underbark, Ginger, Feverfew, and Rosemary. Drink warm with raw honey 3-4 times a day.

For the occasional **sore throat**, time-honored remedies include honey and garlic "syrups" and ginger, Tilden flower, or sage teas. Drink warm with honey and perhaps lemon several times a day. Gargling with warm salt water will also bring relief. Licorice root and honey lozenges are also popular in decreasing painful swallowing.

A study in Israel used a substance found in black elderberries known as Sambucol. The study found that those who were given it had substantially shorter periods of flu symptoms than those given placebos. Sambucol is thought to have strong antioxidant properties and strengthen the immune system. It did not appear to affect those with the common cold, however.

Although the herbs described in this article have all been known to be helpful, it is important to remember that individual response to a particular herbal product differs from person to person. Also, the quality of an essential oil may differ dependent on various factors, including rainfall, soil conditions or the time of year harvested.

Guide to protective masks

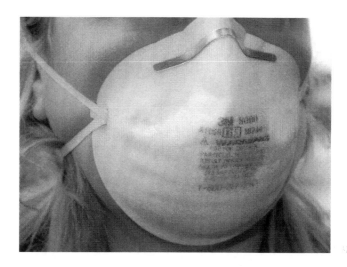

Typical N95 mask

Throughout history, infectious diseases have been part and parcel of the human experience. Ever since the Middle Ages, we have figured out that some infections have the capacity of passing from person to person. Medical personnel have made efforts to protect themselves from becoming the next victim to succumb from the disease.

This makes sense from more than a selfish standpoint: In survival situations, there will be few medically trained individuals to serve a group or community. The medic, therefore, is a valuable resource. It would be a disservice to those they depend upon if they became ill during an epidemic.

Even before we knew there were such things as viruses and bacteria, efforts to protect the healthcare provider were made by the use of masks. Around the year 1900, masks began to be used routinely during surgery to prevent micro-organisms from contaminating the operative field. A secondary purpose was to protect the wearer from blood spatter and other fluids from the patient. These were not always used by all members of the surgical team until later in the century.

Nowadays, the basic surgical mask hasn't changed much in general appearance. No doubt, you've seen photos of people wearing them in areas where there is an epidemic. In Asia, especially, it is considered good etiquette and socially responsible to wear them if you have a cold or flu and are going out in public. Face masks have the added advantage of reminding people to keep their hands away from their nose and mouth, a major source of the spread of infection.

If you will be taking care of your family or survival group in situations where modern medical care is unavailable, you will want a good supply of masks (and gloves) in your medical storage. Without these items, it will be likely that an infectious disease could affect every member, including yourself.

Medical masks are evaluated based upon their ability to serve as a barrier to very small particles (we're talking fractions of microns) that might contain bacteria or viruses. These are tested at an air flow rate that approximates human breathing, coughing or sneezing.

As well, masks are tested for their ability to tightly fit the average human face. The most commonly available face masks use ear loops or ties to fix them in place, although adhesive masks are being developed. Most masks are fabricated of "melt-blown" coated fabric, providing better protection than woven cotton or gauze. Despite this, masks do not confer complete immunity.

Standard medical masks have a wide range of protection based on fit and barrier quality; 3 ply masks (the most common version) are more "breathable", as you can imagine; 6 ply masks likely present more of a barrier. A tight fit is imperative in providing a barrier to infectious droplets.

The upgrade to the basic mask is the **N95** respirator mask. N95 Medical Masks are a class of disposable respirators that have at least 95% efficiency against particulates > 0.3 microns in size. These masks protect against many contaminants but are not 100% protective, although N99 masks (99%) and N100 masks (99.7%) are also available. The N stands for non-oil resistant; there are also R95 (oil resistant) and P95 (oil proof) masks, mostly for industrial and agricultural use.

Many of these masks have a square or round "exhalation valve" in the middle, which helps with breathability. None of these masks, which do not cover the eyes, are protective against gases such as chlorine. For this, you would need a "gas mask", discussed in the section on biological warfare.

So what would be a reasonable strategy? You'll need both standard and N95 masks as part of your medical supplies. I would recommend a significant number of each as the masks will be contaminated once worn and should be discarded.

There are no absolute standards with regards to who wears what in the sick room. I would recommend using the standard surgical masks for those who are ill, to prevent contagion from coughing or sneezing (which can send air droplets several feet) and the N95 masks for the caregivers. In this fashion, you will give maximum protection to the medical personnel. Remember, your highest priority is to protect yourself and the healthy members of your group. Isolate those that might be contagious, have plenty of masks, as well as gloves, aprons, eye wear, and antiseptics, and pay careful attention to every aspect of hygiene. Your survival may depend on it.

FOOD AND WATER-BORNE ILLNESS

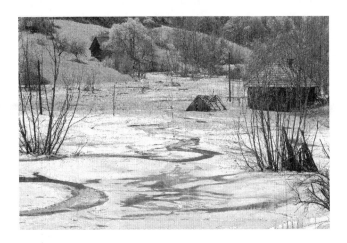

Modern water treatment practices and disinfectant techniques have made drinking water and eating food a lot safer than in the past. Contaminated water was the source of many thousands of deaths in olden times, and still causes epidemics of infectious disease in underdeveloped countries.

It just makes common sense, therefore, that we can expect sanitation issues in the aftermath of a disaster. Aquifers may be contaminated by damage to levees or, more likely, by pollution caused by careless or uninformed citizens.

Any water source that has not been sterilized or any food that hasn't been properly cleaned and cooked could place an entire community at risk. As the designated medic, your duty as Chief Sanitation Officer will be to assure that water is drinkable and that food preparation areas are disinfected.

Sterilizing Water

As we mentioned, water can be contaminated by floods, disruptions in water service and a number of other random events. A dead raccoon upstream from where you collect your water supplies could be a source of deadly bacteria.

Even the clearest mountain brook could be a source of parasites, called protozoa, which can cause disease. A parasite is an organism that, once it is in your body, set up shop and causes you harm. Common parasites that cause illness include Giardia and Entamoeba; they can even affect hikers in the deepest wilderness settings.

If you're starting with cloudy water, it is because there are many small particles of debris in it. There are many excellent commercial filters of various sizes on the market that deal with this effectively. You could also make your own particulate filter by using a length of 4 inch wide PVC pipe and inserting 2 or 3 layers of gravel, sand, zeolite, and/or activated charcoal, with each layer separated by pieces of cloth or cotton. Once flushed out and ready to go, you can run cloudy water through it and see clear water coming out the other side.

This type of filter, with or without activated charcoal, will get rid of particulate matter but will not kill bacteria and other pathogens (disease-causing organisms). It's important to have several ways available to sterilize your water to get rid of organisms. This can be accomplished by several methods:

- **Boiling:** Use a heat source to get your water to a roiling boil. There are bacteria that may survive high heat, but they are in the minority. Using a pressure cooker would be even more thorough.
- **Chlorine:** Household bleach sold for use in laundering clothes is a 3-8% solution of sodium hypochlorite. A 12% solution is widely used in waterworks for the chlorination of water, and a 15% solution is often used for disinfection of waste water in treatment plants. Bleach has an excellent track record of eliminating bacteria and 8-10 drops in a gallon of water will do the trick. If you're used to drinking city-treated water, you probably won't notice any difference in taste.
- **2% Tincture of Iodine:** About 12 drops per gallon of water will be effective. An eyedropper is a useful item to have as part of your supplies. Running water from a stream may need less iodine than still water from, say, a lake.
- **Ultraviolet Radiation:** Exposure to sunlight will kill bacteria! 6-8 hours in direct sunlight (even better on a

reflective surface) Fill your clear gallon bottle and shake vigorously for 20 seconds. The oxygen released from the water molecules will help the process along and, amazingly, even improves the taste.

Sterilizing Food

Anyone who has eaten food that has been left out for too long has probably experienced an occasion when they have regretted it. Properly cleaning food and food preparation surfaces is a key to preventing disease.

Your hands are a food preparation surface. Wash your hands thoroughly prior to preparing your food. Other food preparation surfaces like counter tops, cutting boards, dishes, and utensils should also be cleaned with hot water and soap or a dilute bleach solution before using them. Soap may not kill germs, but it helps to dislodge them from surfaces.

If you have a good supply, use paper towels to clean surfaces. Kitchen towels, especially if kept damp, really accumulate bacteria. If you ever reach a point when paper towels are no longer available, boil your towels before using them.

Wash your fruits and vegetables under running water before eating them. Food that comes from plants that grow in soil may have disease-causing organisms, and that's without taking into account fertilizers like manure. You're not protected if the fruit has a rind; the organisms on the rind will get on your hand and will be transferred to the fruit once you peel it.

Raw meats are notorious for having their juices contaminate food. Prepare meats separately from your fruits and vegetables. A useful item to make certain that meats are safe is a meat thermometer. Assure that meats reach an appropriate safe temperature and remain consistently at that temperature until cooked; this varies by the type of meat:

- Beef: 145 degrees F
- Pork: 150 degrees F
- Lamb: 160 degrees F
- Poultry: 165 degrees F
- Ground Meats: 160 degrees F
- Sauces and Gravy: 165 degrees F
- Soups with Meat: 165 degrees F
- Fish: 145 degrees F

DIARRHEAL DISEASE AND DEHYDRATION

With worsening sanitation and hygiene, there will likely be an increase in infectious disease, none of which will be more common that diarrhea. **Diarrhea** is defined as an increased frequency of loose bowel movements. If a person has 3 liquid stools in a row, it is a red flag that tells you to watch for signs of dehydration. **Dehydration** is the loss of water from the body. If severe, it can cause a series of chemical imbalances that can threaten your life. Over 80,000 soldiers perished in the Civil War, not from bullets, but from dehydration related to diarrheal disease.

Diarrhea is a common ailment and may go away on its own simply by restricting your patient to clear fluids and avoiding solid food for a period of time. I would recommend 12 hours without eating solids to be safe. However, there are some symptoms that may present in association with diarrhea that can be a sign of something more serious. Those symptoms are:

- Fever equal to or greater than 101 degrees Fahrenheit
- Blood or mucus in the stool
- Black or grey-white stool
- Severe vomiting
- Major abdominal distension and pain
- Moderate to severe dehydration
- Diarrhea lasting more than 3 days

All of the above may be signs of serious infection, intestinal bleeding, liver dysfunction, or even surgical conditions such as appendicitis. As well, all of the above will increase the likelihood that the person affected won't be able to regulate their fluid balance.

Epidemics caused by organisms that cause diarrhea have been a part of the human experience since before recorded history. Cholera is one particularly dangerous disease that was epidemic in the past and may be once again in the uncertain future. This infection will produce a profuse watery diarrhea with abdominal pain. Although there is a vaccination, it is not very effective; therefore, I cannot recommend it.

Typhoid fever is another very dangerous illness caused by contaminated food or drink. It is characterized by bloody diarrhea and pain and, like cholera, has been the cause of deadly outbreaks over the centuries. In typhoid cases, fever rises daily and, after a week or more, you may see a splotchy rash and spontaneous nosebleeds. The patient's condition deteriorates from there.

The end result (and most common cause of death) of untreated diarrheal illness is dehydration. 75% of the body's weight is made up of water; the average adult requires 2 to 3 liters of fluid per day to remain in balance. Children become dehydrated more easily than adults: 4 million children die every year in underdeveloped countries from dehydration due to diarrhea and other causes.

The severity of dehydration depends on the percent of water that has been lost. The thirst mechanism is activated when you have lost just 1% of your total body water content. You are still functioning normally but if you fail to replace the fluids, you will begin to feel ill. As the percentage of water lost increases, however, you begin to see additional symptoms and increased risks. Dehydration is often classified as mild, moderate, and severe:

- **Mild dehydration:** 2% of water content lost (5% of body weight). Symptoms include anxiety, loss of appetite and decreased work efficiency. Urine appears darker and is more concentrated. Pulse rate and respiration rate may begin to increase

- **Moderate dehydration:** 4% of water content lost (10% of body weight). In addition to the above symptoms, the patient experiences nausea and vomiting (even if they didn't before), dizziness, fatigue and mood swings. Decreased urine output. Pulse rate and respirations rise and blood pressure drops.

- **Severe dehydration:** 6% of water content lost (more than 10% body weight). In addition to the above symptoms, the patient experiences loss of coordination and becomes incoherent and delirious. Little or no urine output. Vitals signs worsen.

- In severe dehydration, you will notice changes in the skin elasticity, also known as "turgor". To determine skin turgor, pick up the skin on the lower arm or torso between two fingers so that it is "tented" up. The skin is held for a few seconds and then released. If turgor is normal, the skin will return rapidly to its normal position. Skin with decreased turgor remains elevated or returns slowly to normal in a severely dehydrated individual.

- Once a person is severely dehydrated, continued water loss begins to cause the patient to be unable to regulate their own body temperature. Chemical imbalances begin to occur that just replacing water cannot repair. Organs will begin to malfunction and shock ensues. Once they reach approximately 20% water loss, the patient may slip into a coma and die.

Rehydration

Fluid replacement is the treatment for dehydration. Oral rehydration is the first line of treatment, but if this fails, intravenous fluid (IV) may be needed, which requires special skills. Always start by giving your patient small amounts of clear fluids. Clear fluids are easier for the body to absorb; examples include: water, clear broth, gelatin, Gatorade, Pedialyte, etc.

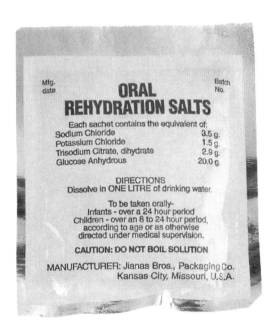

Oral rehydration packets are commercially available, but you can produce your own homemade rehydration fluid very easily: To a liter of water, add:

- 6-8 teaspoons of sugar (sucrose)
- 1 teaspoon of salt (sodium chloride)
- ½ teaspoon of salt substitute (potassium chloride)
- A pinch of baking soda (sodium bicarbonate)

As the patient shows an ability to tolerate these fluids, advancement of the diet to juices, puddings and thin cereals like grits or farina (cream of wheat) is undertaken. It is wise to avoid milk as some are lactose intolerant. Once the patient keeps down thin cereals, you can advance them to solid food.

A popular strategy for rapid recovery from dehydration is the **BRAT** diet, used commonly in children. This diet consists of:

- Bananas
- Rice
- Applesauce
- Plain Toast (or crackers)

The advantage of this strategy is that these food items are very bland, easily tolerated, and slow down intestinal motility (the rapidity of movement of food/fluids through your system). This will slow down diarrhea and, as a result, water loss. In a collapse situation, you will probably not have many bananas, but hopefully you have stored rice and/or applesauce, and have the ability to bake bread.

Of course, there are medicines that can help and you should stockpile these in quantity. Pepto-Bismol and Imodium (Loperamide) will help diarrhea. They don't cure infections, but they will slow down the number of bowel movements and conserve water. These are over the counter medicines, and are easy to obtain. In tablet form, these medicines will last for years if properly stored.

A good prescription medicine for vomiting is Zofran (Ondansetron). Doctors will usually have no qualms about writing this prescription, especially if you are traveling out of the country. Of course, ibuprofen or acetaminophen is good to treat fevers. The higher the fever, the more water is lost. Therefore, anything that reduces the fever will help a person's hydration status.

Various natural substances have been reported to be helpful in these situations. Herbal remedies that are thought to "dry up" the mucous membranes in the intestine include:

- Blackberry leaf
- Raspberry leaf
- Peppermint

Make a tea with the leaves and drink a cup every 2-3 hours.

Half a clove of crushed garlic and 1 teaspoon of raw honey 4 times a day is thought to exert an antibacterial effect in some cases of diarrhea. A small amount of nutmeg may decrease the number of loose bowel movements. Ginger tea is a time-honored method to decrease the abdominal cramps associated with diarrhea.

As a last resort to treat dehydration from diarrhea (especially if there is also a high fever), you can try antibiotics or anti-parasitic drugs. Ciprofloxacin, Doxycycline and Metronidazole are good choices, twice a day, until the stools are less watery. Some of these are available in veterinary form without a prescription (discussed later in this book). These medicines should be used only as a last resort, as the main side effect is usually...diarrhea!

DEALING WITH SEWAGE ISSUES

When our infrastructure is working, we generally are able to provide fresh clean water for drinking and provide food for the table that is free of contamination. We also have ways to flush waste from our immediate surroundings. When that infrastructure is damaged, we will be easy prey for infectious disease. One only has to look back a short time to the earthquakes in Haiti and the subsequent Cholera epidemic there to know that this is true.

A growing number of people are now storing food for use in tough times. To their credit, many are also putting away medical supplies and learning skills to deal with injuries and common medical complaints.

Few, however, have given a great deal of thought to how they will maintain a sanitary environment for their family or survival group in times of trouble. And this is despite daily news reports of hundreds or even thousands of deaths due to this issue in many third world countries. If you can effectively and safely dispose of your waste, you will go a long way to keeping your family healthy.

When electrical power is lost due to a storm, water utilities cannot operate the pumps that maintain water pressure in the pipes that travel to your home. This pressure is one way water utilities ensure that your water is free from harmful bacteria. When the pressure is lost, a "boil water" order is established by the local authorities. In our neck of the woods (South Florida), lessons have been learned the hard way by as a result of hurricanes. This led to the outfitting of waste treatment and distribution facilities with generators. This is admirable, but unlikely to last long in a survival situation.

Therefore, we must realize that human sewage may be a big problem in the aftermath of a storm or a complete collapse. If the water isn't running, a community without a ready supply will have a nightmare on their hands after as little as three days.

There are various examples of this in the recent past. In the grand majority, people were clueless as to what appropriate planning was with regards to simply flushing a toilet. After filling whatever porcelain or ceramic options they had, they proceeded to pick rooms where they would defecate and, as a result, their homes were uninhabitable in less than a week.

Here's where some simple planning pays off. If you have access to water, even water unfit to drink, you can have a working toilet by filling the tank with water before flushing or by pouring a couple of gallons directly into the toilet bowl. This will trigger the siphoning action of the plumbing and send your excrement on its merry way. This also works if you have a septic tank, although probably not forever.

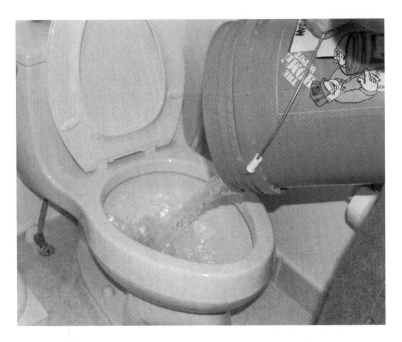

Manual Flush

If you have municipal sewer lines, you have a line known as a "lateral" that goes from your home to the sewer main. Find out if the sewer main is down or not. If the main line is functioning, you can use the process in the above paragraph. If the sewer main is down or blocked, the act of flushing the toilet will eventually back up sewage into the rest of your plumbing (known as backflow). There are backflow prevention valves that can be installed or might already be there; try to find out if you have them.

So how would you deal with human waste when you have no water to spare for the purpose? If you are in your home, empty your toilet as much as possible; then, place two layers of garbage bags (the sturdier the better) inside and lower the lid to hold them in place. Once you have done your duty, pour some sand and some bleach solution over the waste; this will help deodorize it.

If you're a cat person, you have a head start as you've probably stored away some kitty litter to use. Otherwise, consider some of the commercially produced powders that are on the market. After several uses, it will be clear that it's time to dispose of the waste, which you already have conveniently bagged.

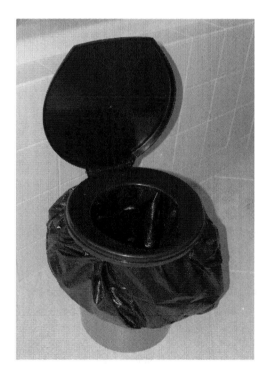

5 gallon bucket with "luggable loo" toilet lid

It might be even wiser to move this bodily function outdoors, as our ancestors did. Here's where a 5 gallon bucket from Home Depot or Lowe's comes in handy. Line it with the same 2 garbage bags (essential items to have stored in quantity) and place your toilet seat, a couple of short length 2 x 4s, or even a commercially produced plastic attachment made for that purpose on top, and you're good to "go". Use sand, dirt, kitty litter, or even quicklime along with some bleach solution until the bag is half full or so. There are even self-composting toilets that are manufactured especially for power-down scenarios, but I have no experience with them. If you do, please let me know how they worked out.

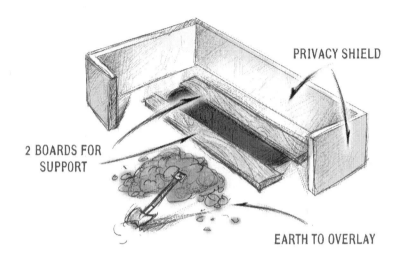

PRIVACY SHIELD

2 BOARDS FOR SUPPORT

EARTH TO OVERLAY

LATRINE

Of course, there is the outdoor latrine for either individual or community use. For those on the move, a single hole dug when the need arises will work, if covered effectively and some important rules are followed (see below). For the long term, you will want to dig a trench latrine A trench latrine is basically just that, a trench dedicated to waste that can be utilized multiple times.

The dimensions of the latrine will depend on the length of time it is needed and the number of people in your group. For a small group, make it 18 inches wide, at least 24 inches deep and at least several feet long. Keep the dirt from the trench in a pile next to it with a shovel, and make sure you cover up the waste after each use to discourage flies, etc.

As an aside, when I was traveling in the third world some years ago, the public restrooms consisted of a hole in the ground that you straddled and bent over. Not very dignified, but it did the job. Consider a longer trench and some kind of partition sheet if your group is big enough to have more than one person utilizing it at a time.

A main concern about any latrine or waste deposited in a hole is contamination of the local water supply. Follow these rules diligently when choosing latrine location and waste disposal outside:

- Don't place a latrine anywhere near your water supply (at least 200 feet away is best)
- Disperse single holes over as wide an area as possible (again, at least 200 feet away from water)
- Don't place latrines anywhere near where rain water runoff occurs
- Don't place latrines near food preparation or eating areas
- Avoid digging single use holes where others are likely to wander
- Dig holes in raised areas; they will be less likely to cause leaching into the water supply
- Consider areas in sunlight as they heat up the soil and speed decomposition

Finally, always be certain to wash your hands after visiting the latrine. We rarely pay enough attention to hand hygiene, and pay the penalty for this by contracting all sorts of illnesses.

Respiratory viruses (colds and flus), E. Coli bacteria (stomach "flus"), Strep throat, Hepatitis A and B, and MRSA are just a few of the ways that you pay the piper by not keeping your hands clean. Some of these bugs can remain alive on your hands for hours.

It is your responsibility as a caregiver to educate your family or group on hand hygiene.

FOOD POISONING

If we find ourselves in a collapse situation, everyone that doesn't have an extensive survival garden up and running will be looking to their environment for edible wild plants. It's likely we'll be less than perfect in our choice of safe, tasty greens. We could easily become ill soon after trying a new plant.

Most food poisoning is actually due to eggs, dairy products and meat that have been contaminated by some type of bacteria. Despite this, most animal meat is not toxic by itself (puffer fish and barracuda are exceptions that come to mind), but there are plenty of plants that have toxins that could seriously harm you. Eating the seeds of an apple, in quantity, will make you sick due to cyanide-like compounds within it. It is just as important to be aware of how to process a particular plant. Many plants that are toxic raw are edible if cooked.

It would be wise to perform some research on what plants grow naturally in your area that have potential for use as food. Some practice "guerilla gardening": That is, they plant seeds for fruits and vegetables in areas that are not normally thought to be farmland. I recently, for example, came across a squash patch on some empty land on a hike near the Great Smoky Mountains National Park.

Some plants send up red flags that tell you to beware. Extreme caution should be taken, for example, with mushrooms and any berries that are white or red unless you have eaten them before without ill effect. Some foods that are fine when cooked are inedible raw.

A survival edibility test can be performed to test whether a substance is safe or not; this test is controversial, with experts recommending both for and against it. It basically involves a stepwise process in which you would first rub the plant against your skin to see if you are allergic to it. Then, you would place it on your lips, in your mouth, and then swallow it in increments; wait a period of time between one step and the next.

You would make sure to try each part of the plant (leaves, flower, stem) separately, using this technique. Certain parts may be safer to eat than others. If done properly, the whole process would take 16 hours for each part of the plant you are testing. This procedure is not foolproof, so

FOOD POISONING

proceed with caution. Symptoms to expect if you have food poisoning would include nausea and vomiting, dizziness, vision disturbances, confusion and palpitations.

When you suspect that you have been poisoned, wash your mouth out immediately to make sure that you don't have any plant material still to be ingested. Then purge yourself, whether it is by pressing down on the back of your tongue with 2 fingers or by using a preparation like Syrup of Ipecac. Most poison control centers will advise against using this substance because it may be difficult to figure out exactly how much will work. The answer is to use the smallest amount of the concoction that will make you vomit. Drink clear fluids to dilute the toxin and help flush it out of your system.

Activated charcoal is another product that is used to treat poisoning. Activated charcoal in your stomach and intestines causes toxins to bind to it, therefore keeping them from entering your system. Some poison control centers don't want you to use this either, due to dosing issues and the fact that it could give you constipation. You may consider taking a laxative when you ingest the charcoal to help move things along. In terms of dosing, there are various pre-measured charcoal products that you can use in liquid or capsule form. Some brand names are SuperChar, Actidote, Liqui-char, InstaChar, and Charcodote.

The best way to prevent food poisoning is by being sure about what you're eating; get a good edible plant guide for your area. Look for one with plenty of photos. A description of which parts are edible and which aren't is important. Foragerpress.com has an assortment of books that might fit the bill. Remember, if there is still modern medical care available to you and you feel sick, get to an emergency room as soon as possible.

In mild cases due to contaminated food sources, you could consider this home remedy: Squeeze 4 lemons, add sugar or honey to sweeten. Take this mixture and drink it twice daily. The idea behind this remedy is to kill any offending bacteria with the acidic lemon juice. Along that same line of thinking is a remedy using 4 tablespoons of apple cider vinegar in 1 big glass of water, with or without a sweetener. Drink this mixture twice a day until improved.

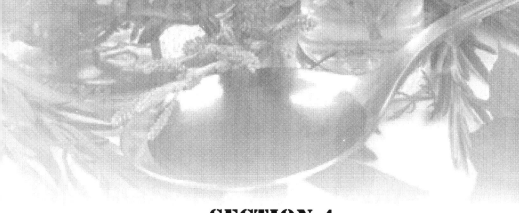

SECTION 4

✚ ✚ ✚

INFECTIONS

In the last section, we discussed infections that usually come as a result of poor sanitation and hygiene, such as diarrheal disease and body lice. There are many other types of bacterial, viral, and parasitic disease that may not necessarily have sanitation and hygiene as a factor, but can be as dangerous. Appendicitis, for example, can occur in anyone regardless of their cleanliness or the conditions at their retreat. A simple ingrown hair may lead to a boil or abscess.

Our bodies' natural ability to fight illness is impressive. There are, however, no organs that are immune to infections; the ability to recognize and treat these illnesses early is essential for the successful survival medic. This section will discuss some of the more common ones that you might see.

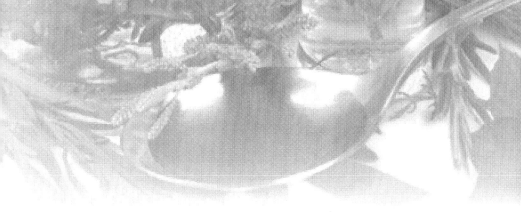

APPENDICITIS AND CONDITIONS THAT MIMIC IT

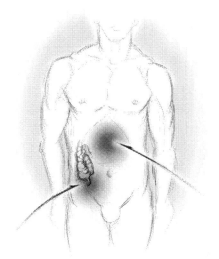

PAIN AREAS LIKELY
IN APPENDICITIS

There are various infections that can cause abdominal pain, some of which can be treated medically and some which are treated surgically. One relatively common issue that could be life-threatening in a long term survival situation, especially to young people, would be appendicitis. Appendicitis (inflammation of the appendix) occurs in approximately 8 out of every 100 people.

Appendicitis can occur in anyone but most likely affects people under 40. The appendix is a tubular worm-shaped piece of tissue 2-4 inches long which connects to the intestine at the lower right side of the abdomen. The inside of this structure forms a pouch that opens to the large intestine. The appendix was once an important organ and still is in some animals (for example, horses), but it is shrunken and nonfunctional in human beings. This is an example of a "vestigial" organ, which means that it exists but serves little useful purpose.

The appendix causes trouble as a result of a blockage. This allows bacteria to multiply and cause inflammation, infection, and even fill up with pus. If the problem is not treated, the appendix can burst, spilling infected matter into the abdominal cavity. This causes a condition called "peritonitis" which can spread throughout the entire abdomen and become very serious. Before the development of antibiotics, it was not unusual to die from the infection; one well-known victim was the silent film star Rudolph Valentino.

Some believe that eating a diet rich in seeds is a cause of appendicitis. Others believe that a lack of fiber in the diet causes small bits of very hard stool to become lodged in the organ. Although these are (rare) possibilities, most cases have no obvious cause.

Appendicitis starts off with vague discomfort in the area of the belly button, but moves down to the lower right quadrant of the abdomen after 12-24 hours. This area, also known as "McBurney's Point", is located about two thirds of the way down from the belly button to the top of the right pelvic bone.

Other likely symptoms may include:

- Nausea and Vomiting
- Loss of appetite
- Fever and Chills
- Abdominal Swelling
- Pain worsening with coughs or walking
- Difficulty passing gas

- Constipation or Diarrhea

A patient may resist using his legs, as that triggers movement of abdominal muscles. Nausea, vomiting, and fever are other common signs and symptoms you may see.

To diagnose this condition, press down on the lower right of the abdomen. Your patient will probably find it painful. Pressing on the left lower quadrant may elicit pain in the lower right quadrant, as well. A sign of a possible ruptured appendix may be what is called "**rebound tenderness**". In this circumstance, pressing down will cause pain, but it will be even more painful when you **remove** your hand.

The patient should be restricted to small amounts of clear liquids as soon as you make the diagnosis. Surgical removal of the appendix is curative here, but will be difficult to carry out without modern medical facilities.

If modern surgical care is unavailable, consider giving the patient antibiotics by mouth in the hope of eliminating an early infection. Of course, intravenous antibiotics, such as Cefoxitin, are more effective than related oral antibiotics, such as Cephalexin (veterinary equivalent: Keflex or FISH-FLEX). Studies in the United Kingdom achieved some success using intravenous antibiotics in early (uncomplicated) cases of appendicitis.

A combination of Ciprofloxacin (veterinary equivalent: FISH-CIN) and Metronidazole (FISH-ZOLE) is an option if intravenous antibiotics or surgical intervention is not available. It is also acceptable in those allergic to Penicillins. Recovery, although slow, may still be possible if treatment is begun early enough or the body has formed a wall around the infection. See the chapter on stockpiling medications for more information on antibiotics.

Can surgery be performed in situations where general anesthesia is unavailable? Most surgeries can't, without the likelihood of losing a patient. Having said that, surgeons in third world countries have, not uncommonly, done appendectomies under local anesthesia

Before surgery is contemplated to deal with an inflamed appendix, you must be certain that you are dealing with that exact problem. Sometimes, different medical problems present with similar symptoms, and you will have to do some detective work to differentiate one from another. This is called making the "differential diagnosis".

There are various conditions which may mimic appendicitis. The following are just a few:

Tubal Pregnancy

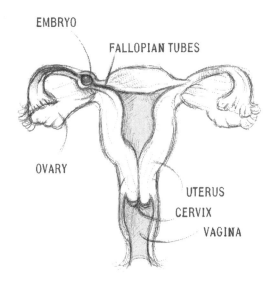

EMBRYO

FALLOPIAN TUBES

OVARY

UTERUS

CERVIX

VAGINA

TUBAL ECTOPIC PREGNANCY

In women of childbearing age, a tubal pregnancy should be ruled out. This is a condition that occurs in 1 in every 125 pregnancies. In this condition, a fertilized egg fails to implant in the normal location (the uterine wall) and implants in the Fallopian tube instead. It grows in this tiny canal until it reaches a size that bursts the tube. This, oftentimes, will cause pain and internal bleeding; in the past, it was not uncommon for a tubal pregnancy to be fatal.

In this case, the pain is due to the presence of blood instead of an infection. If you have women of childbearing age in your family or survival group, have some pregnancy tests in your medical supplies. A woman with a missed period, positive pregnancy test, and severe pain on one side of the lower abdomen is a tubal pregnancy until proven otherwise.

Diverticulitis

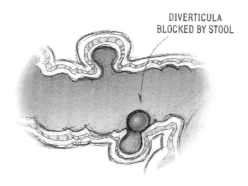

DIVERTICULA
BLOCKED BY STOOL

DIVERTICULITIS

Diverticulitis, unlike appendicitis, is seen mostly in older patients. Diverticula are small pouches in the large bowel that resemble an inner tube peeking out of a defect in an old-timey car tire. These areas may become blocked just like the appendix might. The symptoms are very similar, but most diverticulitis patients will complain of pain in the lower **left** quadrant instead of the right.

Other inflammatory conditions in the bowel, such as Crohn's Disease or Ulcerative Colitis, may present with pelvic pain. These are commonly treated with steroids but may require surgery, as well.

Pelvic Inflammatory Disease

A female pelvic infection often caused by sexually transmitted diseases, such as gonorrhea or chlamydia, may imitate some of the symptoms of an inflamed appendix. This is known as Pelvic Inflammatory Disease (also called "PID"). These patients will, however, usually have pain on **both** sides of the lower abdomen, associated with fever and, sometimes, a foul vaginal discharge.

Pelvic Inflammatory Disease can cause major damage to internal female anatomy. Scarring ensues as the body tries to heal, sometimes causing infertility and chronic discomfort. Serious female infections involving the pelvis are best treated with antibiotics such as Doxycycline, sometimes in combination with Metronidazole twice a day for a week. It is a good idea to treat sexual partners.

Ovarian Cysts

Other female issues in the pelvis, such as large or ruptured ovarian cysts, could also cause pain due to pressure or bleeding. An ovarian cyst is an accumulation of fluid within an ovary that is surrounded by a wall. Many arise from egg follicles, but other can be benign or, less often, cancerous tumors.

Most cysts cause pain by rupturing; a rupture may either cause a painful irritation of the abdominal lining or an episode of internal bleeding. Sometimes, ovarian cysts go away spontaneously, but a ruptured cyst that is actively bleeding will require surgery. A right-sided ruptured cyst could appear similar to appendicitis as the pain is in the same location.

The diagnosis of appendicitis or other causes of abdominal pain without modern diagnostic equipment will be challenging. Despite this, we have to remember that medical personnel, in the past, had only the physical signs and symptoms to help them reach a diagnosis.

Hopefully, we will never be placed in a situation where modern medical care is not available. Many of the conditions described above will represent a possibly fatal result without the ability to perform surgery or give intravenous medications.

Everyone who expects to be responsible for the medical well-being of their family in hard times, however, will have to rely on the skills and knowledge they have learned BEFORE the tribulations began. It may be all we have in the aftermath of a calamity.

URINARY INFECTIONS

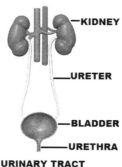

—KIDNEY

—URETER

—BLADDER

—URETHRA

URINARY TRACT

Besides the bowels, our waste is excreted through the urinary tract. The urinary tract includes the kidneys, ureters, bladder, and urethra. It is, essentially, the body's plumbing.

You might find it interesting to know that urine, although a waste product is normally sterile. Most women, at some time of their lives, have experienced a urinary tract infection, or "UTI". An infection of the bladder is known as "**cystitis**", this type of infection usually affects the urethra (the tube that drains the bladder) as well.

Although men are not immune from a bladder infection, the male urethra is much longer. Therefore, it's a much longer trip for bacteria to reach the bladder. Various organisms may cause this infection; E. Coli is the most common.

Some urinary infections are sexually transmitted, such as Gonorrhea. In men, painful urination (also called "**dysuria**") is very common, though most women might only note a yellowish vaginal discharge.

Although painful urination is not uncommon in cystitis, the most common symptom is frequency. Some people notice that the stream of urine is somewhat hesitant ("hesitancy") or may feel an urgent need to go without warning ("urgency"). If not treated, a bladder infection may possibly ascend to the kidneys, causing an infection known as "**pyelo-**

nephritis". This is, again, most commonly caused by the bacterium E. Coli. Once an infections is in the kidney, your patient may experience:

- One-sided back or flank pain
- Persistent fever and chills
- Abdominal pain
- Bloody, cloudy, or foul urine
- Dysuria
- Sweating
- Mental changes (in the elderly)

Once the infection is in the kidneys, antibiotics will be necessary. If the infection is not treated, the condition may progress to "sepsis", where the infection reaches the bloodstream via the kidneys. These patients will show signs of shock, such as rapid breathing, decreased blood pressure, fever and chills, and confusion or loss of consciousness.

Preventative medicine plays a large role in decreasing the likelihood of this problem. Adherence to basic hygienic methods in those at high risk, especially women, is warranted. Standard recommendations include wiping from front to back after urinating or defecating, as well as urinating right after an episode of sexual intercourse. Also, never postpone urinating when there is a strong urge to do so.

Advise your patients to wear cotton undergarments; this will allow better air circulation in areas that might otherwise encourage bacterial or fungal growth. Adequate fluid intake is also a key to remaining free of bladder issues. Consider natural diuretics (substances that increase urine output) to flush out your system. Never postpone urinating when you feel a strong urge to do so.

Treatment revolves around the vigorous administration of fluids. Lots of water will help flush out the infection by decreasing the concentration of bacteria in the bladder or kidney. Applying warmth to the bladder region is soothing for patients with cystitis. Antibiotics are another mainstay of therapy (brand names and veterinary equivalents in parenthesis):

- Sulfamethoxazole-trimethoprim (Bactrim, Septra, Bird-Sulfa)
- Amoxicillin (Amoxil, Fish-Mox)
- Nitrofurantoin (Macrobid)
- Ampicillin (Fish-Cillin)
- Ciprofloxacin (Cipro, Fish-Flox)

An over-the-counter medication that eliminates the painful urination seen in urinary infections is Phenazopyridine (also known as Pyridium, Uristat, Azo, etc.). Don't be alarmed if your urine turns reddish-orange; it is an effect of the drug and is temporary. Vitamin C supplements are thought to reduce the concentration of bacteria in the urine, and should also be considered.

A few natural remedies for urinary tract infections are listed below:

- Garlic or garlic oil (preferably in capsules).
- Echinacea extract or tea.
- Goldenrod tea with 1-2 tablespoons of vinegar.
- Uva Ursi (1 tablet).
- Cranberry tablets (1 to 3 pills).
- Alka Seltzer in 2 ounces warm water (poured directly over the urethra)

Use any one of these remedies three times per day.

One more alternative that may be helpful is to perform an external massage over the bladder area with 5 drops of lavender essential oil (mixed with castor oil) for a few minutes. Then, apply a gentle heat source over the area; repeat this 3 to 4 times daily. The combination of lavender/castor oil and warmth may help decrease bladder spasms and pain.

HEPATITIS

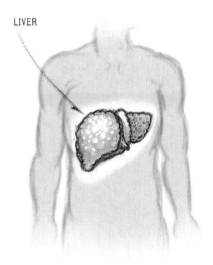

LIVER

CIRRHOSIS

The largest internal organ in the human body is the liver. This organ is extremely important for survival, and any impairment in its function is dangerous. The liver has many duties, including:

- Production of bile to help digestion
- Filtration of toxins from the blood (for example, alcohol)
- Storage of certain vitamins and minerals
- Production of amino acids (for protein synthesis)
- Maintenance of normal levels of glucose (sugar) in the blood
- Conversion of glucose to glycogen for storage purposes.
- Production of cholesterol
- Production of urea (main component in urine)
- Processing of old red blood cells
- Production of certain hormones

Hepatitis is the term used for inflammation of the liver. Mostly caused by viruses, this condition causes the inability of the body to process toxins and perform the other functions listed above, and can be life-threatening.

There are various types of Hepatitis, often called Hepatitis A, Hepatitis B, and Hepatitis C, etc. Hepatitis can also occur due to adverse reactions from drugs and alcohol, among other things.

Hepatitis may be caused by oral/fecal contamination, as well. As such, I was in a quandary regarding whether to put this in the last section on hygiene and sanitation or here. I decided to place it here as some types of liver damage are not hygiene-related, such as those caused by alcohol abuse. Hepatitis can also be spread by sexual contact.

The **hepatitis A** virus is found in the bowel movements of an infected individual. When a person eats food or drinks water that is contaminated with the virus, they develop a flu-like syndrome that can quickly become serious.

This illness could easily go through an entire community in a very short time. Even now, we are at risk; if a restaurant employee with hepatitis A doesn't wash his hands after using the bathroom, everyone that eats there may get sick.

The hallmark of hepatitis is "**jaundice**". You will find that your patient's skin and the whites of their eyes will turn yellow. Their urine becomes darker and their stools turn grey. The liver, which can be found on the right side of the abdomen just below the lowest rib, becomes enlarged or tender to the touch. There is also a sensation of itchiness that is felt all over the body. Add to this a feeling of extreme fatigue, weight loss, vague nausea, and sometimes fever. In some circumstances, people with hepatitis may have no symptoms at all and still pass the illness to others.

Hepatitis B can be spread by exposure to infected blood, plasma, semen, and vaginal fluids. Symptoms are usually indistinguishable from Hepatitis A, although they may lead to a chronic condition known as "**Cirrhosis**" that leads to permanent liver damage.

In cirrhosis, the functioning cells of the liver are replaced by nodules that do nothing to help metabolism. Cirrhosis can also be caused by long-term alcohol and chemical abuse. Possible signs and symptoms of liver cirrhosis include "**ascites**" (accumulation of fluid in the abdomen), varicose veins (enlarged veins, especially in the stomach and esophagus), jaundice and/or swollen ankles. Brain damage is a possibility, due to the accumulation of toxins that are no longer processed by the damaged liver.

About 200 million people are chronically infected with **hepatitis C** virus throughout the world. It is a blood-borne virus contracted by intravenous drug use, transfusion, and unsafe sexual or medical practices. A percentage of these patients will progress to cirrhosis over time.

There are a number of other types of Hepatitis, all the way to Hepatitis X. The ones discussed are the most common.

Other than making your patient comfortable, there isn't very much that you will be able to do in an austere setting regarding this condition.

The drugs used for this condition will be unavailable. Most cases of Hepatitis, however, are self-limited, which means that they will resolve on their own after a period of time. Expect at least 2 – 6 weeks of down time. There is a vaccine available for Hepatitis B.

You can, however, practice good preventive medicine by encouraging the following policies for your family or community:

- Hand washing after using the bathroom and before preparing food.
- Wash dishes with soap in hot water.
- Avoid eating or drinking anything that may not be properly cooked or filtered.
- Make sure children don't put objects in their mouths.

There are a few "detoxifying" and anti-inflammatory herbal remedies that may help support a liver inflicted with hepatitis. Some of these supplements include:

- Milk Thistle
- Artichoke
- Dandelion
- Turmeric

- Licorice
- Red Clover
- Green Tea

Remember these are not cures, but may assist your other efforts by having a restorative effect.

Nutritional strategies that may help:

- Avoid fatty foods and alcohol
- Increase zinc intake
- Decrease protein intake
- Improve hydration status, especially with herbal teas, vegetable broths and diluted vegetable juices.

INFECTIONS CAUSED BY YEAST

In addition to viruses and bacteria, our body may be susceptible to "yeast". Yeast is a fungus that is one-celled and reproduces by budding off the parent. The human body naturally harbors certain types but can be damaged by others.

Fungal infections may be local, as in vaginal infections, "ringworm", or "athlete's foot", or systemic (throughout the entire body). Some people are affected by intestinal fungal infections that can affect digestion. Systemic fungal infections have been blamed for many illnesses, but proven cases seem to occur mostly in the very young or the elderly; those with compromised immune systems can also be affected.

Vaginal Infections

Vaginal yeast infections (also called "**Monilia**") are extremely common and are not an indication of a sexually transmitted disease. A woman with a yeast infection will have an odorless thick white discharge reminiscent of cottage cheese. She will complain of vaginal itchiness.

This infection is often easily treated with short courses of over-the-counter creams or vaginal suppositories such as Monistat (miconazole), but may recur. Resistant infections may be treated with prescription Fluconazole (Diflucan) 150mg orally once. Repeat in 3 days if symptoms persist.

Non-yeast vaginal infections, those caused by bacteria or protozoa, also exist and are called "**bacterial vaginosis**" and "**trichomoniasis**", respectively. These tend to have a foul odor and are treated with a prescription antibiotic/anti-parasitic medication called Metronidazole (veterinary equivalent: FISH-ZOLE), which is taken orally.

The time-honored vinegar and water douche, performed once a day, is very effective in eliminating minor vaginal infections.

Douche with 1 tablespoon of vinegar to a quart of water. Use this method only until your patient feels better. Women who douche often are, paradoxically, **MORE** likely to get yeast infections. This occurs because douching disrupts the normal balance of pH and allows naturally occurring yeast organisms in the vagina to overrun their environment.

Acidophilus supplements, in powder or capsule form, may be a good oral treatment. Cranberry juice and yogurt are good foods for vaginal infections because they change the pH of the organ to a level inhospitable to yeast.

As garlic has both antibacterial and anti-fungal action, you might consider inserting a clove of garlic wrapped in gauze and placing it in the vagina for no more than 8 hours. Make sure you leave a "tail" of gauze that you can easily reach to remove the garlic.

To relieve itching, sit in a bath of warm water with a few drops of lavender or tea tree oil for 15 minutes. Repeat as needed.

Oral Infections

A related yeast infection may be seen in the mouth of some infants and others. This infection is known as "**Thrush**" and is identified by white patches on the inside of the cheeks, the roof of the mouth, and other areas of the oral cavity. Thrush can cause irritation and the white patches are adherent, causing bleeding if wiped off. Occasionally, nipple tissue is affected in breastfeeding mothers.

Oral thrush may be treated conventionally with liquid Fluconazole (Diflucan) once a day for a week. Nystatin, another antifungal, is available as a "swish-and-swallow" version for oral thrush or can be applied topically four times a day to infected nipples for approximately five to seven days.

Alternative remedies reported to be effective for oral yeast infections include:

- Swabbing the oral cavity with yogurt.
- Applying acidophilus to nipples or other items likely to go in an infant's mouth.
- Applying white vinegar (distilled) or very dilute baking soda solutions (1 teaspoon to 8 ounces of water) to nipples.
- Swabbing the oral area with coconut oil (virgin).

Athlete's Foot

Athlete's foot (also known as "**tinea pedis**") is an infection of the skin caused by a type of fungus. This condition may be a chronic issue, lasting for years if not treated. Although usually seen between the toes, you might see it also on other parts of the feet or even on the hands (often between fingers). It should be noted that this problem is contagious, passed by sharing shoes or socks and even by wet surfaces.

Any fungal infection is made worse by moist conditions. People who are prone to Athlete's foot commonly:

- Spend long hours in closed shoes
- Keep their feet wet for prolonged periods
- Have had a tendency to get cuts on feet and hands
- Perspire a lot
- To make the diagnosis, look for:
- Flaking of skin between the toes or fingers.
- Itching and burning of affected areas
- Reddened skin
- Discolored nails
- Fluid drainage from surfaces traumatized by repeated scratching

If the condition is mild, keeping your feet clean and dry may be enough to allow slow improvement of the condition. Oftentimes, however, topical antifungal ointments or powders such as miconazole or clotrimazole are required for elimination of the condition. In the worst cases, oral prescription antifungals such as fluconazole (Diflucan) are needed. Don't use anti-itching creams very often, as it keeps the area moist and may delay healing.

A favorite home remedy for Athlete's Foot involves placing Tea Tree Oil liberally to a foot bath and soak for 20 minutes or so. Dry the feet well and then apply a few drops onto the affected area. Repeat this process twice daily. Try to keep the area as dry as possible between treatments.

For prevention of future outbreaks of Athlete's Foot, apply tea tree oil once a week before putting on socks and shoes.

Ringworm

Ringworm is just another word for "**tinea**". It represents a fungal infection on the surface of the skin. Oftentimes, a second word is added to denote the location of the infection. Therefore, "tinea pedis" is a fungal infection of the foot, or Athlete's Foot.

The fungus that causes Athlete's foot is just as likely to affect any other area of the skin. Often, it will appear as a raised, itchy patch that is darker on the outside. As such, it may resemble a sharply-defined ring, and is called "Ringworm". Ringworm has nothing to do with worms, however.

If Ringworm occurs in a hairy area, it will likely cause bald patches. Consistent scratching at the patches will cause blistering and oozing. Treatment, both conventional and natural, follows a similar process as that described for Athlete's Foot.

Make sure to:

- Keep skin as dry as possible.
- Antifungal (Miconazole, Clotrimazole) or drying powders or creams.
- Avoid tight-fitting clothing on irritated areas
- Wash regularly.
- Wash sheets daily.

CELLULITIS

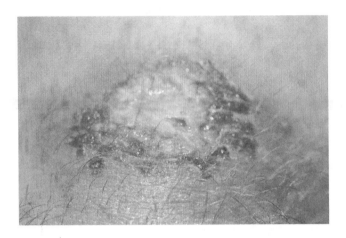

Any soft tissue injury carries with it a degree of risk when it comes to infection. Infections from minor wounds or insect bites are relatively easy to treat today, due to the wide availability of antibiotics. With major wounds, these medications may actually save a life.

In a survival situation, antibiotics will be precious commodities; they should be dispensed only when absolutely necessary. The misuse of antibiotics, along with their frequent use in livestock, is part of the reason that we're beginning to see resistant strains of bacteria.

80% of all the antibiotics in use today are given to livestock. Amazingly, this is not to treat infection, but to speed up growth and get meat to market sooner.

Despite your best efforts to care for a wound, there is always a chance that an infection will occur. Infection in the soft tissues below the superficial level of the skin (the "**epidermis**") is referred to as "**cellulitis**". Below the epidermis, the main layers of soft tissue are the "**dermis**" (you've seen this area when you scraped your knee as a kid), the subcutaneous fat, and the muscle layers.

Cellulitis is significant to the preparedness community because it will be very commonly seen in a collapse. Although preventable, the sheer number of cuts, scrapes, and burns will make it one of the most prevalent medical problems. This infection can easily reach the bloodstream, and, without antibiotics, can cause a life-threatening condition known as "**sepsis**". Once sepsis has set in, inflammation of the spinal cord ("**meningitis**") or bony structures ("**osteomyelitis**") can further complicate the situation. In the past, people who became septic frequently died.

The bacteria that can cause cellulitis are on your skin right now. Normal inhabitants of the surface of your skin include Staphylococcus and Group A Streptococcus. They do no harm until the skin is broken. Then, they invade deeper layers where they are not normally seen and start causing inflammation.

Cuts, bites, blisters, or cracks in the skin can all be entry ways for bacteria to cause infections that could be life-threatening if not treated.

Cellulitis, as an aside, has nothing to do with the dimpling on the skin called cellulite. The suffix "-itis" simply means "inflammation", so cellul-itis simply means "inflammation of the cells", appendicitis means "inflammation of the appendix" and so on...

Conditions that might cause cellulitis are:

- Cracks or peeling skin between the toes
- Varicose veins/poor circulation
- Injuries that cause a break in the skin
- Insect bites and stings, animal bites, or human bites
- Ulcers from chronic illness, such as diabetes
- Use of steroids or other medications that affect the immune system
- Wounds from previous surgery
- Intravenous drug use

The symptoms and signs of cellulitis are:

- Discomfort/pain in the area of infection
- Fever and Chills
- Exhaustion (**fatigue**)
- General ill feeling (**malaise**)
- Muscle aches (**myalgia**)
- Heat in the area of the infection
- Drainage of pus/cloudy fluid from the area of the infection

- Redness, usually spreading towards torso
- Swelling in the area of infection (causing a sensation of tightness)
- Foul odor coming from the area of infection

Other, less common, symptoms that can occur with this disease:

- Hair loss at the site of infection
- Joint stiffness caused by swelling of the tissue over the joint
- Nausea and vomiting

Although the body can sometimes resolve cellulitis on its own, treatment usually includes the use of antibiotics; these can be topical, oral or intravenous. Most cellulitis will improve and disappear after a 10 – 14 day course of therapy with medications in the Penicillin, Eythromycin, or Cephalosporin (Keflex) families. Amoxicillin and Ampicillin are particularly popular. If the cellulitis is in an extremity, it is helpful to keep the limb elevated.

Many of these are available in veterinary form without a prescription (see our section on stockpiling medications later in this volume). Acetaminophen (Tylenol) or Ibuprofen (Advil) is useful to decrease discomfort. Warm water soaks have been used for many years, along with elevation of infected extremities, for symptomatic relief. Over several days, you should see an improvement. It would be wise to complete the full 10-14 days of antibiotics to prevent any recurrences.

ABSCESSES (BOILS)

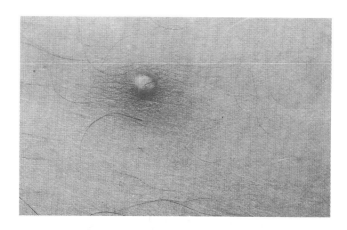

An **abscess** is a form of cellulitis that is, essentially, a pocket of pus. Pus is the debris left over from your body's attempt to eliminate an infection; it consists of white and red blood cells, live and dead organisms, and inflammatory fluid.

If the abscess was not caused by an infected wound or diseased tooth, it is possible that it originated in a "**cyst**", which is a hollow structure filled with fluid. There are various types of cysts that can become infected and form abscesses:

Sebaceous: skin glands often associated with hair follicles, they are concentrated on the face and trunk. These cysts produce oily material known as "sebum".

Inclusion: These occur when skin lining is trapped in deeper layers as a result of trauma. They continue to produce skin cells and grow.

Pilonidal: These cysts are located over the area of the tailbone, and are due to a malformation during fetal development. They easily become infected and require intervention.

The body's attempt to cure an infection is a good thing. However, abscesses or boils have a tendency to wall off the infection, which also makes it hard for medications like antibiotics to penetrate. As such, you may have to intervene by performing a procedure.

To deal with an abscess, a route must be forged for the evacuation of pus. The easiest way to facilitate this is to place warm moist compresses over the area. This will help bring the infection to the surface of the skin, where it will form a "head" and perhaps drain spontaneously. This is called "ripening" the abscess. The abscess will go from firm to soft, and have a "whitehead" pimple at the likely point of exit.

If this fails to happen by itself over a few days, you may have to open the boil by a procedure called "**incision and drainage**" First, apply some ice to the area to help numb the skin. Then, using the tip of a scalpel (a number 11 blade is best), pierce the skin over the abscess where it is closest to the surface. The pus should drain freely, and your patient will probably experience immediate relief from the release of pressure.

Finally, apply some triple antibiotic ointment to the skin surrounding the incision and cover with a clean bandage. Alternatives to triple antibiotic ointment could be:

- Lavender essential oil
- Tea Tree essential oil
- Raw Honey

Incision and drainage may be helpful for dental abscesses as well, but may not save overlying teeth. Information about how to extract a tooth may be found in the dental section of this book.

TETANUS

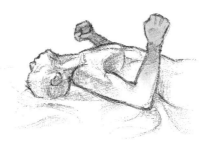

TETANUS

Classic position associated with Tetanus

Most of us have dutifully gone to get a tetanus shot when we stepped on a rusty nail, but few have any real concept of what Tetanus is and why it is dangerous. The role of the survival medic is to know the answers to these questions. Knowledge of risks, prevention, and treatment will be the armor plate in your medical defense.

Tetanus (from the Greek word tetanos, meaning tight) is an infection caused by a bacteria called Clostridium Tetani. The bacteria produces spores (inactive bacteria-to-be) that primarily live in the soil or the feces of animals. These spores are capable of living for years and are resistant to extremes in temperature.

Tetanus is relatively rare in the United States, with about 50 reported cases a year. Worldwide, however, there are more than 500,000 cases a year. Most victims are found in developing countries in Africa and Asia that have poor immunization programs.

Why should this fact have significance for you and your family? Citizens of developed countries may be thrown into third world status in the aftermath of a mega-catastrophe. Therefore, it's important to be prepared for third world medical issues. Tetanus is one.

Most tetanus infections occur when a person has experienced a break in the skin. The skin is the most important barrier to infection, and any chink in the armor leaves a person open to infection. The most common cause is some type of puncture wound, such as an insect or animal bite, a splinter, or even that rusty nail. This is because the tetanus bacterium doesn't like oxygen, and deep, narrow wounds give less access to it. Any injury that compromises the skin, however, is eligible: Burns, crush injuries, and lacerations can be entryways for Tetanus bacteria.

When a wound becomes contaminated with Tetanus spores, the spore becomes activated as a full-fledged bacterium and reproduces rapidly. Damage to the victim comes as a result of a strong toxin excreted by the organism known as Tetanospasmin. This toxin specifically targets nerves that serve muscle tissue.

Tetanospasmin binds to motor nerves, causing "misfires" that lead to involuntary contraction of the affected areas. This neural damage could be localized or can affect the entire body. You would possibly see the classical symptom of "**Lockjaw**", where the jaw muscle is taut; any muscle group, however, is susceptible to the contractions if affected by the toxin. This includes the respiratory musculature, which can inhibit normal breathing and become life-threatening.

The most severe cases seem to occur at extremes of age, with newborns and those over 65 most likely to succumb to the disease. Death rates from generalized Tetanus hover around 25-50%, higher in newborns.

You will be on the lookout for the following early symptoms:

- Sore muscles (especially near the site of injury)
- Weakness
- Irritability
- Difficulty swallowing
- Lockjaw (also called "Trismus"; facial muscles are often the first affected)

Initial symptoms may not present themselves for up to 2 weeks. As the disease progresses, you may see:

- Progressively worsening muscle spasms (may start locally and become generalized over time)
- Involuntary arching of the back (sometimes so strong that bones may break or dislocations may occur!)

- Fever
- Respiratory distress
- High blood pressure
- Irregular heartbeats

The first thing that the survival medic should understand is that, although an infectious disease, Tetanus is not contagious. You can feel confident treating a Tetanus victim safely, as long as you wear gloves and observe standard clean technique. Begin by washing your hands and putting on your gloves. Then, wash the wound thoroughly with soap and water, using an irrigation syringe to flush out any debris. This will, hopefully, limit growth of the bacteria and, as a result, decrease toxin production.

You will want to administer antibiotics to kill off the rest of the bacteria in the system. Metronidazole (veterinary equivalent: Fish-Zole) 375-500mg twice a day or Doxycycline (Bird-Biotic) 100 mg twice a day are known to be effective. The earlier you begin antibiotic therapy, the less toxin will be produced. IV rehydration, if you have the ability to administer it, is also helpful. The patient will be more comfortable in an environment with dim lights and reduced noise.

Late stage Tetanus is difficult to treat with modern technology. Ventilators, Tetanus Antitoxin, and muscle relaxants/sedatives such as Valium are used to treat severe cases but will be unlikely to be available to you in a long term survival situation. For this reason, it is extraordinarily important for the survival medic to watch anyone who has sustained a wound for the early symptoms listed above.

As medic, you must obtain a detailed medical history from anyone that you might be responsible for in times of trouble. This includes immunization histories where possible. Has the injured individual been immunized against Tetanus? Most people born in the U.S. will have gone through a series of immunizations against Diptheria, Tetanus, and Whooping Cough early in their childhood. If not, encourage them to get up to date with their immunizations against this dangerous disease as soon as possible. Booster injections are usually given every 10 years.

Tetanus vaccine is not without its risks, but severe complications such as seizures or brain damage occur is less than one in a million cases. Milder side effects such as fatigue, fever, nausea and vomiting, headache, and inflammation in the injection site are more common.

Given the life-threatening nature of the disease, this is one vaccine that you should encourage your people to receive, regardless of your feelings about vaccines in general. If not caught early, there may be little you can do to treat your patient in an austere setting.

MOSQUITO BORNE ILLNESSES

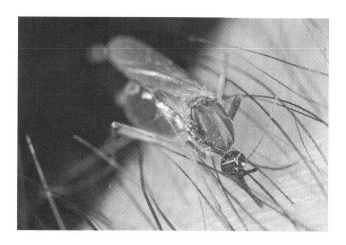

Unlike the stings of bees or wasps, mosquito bites are common vectors of various infectious diseases. Anaphylaxis (severe allergic reaction) is rarely an issue with mosquitos and is covered in another part of this book.

The increased amount of time we will spend outside in a survival situation will increase the chances of exposure to one or more mosquito-borne illnesses. One of the most notorious diseases caused by mosquito vectors is Malaria.

Malaria is caused by a microscopic organism called a protozoan. When mosquitos get a meal by biting you, they inject these microbes into your system. Once in the body, they colonize your liver. From there, they go to your blood cells and other organs. By the way, only female mosquitos bite humans.

Symptoms of Malaria appear flu-like, and classically present as periodic chills, fever, and sweats. The patient becomes anemic as more blood cells are damaged by the protozoa. With time, periods between episodes become shorter and permanent organ damage may occur.

Diagnosis of malaria cannot be confirmed without a microscope, but anyone experiencing relapsing fevers with severe chills and sweating should be considered candidates for treatment. The medications, among others, used for Malaria are Chloroquine, Quinine, and Quinidine.

Sometimes, an antibiotic such as Doxycycline or Clindamycin is used in combination with the above. Physicians are usually sympathetic towards prescribing these medications to those who are contemplating trips to places where mosquitos are rampant, such as some underdeveloped countries.

Other mosquito-borne diseases include Yellow Fever, Dengue Fever, and West Nile Virus. The fewer mosquitos near your retreat, the less likely you will fall victim to one of these diseases. You can decrease the population of mosquitos in your area and improve the likelihood of preventing illness by:

- Looking for areas of standing water that could serve as mosquito breeding grounds. Drain all water that you do not depend on for survival.
- Monitoring the screens on your retreat windows and doors and repairing any holes or defects.
- Being careful to avoid outside activities at dusk or dawn. This is the time that mosquitos are most active.
- Wear long pants and shirts whenever you venture outside.
- Have a good stockpile of insect repellants.

If you are reluctant to use chemical repellants, you may consider natural remedies. Plants that contain Citronella may be rubbed on your skin to discourage bites. Lemon balm, despite having a fragrance similar to citronella, does not have the same bug-repelling properties. Despite its name, lemon balm is actually a member of the mint family.

When you use an essential oil to repel insects, re-apply frequently and feel free to combine oils as needed. Besides Citronella oil, you could use:

- Lemon Eucalyptus oil
- Cinnamon oil
- Peppermint oil
- Geranium oil
- Clove oil
- Rosemary oil

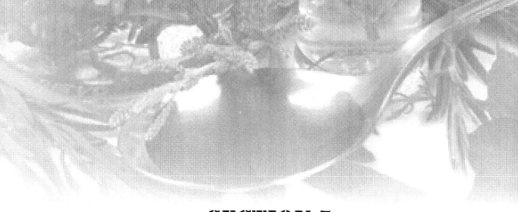

SECTION 5

+ + +

ENVIRONMENTAL FACTORS

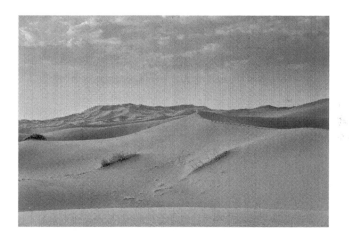

A creature's habitat is the place where it lives. This could be a forest, a lake, the branches of a tree or the underside of a leaf. If you're a human being, your habitat is likely a town; few humans can call the wilderness their home. When you are in an environment that is not your own, careful planning is necessary to avoid running afoul of the elements.

THE SURVIVAL MEDICINE HANDBOOK

The focus of your medical training should be general, but also take into account the type of environment that you expect to live in if a societal collapse occurs. If you live in Miami, it's unlikely you'll be treating a lot of people with hypothermia. If you live in Siberia, it's unlikely you'll be treating a lot of people with heat stroke. Learn how to treat the likely medical issues for the area and situation that you expect to find yourself in.

One major environmental risk is the effect of ambient temperature. Humans tolerate a very narrow range and are susceptible to damage as a result of being too cold or too hot. Your body has various methods it uses to control its internal "core" temperature, either raising it or lowering it to appropriate levels. The body "core" refers to the major internal organ systems that are necessary to maintain life, such as your brain, heart, liver, and others. The remainder (your skin, muscles and extremities) is referred to as the "periphery".

Your body regulates its core temperature in various ways:

- **Vasoconstriction** – blood vessels tighten to decrease flow to periphery, thereby decreasing heat loss.
- **Vasodilation** – blood vessels expand to increase flow, thereby increasing heat loss.
- **Perspiration** – sweat evaporates, causing a cooling effect.
- **Shivering** – muscles produce heat by movements which create warmth.
- **Exertion** – increasing work levels produce heat, decreasing work levels decrease heat.

Your body also regulates its temperature by common sense, adding or subtracting layers of clothing to match the environment.

Illness related to exposure to extreme cold is referred to as "**Hypothermia**". Illness related to exposure to excessive heat is called "**Hyperthermia**", but is better known by the terms "Heat Exhaustion" and "Heat Stroke".

Many environmental causes of illness are preventable with some planning. If you are in a hot environment, don't schedule major outdoor work sessions in the middle of the day. If you absolutely must work in the heat, provide a canopy, hats, or other protection against the sun. Be certain that everyone arrives well-hydrated and gets plenty of water throughout. Expect each person to require a pint of water an hour while working in the heat. Failure to take the above precautions could lead to dehydration (discussed in the section on diarrheal disease), sunburns, and increased likelihood of work injury.

Likewise, those in cold environments should take the weather into account when planning outdoor activities in order to avoid hypothermia issues, such as frostbite. Youngsters especially will run out into the cold without paying much attention to dressing warmly. Adults will often ignore the wind chill factor. Likewise, if an adult has had too much to drink, impaired judgment may put them in jeopardy of suffering a cold-related event.

Part of the healthcare provider's role is to educate each and every member of their family or group on proper planning for outdoor activities. Monitor weather conditions as well as the people you're sending out in the heat or cold. If you don't, your environment becomes your enemy (a formidable one).

HEAT-RELATED MEDICAL ISSUES HYPERTHERMIA (HEAT STROKE)

In the aftermath of storms or in the wilderness, you may find yourself without shelter to protect you from the elements. In the heat of summer, a common condition you'll encounter might be heat stroke, otherwise known as **hyperthermia**. Even in cold weather, significant physical exertion in an over-clothed and under-hydrated individual could lead to significant heat-related injury. The elderly are particularly prone to issues relating to overheating, and must be watched closely if exposed to the sun.

The ill effects due to overheating are called "heat exhaustion" if mild to moderate; if severe, these effects are referred to as "heat stroke". Heat exhaustion usually does not result in permanent damage, but heat stroke does; indeed, it can permanently disable or even kill its victim. It is a medical emergency that must be diagnosed and treated promptly.

The risk of heat stroke correlates strongly to the "heat index", a measurement of the effects of air temperature combined with high humidity. Above 60% relative humidity, loss of heat by perspiration is impaired, increasing the chances of heat-related illness. Exposure to full sun increases the reported heat index by as much as 10-15 degrees F.

Simply having muscle cramps or a fainting spell does not necessarily signify a major heat-related medical event. You will see "heat cramps" often in children that have been running around on a hot day. Getting them out of the sun, massaging the affected muscles, and providing hydration will usually resolve the problem.

To make the diagnosis of heat exhaustion, a significant rise in the body's core temperature is required. As many heat-related symptoms may mimic other conditions, a thermometer of some sort should be a component of your medical supplies.

In addition to muscle cramps and/or fainting, heat exhaustion is characterized by:

- Confusion
- Rapid pulse
- Flushing

- Nausea and Vomiting
- Headache
- Temperature elevation up to 105 degrees F

If no action is taken to cool the victim, heat stroke may ensue. Heat stroke, in addition to all the possible signs and symptoms of heat exhaustion, will manifest as loss of consciousness, seizures or even bleeding (seen in the urine or vomit). Breathing becomes rapid and shallow.

If not dealt with quickly, shock and organ malfunction may ensue, leading to your patient's demise. The skin is likely to be hot to the touch, but dry; sweating might be absent. The body makes efforts to cool itself down until it hits a temperature of 106 degrees or so. At that point, thermoregulation breaks down and the body's ability to use sweating as a natural temperature regulator fails. In heat stroke, the body core can rise to 110 degrees Fahrenheit or more.

You'll notice that the skin becomes red, not because it is burned, but because the blood vessels are dilating in an effort to dissipate some of the heat.

In some circumstances, the patient's skin may actually seem cool. It is important to realize that it is the body CORE temperature that is elevated. A person in shock may feel "cold and clammy" to the touch. You could be misled by this finding, but simply taking a reading with your thermometer will reveal the patient's true status.

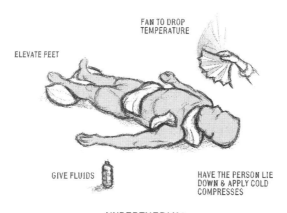

FAN TO DROP TEMPERATURE

ELEVATE FEET

GIVE FLUIDS

HAVE THE PERSON LIE DOWN & APPLY COLD COMPRESSES

HYPERTHERMIA

When overheated patients are no longer able to cool themselves, it is up to their rescuers to do the job. If hyperthermia is suspected, the victim should immediately:

- Be removed from the heat source (for example, out of the sun).
- Have their clothing removed.
- Be drenched with cool water (or ice, if available)
- Have their legs elevated above the level of their heart (the shock position)
- Be fanned or otherwise ventilated to help with heat evaporation
- Have moist cold compresses placed in the neck, armpit and groin areas

Why the neck, armpit and groin? Major blood vessels pass close to the skin in these areas, and you will more efficiently cool the body core. In the wilderness, immersion in a cold stream may be all you have in terms of a cooling strategy. This is a worthwhile option as long as you are closely monitoring your patient.

Oral rehydration is useful to replace fluids lost, but ONLY if the patient is awake and alert. If your patient has altered mental status, he or she might "swallow" the fluid into their airways; this causes damage to the lungs and puts you in worse shape than when you started.

You might think that acetaminophen or ibuprofen could help to lower temperatures, but this is actually not the case. These medications are meant to lower fevers caused by an infection, and they don't work as well if the fever was not caused by one.

Wear clothing appropriate for the weather. Tightly swaddling an infant with blankets, simply because that is "what's done" with a baby, is a recipe for disaster in hot weather. Have everyone wear a head covering. A bandanna soaked in water, for example, would be effective against the heat. Much of the sweating we do comes from our face and head, so towel off frequently to aid in heat evaporation.

If you can avoid dehydration, you will likely avoid heat exhaustion or heat stroke. Work or exercise in hot weather (especially by someone in poor physical condition) will easily cause a person to lose body water content.

A loss of just 1% of your total water initiates the thirst mechanism. You'll need a pint of water an hour to stay hydrated. If thirst is not quenched, as little as 2% water loss begin to affect work efficiency, mood, and other parameters. At 6%, you're as delirious and unco-ordinated as if you've been crawling for miles through Death Valley.

Carefully planning your outdoor work in the summer heat and keeping up with fluids will be a major step in keeping healthy and avoid-ing heat-related illness. Monitor the workload (and the workers) and you'll stay out of trouble.

COLD-RELATED MEDICAL ISSUES
HYPOTHERMIA

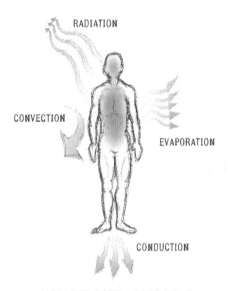

HOW THE BODY LOSES HEAT

Hypothermia is a condition in which body core temperature drops below the temperature necessary for normal body function and metabolism. The normal body core temperature is defined as between 97.5-99.5 degrees Fahrenheit (36.0-37.5 degrees Celsius). Here are some common temperatures converted from Fahrenheit to Celsius:

Fahrenheit	Celsius
32	0
50	10
68	20
77	25
86	30
87.8	31
89.6	32
91.4	33
93.2	34

95	35
96.8	36
98.6	37
100.4	38
102.2	39
104	40
105.8	41
107.6	42
109.4	43

The body loses heat in various ways:

Evaporation – the body perspires (sweats), which releases heat from the core.

Radiation – the body loses heat to the environment anytime that the ambient (surrounding) temperature is below the core temperature (say, 98.6 degrees Fahrenheit). For example, you lose more heat if exposed to an outside temperature of 20 degrees F than if exposed to 80 degrees F.

Conduction – The body loses heat when its surface is in direct contact with cold temperatures, as in the case of someone falling from a boat into frigid water. Water, being denser than air, removes heat from the body much faster.

Convection – Heat loss where, for instance, a cooler object is in motion against the body core. The air next to the skin is heated and then removed, which requires the body to use energy to re-heat. **Wind Chill** is one example of air convection: If the ambient temperature is 32 degrees F but the wind chill factor is at 5 degrees F, you lose heat from your body as if it were actually 5 degrees F.

Most heat is lost from the head area, due to its large surface area and tendency to be uncovered. Direct contact with anything cold, especially over a large area of your body, will cause rapid cooling of your body core temperature. The classic example of this would be a fall into cold water. In the Titanic sinking of 1912, hundreds of people fell into near-freezing water. Within 15 minutes, they were probably beyond medical help.

The body, once it is exposed to cold, kicks into action to produce heat once the core cools down below 95 degrees Fahrenheit (35 degrees Celsius), the temperature below which hypothermia occurs. The main mechanism to produce heat is shivering. Muscles shiver to produce heat, and this will be the first symptom you're likely to see. As hypothermia worsens, more symptoms will become apparent if the patient is not warmed.

Aside from shivering, the most noticeable symptoms of hypothermia will be related to mental status. The person may appear confused, uncoordinated, and lethargic. As the condition worsens, speech may become slurred; the patient will appear apathetic and uninterested in helping themselves, or may fall asleep. This occurs due to the effect of cooling temperatures on the brain; the colder the body core gets, the slower the brain works. Brain function is supposed to cease at about 68 degrees Fahrenheit, although I have read of exceptional cases in which people (usually children) have survived even lower temperatures.

Prevention of Hypothermia

An ounce of prevention is worth a pound of cure. To prevent hypothermia, you must anticipate the climate that you will be traveling through, including wind conditions and wet weather. Condition yourself physically to be fit for the challenge. Travel with a partner if at all possible, and have enough food and water available for the entire trip.

It may be useful to remember the simple acronym C.O.L.D. This stands for: Cover, Overexertion, Layering, and Dry:

- Cover. Protect your head by wearing a hat. This will prevent body heat from escaping from your head. Instead of using gloves to cover your hands, use mittens. Mittens are more helpful than gloves because they keep your fingers in contact with one another. This conserves heat.
- Overexertion. Avoid activities that cause you to sweat a lot. Cold weather causes you to lose body heat quickly, and wet,

sweaty clothing accelerates the process. Rest when necessary; use rest periods to self-assess for cold-related changes. Pay careful attention to the status of your elderly or juvenile group members.

- Layering. Loose-fitting, lightweight clothing in layers insulate you well. Use clothing made of tightly woven, water-repellent material for protection against the wind. Wool or silk inner layers hold body heat better than cotton does. Some synthetic materials work well, also. Especially cover the head, neck, hands and feet.

- Dry. Keep as dry as you can. Get out of wet clothing as soon as possible. It's very easy for snow to get into gloves and boots, so pay particular attention to your hands and feet.

As with many other situations, the very young and the elderly are most at risk for hypothermia. Diabetics and those who suffer from low thyroid levels are also more at risk.

One factor that most people don't take into account is the use of alcohol. Alcohol may give you a "warm" feeling, but it actually causes your blood vessels to expand, resulting in more rapid heat loss from the surface of your body. The body reacts to cold by constricting the blood vessels, so expansion would negate the body's efforts to stay warm. Alcohol also causes impaired judgment, which might cause those under the influence to choose clothing that would not protect them in cold weather. This also goes for various "recreational" drugs.

The diagnosis of hypothermia may be difficult to make with a standard glass thermometer, which doesn't register below 94 degrees Fahrenheit. Unless you have a thermometer that can measure low ranges, it may be difficult to know for certain that you're dealing with this problem. However, if you encounter a person in a cold environment who is unconscious, confused or lethargic, and whose temperature does not register, you should always assume the patient is hypothermic until proven otherwise.

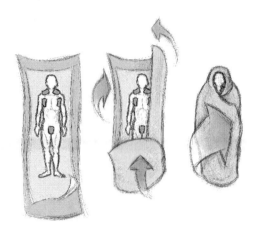

HYPOTHERMIA WRAP

Immediate action must be taken to reverse the ill effects of hypothermia. Important measures to take are:

- **Get the person out of the cold** and into a warm, dry location. If you're unable to move the person out of the cold, shield him or her from the cold and wind as much as possible.
- **Take off wet clothing.** If the person is wearing wet clothing, remove them gently. Cover them with layers of dry blankets, including the head (leave the face clear). If you are outside, cover the ground to eliminate exposure to the cold surface.
- **Monitor breathing.** A person with severe hypothermia may be unconscious. Verify that the patient is breathing and check for a pulse. Begin CPR if necessary.
- **Share body heat.** To warm the person's body, remove your clothing and lie next to the person, making skin-to-skin contact. Then cover both of your bodies with blankets. Some people may cringe at this notion, but it's important to remember that you are trying to save a life. Gentle massage or rubbing may be helpful, but vigorous movements may traumatize the patient
- **Give warm oral fluids.** If the affected person is alert and able to swallow, provide a warm, nonalcoholic, non-caffeinated beverage to help warm the body. Remember, alcohol does not warm you up!

- **Use warm, dry compresses.** Use a first-aid warm compress (a fluid-filled bag that warms up when squeezed), or a makeshift compress of warm (not hot) water in a plastic bottle. Apply a compress only to the neck, chest wall or groin. These areas will spread the heat much better than putting warm compresses on the extremities, which sometimes worsens the condition.
- **Avoid applying direct heat.** Don't use hot water, a heating pad or a heating lamp to warm the person. The extreme heat can damage the skin, cause strain on the heart or even lead to cardiac arrest.

If left untreated, hypothermia leads to complete failure of various organ systems and to death. People who develop hypothermia due to exposure to cold are also vulnerable to other cold-related injuries, such as frostbite and immersion foot.

Frostbite and Immersion (trench) Foot

Frostbite, or freezing of body tissues, usually occurs in the extremities and sometimes the ears and nose. Initial symptoms include a "pins and needles" sensation and numbness. Skin color changes from red to white to blue. If the color then changes to black, a condition known as "**gangrene**" has set in. Gangrene is the death of tissue resulting from loss of circulation. This usually results in the loss of the body part affected.

Immersion foot (formerly known as Trench Foot) causes damage to nerves and small blood vessels due to prolonged immersion in water. When seen in areas other than the feet, this condition is referred to as "chilblains". Immersion foot appears similar to frostbite, but might have a more generally swollen appearance.

Frostbite or Immersion Foot is treated with a warm water (no more than 104 degrees F) soak of the affected extremity. Follow these tips when treating these conditions:

1. Don't allow thawed tissue to freeze again. The more often tissue freezes and thaws, the deeper the damage (think about what happens to a steak that goes from the freezer to outside and back

again). If you can't prevent your patient from being exposed to freezing temperatures again, you should wait before treating, but not more than a day.

2. Don't rub or massage frostbitten tissue. Rubbing frostbitten tissue will result in damage to already injured tissues.

3. Don't use heat lamps or fires to treat frostbite. Your patient is numb and cannot feel the frostbitten tissue. Significant burns can ensue.

4. You can use body heat to thaw mild frostbite. You can put mildly frostbitten fingers under your arm, for example, to warm them up.

Cold Water Safety

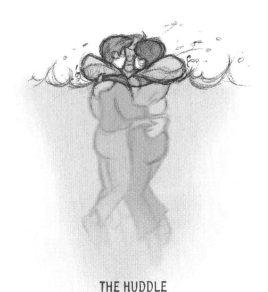

THE HUDDLE

Water doesn't have to be cold to cause hypothermia. Any water that's cooler than normal body temperature will cause heat loss. You could die of hypothermia off a tropical coast if immersed long enough.

In the event that you find yourself in cold water, you'll need to have a strategy that will keep you alive until you're rescued. First, we'll talk about falling into the water when your boat capsizes, and then we'll talk about falling through the ice during a winter hike.

To increase your chances of survival in cold water, do the following:

- **Wear a life jacket.** Whenever you're on a boat, wear a life jacket. A life jacket can help you stay alive longer by enabling you to float without using a lot of energy and by providing some insulation. The life jackets with built-in whistles are best, so you can signal that you're in distress.
- **Keep your clothes on.** While you're in the water, don't remove your clothing. Button or zip up. Cover your head if at all possible. The layer of water between your clothing and your body is slightly warmer and will help insulate you from the cold. Remove your clothing only after you're safely out of the water and then do whatever you can to get dry and warm.
- **Get out of the water, even if only partially.** The less percentage of your body exposed to cold, the less heat you will lose. Climbing onto a capsized boat or grabbing onto a floating object will increase your chances of survival, even if you can only partially get out of the water. However, don't use up energy swimming unless you have a dry place to swim to.
- **Position your body to lessen heat loss.** Use a body position known as the Heat Escape Lessening Position (think **H.E.L.P.**) to reduce heat loss while you wait for help to arrive. Just hold your knees to your chest; this will help protect your torso (the body core) from heat loss.
- **Huddle together.** If you've fallen into cold water with others, keep warm by facing each other in a tight circle and holding on to each other.

Falling Through The Ice

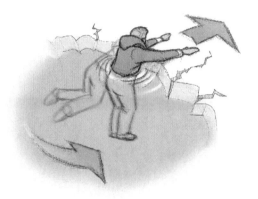

FALL THROUGH THE ICE

What if you're hiking in the wilderness and that snow field turns out to be the icy surface of a lake? Whenever you're out in the wild, it makes sense to take a change of clothes in a waterproof container so that you'll have something dry to wear if the clothes you're wearing get wet. Also have a fire starter that will work even when wet.

You might be able to identify weak areas in the ice. If a thin area of ice on a lake is covered with snow, it tends to look darker than the surrounding area. Interestingly, thin areas of bare ice without snow appear lighter. Beware of areas of contrasting color as you're walking.

Your body will react to a sudden immersion in cold water by an increased pulse rate, blood pressure, and respirations. Although it won't be easy, make every effort to keep calm. You have a few minutes to get out before you succumb to the effects of the cold. Panic is your enemy.

Get your head out of the water by breathing in and bending backward. Tread water and quickly get rid of any heavy objects that are weighing you down. Turn your body in the direction of where you came from; you know the ice was strong enough to hold you there.

Now, try to lift up out of the ice using your hands and arms. Keep them spread in front of you. Kick with your feet to give you some forward momentum and try to get more of your body out of the water. Lift a leg onto the ice and then lift and roll out onto the firmer surface. Do not stand up! Keep rolling in the direction that you were walking before you feel through. This will spread your weight out, instead of concentrating it on your feet. Then crawl away until you're sure you're safe. Start working to get warm immediately.

I would like to mention a brand new item that would be helpful for falls through the ice or avalanche protection. An air bag accessory is now available for those who are traveling in snow country. It can be easily deployed to achieve buoyancy in the water or to help prevent from being deeply buried in the snow. Upon burial in an avalanche, hypothermia will set in quickly. The air bag causes the victim to become a larger object; these seem to stay towards the top of the snow in avalanche scenarios.

ALTITUDE SICKNESS

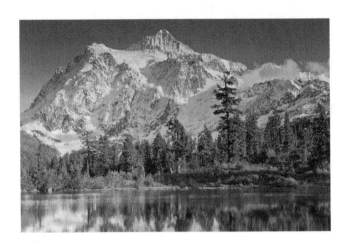

In any survival situation, we might find ourselves having to relocate from a home at sea level to a retreat or "bug-out" location in the mountains. When this becomes necessary, it's likely that you will be moving fast. The rapid change in elevation will, for some, cause a condition known as **Altitude sickness** or Acute Mountain Sickness (AMS). This occurs as a result of entering an area with lower oxygen availability and reduced air pressures without first acclimating oneself.

Altitude sickness occurs most commonly at elevations approaching 8,000 feet above sea level, and is aggravated by exerting oneself.

Although Altitude Sickness is usually a temporary condition, some patients may develop complications in the form of "**edema**" of certain organs. Edema is the accumulation of fluid; in altitude sickness, it may occur in the lungs (called "pulmonary edema") or brain (called "cerebral edema"). Either of these conditions can be life-threatening.

Like many illnesses, the best strategy against altitude sickness is prevention. Choose your route to your retreat so that the ascent is as gradual as possible. Do not attempt more than 2,000 feet of ascent per day. Ensure that your personnel do not over-exert themselves as they ascend, and provide lots of fresh water. Avoid the consumption of alcohol on the way.

Some normal people may be susceptible to AMS at lower elevations than others. If you have no choice but to make a rapid ascent, close monitoring of every member of your party will be needed. You will usually see patients present to you with symptoms similar to a hangover or influenza. If mild, you will commonly see:

- Fatigue
- Insomnia
- Dizziness
- Headaches
- Nausea and Vomiting
- Lack of appetite
- Tachycardia (fast heart rate)
- "Pins and Needles" sensations
- Shortness of breath

Those who will have major complications of altitude sickness will present with the following:

- Severe shortness of breath
- Confused and apathetic behavior
- Cough and chest congestion (not nasal)
- Cyanosis (blue or gray appearance of the skin, especially the fingertips and lips)
- Loss of coordination
- Dehydration
- Hemoptysis (coughing up blood)
- Loss of consciousness
- Fever (less likely)

Treating altitude sickness first requires rest, if only to stop further ascent and allow more time to acclimate. If available, a portable oxygen tank will be useful upon onset of symptoms.

A diet high in carbohydrates is thought to reduce ill effects.

A medication commonly used for both prevention and treatment is Acetazolamide (Diamox). It has a "**diuretic**" effect, which means that it speeds the elimination of excess fluid from the body by urination. Therefore, it will help prevent the accumulation of fluid in the lungs or brain.

Acetazolamide is superior to many other diuretics in that it also forces the kidneys to excrete bicarbonate. By increasing the amount of bicarbonate excreted, it makes the blood more acidic. Acidifying the blood stimulates ventilation, which increases the amount of oxygen in the blood. This effect may not be immediate, but will speed up acclimatization, at the very least.

Usual dosages of Acetazolamide are 125 to 1,000 mg/day, usually starting a couple of days before the planned ascent. The medicine can serve to prevent as well as to treat altitude sickness.

Other medicines known to have a beneficial effect include the blood pressure medication Nifedipine and the steroid Decadron, especially in those with edema in the lungs and brain.

When you visit your physician, notify him that you are planning a trip into high elevations and would like to avoid altitude sickness. Usually, you will be given an Acetazolamide prescription in case of emergency. The other medications mentioned will be more difficult to obtain, however, as they may have more side effects.

There is some evidence that Gingko Biloba may be helpful in the natural prevention of altitude sickness. A small amount of an extract of this substance has been shown to allow the brain to tolerate lower oxygen levels. Native Americans have used Gingko for Acute Mountain Sickness for centuries with beneficial effect.

WILDFIRE PREPAREDNESS

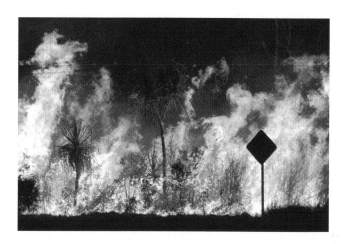

Many in the preparedness community either already have or are planning to have a rural retreat for when things go south. This means that, if you expect to live or at least spend time in a remote location, you'll have the responsibility to not only defend it from hordes of marauding zombies, but also acts of nature such as the occasional wildfire.

Fire is one of nature's ways to renew the land. Some seeds, such as those of the lodge pole pine, actually require fire to help them germinate. Despite the long-term beneficial effect to the forest, fire is an issue that presents a danger to the humans in it. Although wildfires may occur at any time of year, summertime in drought-prone areas is a particularly dangerous time.

Once you are in your homestead or long-term retreat, you'll have to take a look around to evaluate the risk level of natural as well as man-made catastrophes.

One thing that's important is what we call "vegetation management". Your goal is to direct fires away from your shelter. There are a few ways to do this: you'll want to clean up dead wood lying on the ground close to your buildings and off the roofs. Keep woodpiles and other flammables away from structures.

Also, you'll have to remove some of the living vegetation from around your home. This is counter to some advice you'll get regarding keeping your home invisible, and it means that you'd have to remove those thorny bushes you've planted under your windows for defense purposes. This can be a tough decision, but you just might have to make a choice between fire protection and privacy.

Another factor to consider is the material that your retreat is made of. How much fire resistance does your structure have? A wood frame home with wooden shingles will go up like a match in a wildfire. If you are constructing a place to live in times of trouble, you should try to build as much flame resistance into your home as possible.

So, let's create a **defensible space**. A defensible space is an area around a structure where wood and vegetation are treated, cleared or reduced to slow the spread of wildfire towards a structure. Having a defensible space will also provide room to work for those fighting the fire.

The amount of defensible space you'll need depends on whether you're on flat land or on a steep slope. Flatland fires spread more slowly than a fire on a slope (hot air and flames rise). A fire on a steep slope with wind blowing uphill will spread quickly and produces "**spot fires**". These are small fires that ignite vegetation ahead of the main burn, due to small bits of burning debris in the air.

Some landscaping may be necessary to decrease the chance of fire spreading in your direction. You'll want to thin out those thick canopied trees near your house. Any nearby tree within 50 feet on flatland, or 200 feet if downhill from your retreat on top of the mountain, needs to be thinned. You will prune branches off below 10-12 feet high, and separate them by 10-20 feet. Also, eliminate all shrubs at the base of the trunks.

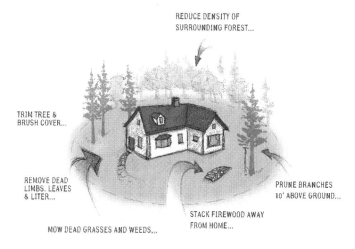

REDUCE DENSITY OF
SURROUNDING FOREST...

TRIM TREE &
BRUSH COVER...

REMOVE DEAD
LIMBS, LEAVES
& LITER...

PRUNE BRANCHES
10' ABOVE GROUND...

MOW DEAD GRASSES AND WEEDS...

STACK FIREWOOD AWAY
FROM HOME...

WILD FIRE SAFETY

Other things you should do:

- Clean up all dead wood in the area.
- Stack firewood at least 20 feet from any building.
- Keep gardening tools and other items stored away.

Of course, once you have a defensible space, the natural inclination is to want to defend it, even against a forest fire. Unfortunately, you have to remember that you'll be in the middle of a lot of heat and smoke. Unless you're a 22 year old Navy Seal in full fire gear and mask, you're probably not going to be able to function effectively.

Even if you ARE a 22 year old Navy Seal, you'll have to take the others under your care into account. The safest option for all involved would be to hit the road if there's a way out. It's a personal decision, but it should also be a realistic one.

If you're leaving, have your supplies already in the car, as well as any important papers you might need to keep and some cash. If you have electricity, make sure you shut off any air conditioning system that draws air into the house from outside. Turn off all your appliances, close all your windows and lock all your doors. Like any other emergency, you should have some form of communication open with your loved ones so that you can contact each other.

If there is any possibility that you might find yourself in the middle of a fire, make sure you're dressed in long pants and sleeves and heavy boots. A wool blanket is very helpful as an additional outside layer because wool is relatively fire-resistant. If you don't have wool blankets, this is a good time to add some to your storage, or keep some in your car.

If you're in a building, stay on the side of the building farthest from the fire outside. Choose a room with the least number of windows –(windows transfer heat to the inside). Stay there unless you have to leave due to smoke or the building catching fire.

If that's the case and you have to leave, wrap yourself in that blanket, leaving only your eyes uncovered. Some people think it's a good idea to wet the blanket first. Don't. Wet materials transfer heat much faster than dry materials and will cause more severe burns.

If you're having trouble breathing because of the smoke, stay low, and crawl out of the building if you have to. There's less smoke and heat the lower you go. Keep your face down towards the floor. This will protect your airway. Don't forget to have some eye wash in your supplies; the smoke will irritate your eyes.

If you ever encounter a person that is actually on fire, you have to act quickly. In circumstances where a person's clothes are on fire, remember the old adage "Stop, Drop, and Roll".

- **Stop:** Your patient will be panicked and likely running around trying to put out the flames. This generates wind which will fan the flames. Stop the patient from running away.
- **Drop:** Knock the patient to the ground and wrap tightly with a wool blanket. Heavy fabrics are best.
- **Roll:** Roll the patient on the floor until the flames are extinguished. Immediately cool any burned areas of skin with copious amounts of water.

Smoke Inhalation

Other than burns, which are discussed in another part of this book, you can become seriously ill or even die simply from inhaling too much smoke. Remember, you can heal from burns on your skin, but you can't heal from burns in your lungs. The scars from the burns will damage the lungs' ability to absorb oxygen and could cause permanent damage. Common causes include:

- **Simple Combustion:** Combustion uses up oxygen near a fire and can kill a person simply from oxygen deficit. This is called "hypoxia". The larger the fire, the more oxygen it removes from the area. This is particularly troublesome in a closed space, such as a building fire.
- **Carbon Dioxide:** Some by-products of smoke may not directly kill a person, but could take up the space in the lungs that Oxygen would ordinarily use. Even the expulsion of a large bubble of Carbon Dioxide can kill wildlife near it, such as in the example of "swamp gas".
- **Chemical irritants:** Many chemicals founds in smoke can cause irritation injury when they come in contact with the lung. This amounts to a burn inside the lung tissue, which causes swelling and airway obstruction. Chlorine gas used in World War I is an example of a deadly chemical irritant.
- **Other asphyxiants:** Carbon Monoxide, Cyanide, and some Sulfides may interfere with the body's ability to utilize oxygen. Carbon monoxide is the most common of these.

Symptoms may include:

- Cough
- Shortness of breath
- Hoarseness
- Upper airway spasm
- Eye irritation
- Headaches
- Pale, bluish or even bright red skin
- Loss of consciousness leading to coma or death

Your evaluation of the patient with smoke inhalation may show soot around the mouth, in the throat, and in nasal passages. Both of these areas may be swollen and irritated. The victim will likely be short of breath and have a hoarse voice.

Of course, you will want to get your patient out of the smoky area and into an environment where there is clean air. This may not be as easy as it seems in a major fire. You must be very careful not to put yourself in a situation where you are likely to succumb to smoke inhalation yourself. Always consider a surgical mask or even a gas mask before entering a conflagration to rescue a victim. Be prepared to use CPR if necessary.

It is important to have some way to deliver oxygen to your patient if needed. There are many portable commercially-available canisters which would be useful to get oxygen quickly into the lungs.

Don't expect a rapid recovery from significant smoke inhalation. Your patient will be short of breath with the slightest activity and will be very hoarse. These symptoms may go away with time, or may be permanent disabilities.

Prevention by planning escape routes and having regular drills will allow your people to get out of dangerous situations quickly. Make sure everyone knows what to do in advance.

STORM PREPAREDNESS

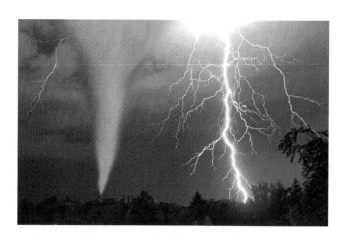

There are few people who haven't been in the path of a major storm at one point or another. Most of those in the path of an oncoming storm will not have planned for its arrival. Some will even openly flaunt their disregard by seeking exposed areas. This is an instance where a lack of common sense can have dire consequences.

If you fail to plan ways to protect yourself and your family, you may find yourself having to treat significant traumatic injuries in the immediate aftermath. Loss of your shelter may expose your family to hypothermia or heat stroke. Later, flooding may contaminate your water supplies and expose you to serious infectious disease. Preparing to weather the storm safely will avoid major medical problems for you, as medic, later on.

TORNADO PREPAREDNESS

A tornado is a violently rotating column of air that is in contact with both the surface of the earth and the thunderstorm (sometimes called a "supercell") that spawned it. From a distance, tornadoes usually appear in the form of a visible dark funnel with all sorts of flying debris in and around it. Because of rainfall, they may be difficult to see when close up.

A tornado (also called a "twister") may have winds of up to 300 miles per hour, and can travel for a number of kilometers or miles before petering out. They may be accompanied by hail and will emit a roaring sound that will remind you of a passing train. I have personally experienced this, and I can tell you that it is terrifying.

There are almost a thousand tornadoes in the United States every year, more than are reported in any other country. Most of these occur in "Tornado Alley", an area that includes Texas, Oklahoma, Missouri, Kansas, Arkansas, and neighboring states. Spring and early summer are the peak seasons.

Injuries from tornadoes usually come as a result of trauma from all the flying debris that is carried along with it. Strong winds can carry large objects and fling them around in a manner that is hard to believe. Indeed, there is a report that, in 1931, an 83 ton train was lifted and thrown 80 feet from the tracks.

Tornadoes are categorized by something called the Fujita Scale, from level 0-5, based on the amount of damage caused:

- F0 Light: Broken tree branches, mild structural damage, some uprooted
- F1 Moderate: Broken windows, small tree trunks broken, overturned mobile homes, destruction of carports or toolsheds, roof tiles missing
- F2 Considerable: Mobile homes destroyed, major structural damage to frame homes due to flying debris, some large trees snapped in half or uprooted
- F3 Severe: Roofs torn from homes, small frame homes destroyed, most trees snapped and uprooted

- F4 Devastating: Strong-structure buildings damaged or destroyed or lifted from foundations, cars lifted and blown away, even large debris airborne
- F5 Incredible: Larger buildings lifted from foundations, trees snapped, uprooted and debarked, objects weighing more than a ton become airborne missiles

Although some places may have sirens or other methods of warning you of an approaching twister, it is important to have a plan for your family to weather the storm. Having a plan BEFORE a tornado approaches is the most likely way you will survive the event. Children should be taught where to find the medical kits and how to use a fire extinguisher. If possible, teach everyone how to safely turn off the gas and electricity.

If you see a twister funnel, take shelter immediately. If your domicile is a mobile home, leave! They are especially vulnerable to damage from the winds. If you live in a mobile home and there is time, get to the nearest building that has a tornado shelter; underground shelters are best. If you live in Tornado Alley, consider putting together your own underground shelter.

Unlike bunkers and other structures built for long-term protection, a tornado shelter has to provide safety for a short period of time. As such, it doesn't have to be very large; 8-10 square feet per person would be acceptable. Despite this, be sure to consider ventilation and the comfort or special needs of those using the shelter.

If you don't have a shelter, find a place where family members can gather if a tornado is headed your way. Basements, bathrooms, closets or inside rooms without windows are the best options. Windows can easily shatter from impact due to flying debris.

For added protection, get under a heavy object such as a sturdy table. Covering up your body with a sleeping bag or mattress will provide an additional shield. Discuss this plan of action with each and every member of your family or group in such a way that they will know this process by heart.

If you're in a car and can drive to a shelter, do so. Although you may be hesitant to leave your vehicle, remember that they can be easily tossed around by high winds; you may be safer if there is a culvert or other area lower than the roadway.

In town, leaving the car to enter a sturdy building is appropriate. If there is no other shelter, however, staying in your car will protect you from some of the flying debris. Keep your seat beat on, put your head down below the level of the windows, and cover yourself if at all possible.

If you are, say, on a hike and caught outside when the tornado hits, stay away from wooded areas. Torn branches and other debris become missiles, so an open field or ditch may be safer. Lying down flat in a low spot in the ground will give you some protection. Make sure to cover your head if at all possible, even if it's just with your hands.

HURRICANE PREPAREDNESS

A hurricane is a large tropical storm with winds that have reached a constant speed of 74 miles per hour or more. In the United States, hurricanes regularly ravage the Gulf or East Coast, causing billions of dollars of damage. Even in high-risk hurricane zones, most people are completely unprepared for the severe rain, winds, flooding, and general mayhem that these storms can cause.

Certainly, these storms can be severe, but they don't have to be life-threatening. Unlike tornados, which can pop up suddenly, hurricanes are first identified when they are hundreds, if not thousands of miles away. We can watch their development and have a good idea of how bad it might get and how much time we have to get ready.

Like tornados, hurricanes are categorized based on severity using the Saffir-Simpson Hurricane Wind Scale. Wind speeds below are "maximum sustained", meaning continuously reaching up to the numbers below when the storm hits:

- Category 1: 74-95 miles per hour
- Category 2: 96-110 miles per hour
- Category 3: 111-130 miles per hour
- Category 4: 131-155 miles per hour
- Category 5: Greater than 155 miles per hour

Higher category storms may cause incredible damage and loss of life, such as occurred in Hurricane Katrina in 2005. You will have to put together an effective plan of action with regards to shelter, food, power, and other important issues. You may also have to make a decision regarding evacuation. Unlike some disaster scenarios, you can actually outrun one of these storms if you get enough of a head start.

If you live on the coast or in an area that has flooding, there will be rising waters (known as the "storm surge") that might be enough of a reason to leave. The authorities will issue an evacuation order in many cases. If you live in pre-fabricated housing, such as a trailer, or near the coast, it just might be a good idea. Cities may no longer have plans for civil defense, but they still do for hurricanes in regions at risk. Oftentimes, the municipality will assign a hurricane-resistant public building in your own community as a designated shelter.

If you do choose to leave town, plan to go as far inland as possible. Hurricanes get their strength from the warm water temperatures over the tropical ocean; they lose strength quickly as they travel over land. One caveat here: If you live on the Florida peninsula, you might want to head north. The southern part of the state is relatively thin and might provide less protection than other areas.

Speaking from personal experience, Hurricane Wilma in 2005 hit Florida's West Coast and still caused damage to our home just a few miles from Florida's East Coast. It might be a wise move to make reservations at a hotel early; there will be little room at the inn for latecomers.

In any case, this is the time to check out that "bug-out bag" of yours to make sure it's ready to go. Although most people pack for 72 hours off the grid, that number is relatively arbitrary; be prepared to at least have a week's supply of food and drinking water, as well as medical supplies.

Usually, you will not be told to leave your homes (except in the cases mentioned above). As such, your planning will determine how much damage you sustain and how much risk you place yourself in. You should have an idea of what your home's weak spots are. For instance, do you know what amount of sustained wind your structure can withstand?

Since South Florida was devastated by Hurricane Andrew in 1992, new homes in South Florida must have the strength to withstand 125 mph winds. Most homes, however, are made to handle 90 mph (hurricane strength is >74 mph). If the coming storm has sustained winds over that level, you may not be able to depend on the structural integrity of your home.

If you decide to stay, make sure you designate a safe room somewhere in the interior of the house. It should be in a part of the home most downwind from the direction of the oncoming hurricane. Figure out who's coming to ride out the storm with you, and plan for any special needs they may have.

Make provisions for any animals you will be sheltering and move all outdoor furniture and potted plants either inside the house or up against the outside wall, preferably secured with chains. Don't forget to put up the hurricane shutters if you have them.

One special issue for South Floridians is coconuts: They turn into cannonballs in a hurricane. Cut them off the tree before the winds come. Interestingly, the palm trees themselves, as they don't have a dense crown, seem to weather most high winds without a problem.

Indoor planning is important, as well. Communications may be out in a major storm, so have a NOAA weather radio and lots of fresh batteries. You will likely lose power, so fill up your gas and propane tanks early in every hurricane season. Install foot and head bolts on double entry doors.

As the storm approaches, you'll want to fill up bathtubs and other containers with water. Turn your refrigerator and freezer down to their coldest settings, so that food won't spoil right away if the power fails. Make sure you know how to shut off the electricity, gas and water, if necessary.

There's another kind of power you should be concerned about. In the aftermath of a storm, credit card verification may be down; without cash, you may have no purchasing power at all.

Of course, have some waterproof tarps available, in case of lost shingles, etc. The roofers are going to be pretty busy after a major storm, and might not get to you right away. In South Florida after Hurricane Wilma in 2005, there were still blue tarps on roofs more than a year later.

If you've hunkered down in your home during the storm, make sure that you've got books, board games, and light sources for when the power goes down. Kids (and most adults) go stir crazy when stuck inside, especially if they don't have TVs or computers in service. Here's where you will finally be thankful for those battery-powered hand-held gaming devices.

Take time to discuss the coming storm in advance; this will give everyone an idea of what to expect, and keep fear down to a minimum. Give the kids some responsibility, as well. Give them the opportunity to pack their own bag or select games to play. This will keep their minds busy and their nerves calm.

After the storm, inland flood water may be polluted. Do not walk around in, drink nor bathe in this water. Thorough sterilization is required. Do not eat fresh food that has come in contact with floodwater; if cans of food have been exposed to the water, wash them off with soap and clean hot water before opening.

Also, watch for downed power lines; they have been the cause of a number of electrocutions. In some cases, entire families have lost their lives jumping into electrified water to save a relative. You should never touch someone who has been electrocuted without first shutting off the power source; if you can't shut off the power, you will have to move the victim. Use a nonmetal object, such as a wooden broom handle or dry rope. If you don't, the current could pass through the individual's body and shock you.

EARTHQUAKES

Hurricanes are more significant for residents of the Gulf or East Coasts of the United States, but the West Coast and even some areas of the Midwest have their own disaster to worry about: Earthquakes. Some populated areas are near "fault lines". A **fault** is a fracture in a volume of base rock. This is an area where earth movement releases energy that can cause major surface disruptions or "earthquakes". This movement is sometimes called a "seismic wave".

The strength of an earthquake is measuring using the Richter Scale. This measurement (from 0-10 or more) identifies the magnitude at a certain location. Quakes less than 2.0 on the Richter Scale may occur every day, but are unlikely to be noticed by the average person. Each increase of 1.0 magnitude increases the strength by a factor of 10. The highest registered earthquake was The Great Chilean Earthquake of 1960 (9.5 on the Richter Scale).

If the energy is released offshore, a "**tsunami**" or tidal wave may develop. In Fukushima, Japan, a powerful earthquake (8.9 on the Richter Scale) and tsunami wreaked havoc in 2011, causing major damage, loss of life, and meltdowns in local nuclear reactors.

A major earthquake is especially dangerous due to the lack of notice given beforehand. Make sure each member of your family knows what to do no matter where they are when an earthquake occurs. Unless it happens in the dead of night, it's unlikely you will all be in the house together. Planning ahead will give you the best chance of keeping you family together and make the best of a bad situation.

To be prepared, you'll need, at the very least, the following:

- Food and water
- Power sources
- Alternative shelters
- Medical supplies
- Clothing appropriate to the weather
- Fire extinguishers
- Means of communication

- Money (don't count on credit or debit cards being good if the power's down)
- An adjustable wrench to turn off gas or water

Figure out where you'll meet in the event of tremors. Find out the school system's plan for earthquakes so you'll know where to find your kids. It would be appropriate to always have a "get-home" bag put together. Some food, liquids, and a pair of sturdy, comfortable shoes are useful items to keep in your car.

Especially important to know is where your gas, electric and water main shutoffs are. Make sure that everyone has an idea of how to turn them off if there is a leak or electrical short. Know where the nearest medical facility is, but be aware that you may be on your own; medical responders are going to have their hands full and may not get to you quickly.

Look around your house for fixtures like chandeliers and bookcases that might not be stable enough to withstand an earthquake. Flat screen TVs, especially large ones, could easily topple. Especially be sure to check out kitchen and pantry shelves; it's probably not a great idea to hang that big mirror over the headboard of your bed, either.

What should you do when the tremors start? If you're indoors, get under a table, desk, or something else solid or get into an inside hallway. You should stay clear of windows, shelves, and kitchen areas. While the building is shaking, don't try to run out; you could easily fall down stairs or get hit by falling debris. I had always thought you should stand in the doorway because of the frame's sturdiness, but it turns out that, in modern homes, doorways aren't any more solid than any other part of the structure.

Once the initial tremors are over, you can go outside. Once there, stay as far away from power lines, chimneys, and anything else that could fall on top of you.

You could, possibly, be in your automobile when the earthquake hits. Get out of traffic as quickly as possible; other drivers are likely to be less level-headed than you are. Don't stop under bridges, trees, overpasses, power lines, or light posts. Don't leave your vehicle while the tremors are active.

One issue to be concerned about is gas leaks; make sure you don't use your camp stoves, lighters, or even matches until you're certain all is clear. Even a match could ignite a spark that could lead to an explosion. If you turned the gas off, you might consider letting the utility company turn it back on.

Don't count on telephone service after a natural disaster. Telephone companies only have enough lines to deal with 20% of total call volume at any one time. It's likely all lines will be occupied. Interestingly, this doesn't seem to include texts; you'll have a better to chance to communicate by texting than by voice due to the wavelength used.

ALLERGIC REACTIONS AND ANAPHYLAXIS

In a survival situation, we may have to vacate our home and head to unfamiliar territory. During our sojourn, we will expose ourselves to insect stings, poison oak and ivy, and strange food items that we aren't accustomed to. When a negative physical response occurs due to a particular substance, we call it an "**allergy**". This substance is greatly hazardous only to those who are allergic.

Foreign substances that cause allergies are called "**allergens**". Our response to them can be negligible or it can be life-threatening. If severe enough, we refer to it as "**anaphylaxis**" or "anaphylactic shock". Anaphylaxis is the word used for serious and rapid allergic reactions usually involving more than one part of the body which, if severe enough, can be fatal.

Minor and Chronic Allergies

Mild allergic reactions usually involve local itching and the development of a patchy, raised rash on the skin. These types of reactions can be transient and go away by themselves or with medications such as Diphenhydramine (Benadryl).

Chronic allergies may manifest as a skin condition known as "**eczema**". This will be a red patchy rash in different places which is itchy and flaky. This type of rash usually responds well to 1% hydrocortisone cream (non-prescription), although sometimes a stronger steroid cream such as Clobetasol (prescription) may be necessary. In the very worst cases, chronic dermatitis (inflammation of the skin) may require oral steroids such as Prednisone.

If the allergic reaction is minor, there are various essential oils you can apply to relieve symptoms such as itching:

- Peppermint
- Lavender
- Chamomile (German or Roman)
- Calendula
- Myrrh

- Cypress
- Helichrysum
- Wintergreen
- Eucalyptus
- Blue Tansy

To use the above oils, you would dilute 50/50 with carrier oil (olive or coconut, for example) and apply 2 drops to the affected area.

Other natural substances that you could apply to a rash include witch hazel, oatmeal baths or compresses, Aloe Vera, Shea butter and vitamin E oil. Apply to the affected area as needed.

Hay Fever

Hay Fever, also known as "allergic rhinitis" or "seasonal allergy", is a collection of symptoms, mostly affecting the eyes and nose, which occur when you breathe in something you are allergic to. Examples of allergens would include dust, animal dander, insect venom, fungi, or pollens. Sufferers of allergic rhinitis would present with:

- Nasal congestion
- Sneezing
- Red eyes with tearing
- Itchy throat, eyes, and skin

Antihistamines such as Claritin and Benadryl are old standbys for this type of allergy. Alternative therapies for hay fever include essential oils for use on the skin:

- German chamomile
- Roman chamomile
- lavender
- eucalyptus
- ginger.

Apply 2 drops to each temple, 2-4 times per day. Steam inhalation, 1 drop of the oil to a bowl of steaming water, involves covering the head with a towel and inhale slowly for 15 minutes. A number of teas to drink that may be useful are licorice root, stinging nettle, and St. John's Wort. Drink 1 cup daily 3 times a day.

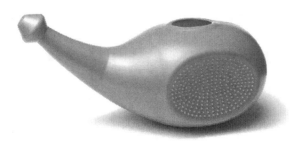

Neti pot

A Neti Pot is a useful item to have to deal with allergic reactions affecting the nasal passages. It looks like a small teapot. Neti pots wash out pollen, clears congestion and mucus, and decreases nasal inflammation. Use with sterile saline (salt water) solution daily in the following fashion:

- Bend over a sink.
- Tilt your head to one side.
- Keep your forehead and chin are at the same level to keep water out of your mouth.
- Breathe through your mouth during the procedure.
- Insert the spout gently into your uppermost nostril.
- Pour the solution so that it drains through the lower nostril.
- Blow your nose to clear your nostrils.
- Change head position and repeat with the other nostril.

Recently, there have been concerns about neti pots from the The Food and Drug Administration (FDA). They warn that, if not used properly, the patient runs the risk of developing serious (even life-threatening) infections. Neti pots are meant to be used with STERILIZED saline; in 2011, two people lost their lives after using contaminated tap water.

Asthma

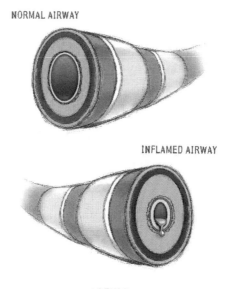

Asthma is a chronic condition that affects your ability to breathe. It affects the airways, which are the tubes that transport air to your lungs. When people with asthma are exposed to a substance that they are allergic to (an "**allergen**"), these airways become inflamed. As the airways become swollen, the diameter of the airway decreases and less air gets to the lungs. As such, you will develop shortness of breath, tightness in your chest, and start to wheeze and cough. This is referred to as an "asthma attack".

In rare situations, the airways can become so constricted that a person could suffocate from lack of oxygen. This extreme condition is sometimes referred to as "Status Asthmaticus". Here are common allergens that trigger an asthmatic attack:

- Pet or wild animal dander
- Dust or the excrement of dust mites
- Mold and mildew
- Smoke
- Pollen

- Severe stress
- Pollutants in the air
- Some medicines
- Exercise

There are many myths associated with asthma; the below are just some:

- Asthma is contagious. (False)
- You will grow out of it. (False-it might become dormant for a time but you are always at risk for it returning)
- It's all in your mind. (False)
- If you move to a new area, your asthma will go away. (False – it may go away for a while, but eventually you will become sensitized to something else and it will likely return)

Here's a "true" myth: Asthma is, indeed, hereditary. If both parents have asthma, you have a 70% chance of developing it compared to only 6% if neither parent has it.

Asthmatic symptoms may be different from attack to attack and from individual to individual. Some of the symptoms are also seen in heart conditions and other respiratory illnesses, so it's important to make the right diagnosis. Symptoms may include:

- Cough
- Shortness of Breath
- Wheezing (usually sudden)
- Chest tightness (sometimes confused with coronary artery spasms/ heart attack)
- Rapid pulse rate and respiration rate
- Anxiety

Besides these main symptoms, there are others that are signals of a life-threatening episode. If you notice that your patient has become "cyanotic", they are in trouble. Someone with **cyanosis** will have blue/ gray color to their lips, fingertips, and face.

You might also notice that it takes longer for them to exhale than to inhale. Their wheezing may take on a higher pitch. Once the patient has spent enough time without adequate oxygen, they will become confused, then drowsy, and then possibly lose consciousness.

To make the diagnosis, use your stethoscope to listen to the lungs on both sides. Make sure that you listen closely to the bottom, middle, and top lung areas. In a mild asthmatic attack, you will hear relatively loud, musical noises when the patient breathes for you. As the asthma worsens, less air is passing through the airways and the pitch of the wheezes will be higher and perhaps not as loud. If no air is passing through, you will hear nothing, not even when you ask the patient to inhale forcibly. This person is in trouble.

You can measure how open your airways are with a simple diagnostic instrument known as a **peak flow meter**. It can help you identify if a patient's cough is part of an asthma attack or not, or whether they are having a panic attack instead. It also identifies the severity of respiratory compromise.

This is what you do: Take your patient's peak flow meter instrument and then (forcefully) exhale into it. This will give you a baseline reading of their normal baseline air flow. Then, when they're having an attack, have them blow into it again.

In moderate asthma, peak flow will be reduced 20-40%. Greater than 50% is a sign of a severe episode. In a non-asthma related cough or upper respiratory infection, your peak flow will be close to normal. The same goes for a panic attack; even though you may feel short of breath, your peak flow is still about normal.

The cornerstones of asthma treatment are the avoidance of "trigger" allergens and the maintenance of open airways. Medications come in one of two forms: drugs that give quick relief from an attack and drugs that control the frequency of asthmatic episodes.

Quick relief drugs include inhalers that open airways (known as bronchodilators), such as Albuterol (Ventolin, Proventil), among others. These drugs should open airways in a very short period of time and give significant relief. These drugs are sometimes useful for people going into a situation where they are exposed to a known "trigger", such as before strenuous exercise. Don't be surprised if you notice a rapid heart rate on these medications; it's a common side effect.

If you find yourself using quick-relief asthmatic medications more than twice a week, you are a candidate for daily control therapy. These drugs work (when taken daily) to decrease the number of episodes and are usually some form of inhaled steroid. There are long-acting bronchodilators as well, such as ipratropium bromide (Atrovent). Another family of drugs known as Leukotriene Modifiers prevents airway swelling before an asthma attack even begins. These are usually in pill form and may make sense for storage purposes. The most popular is Montelukast (Singulair).

Often, medications will be used in combination, and you might find multiple medications in the same inhaler. U.S. commercial product Advair, for example, contains both a steroid and an airway dilator. Remember that inhalers lose potency over time. An expired inhaler, unlike many pills or tablets, will lose potency relatively quickly.

It's important to figure out what allergens trigger your asthma attacks and work out a plan to avoid them as much as possible. Furthermore, make sure to stockpile as much of your asthma medication as possible in case of emergency. Physicians are usually sympathetic to requests for extra prescriptions from their asthmatic patients.

In mild to moderate cases, you might consider the use of natural remedies. There are actually quite a few substances that have been reported to be helpful:

- **Ginger and Garlic Tea:** Put four minced garlic cloves in some ginger tea while it's hot. Cool it down and drink twice a day. Some have reported a beneficial effect with just the garlic.
- **Other herbal teas:** Ephedra, Coltsfoot, Codonopsis, Butterbur, Nettle, Chamomile, and Rosemary all have the potential to improve an asthmatic attack.
  Coffee: Black unsweetened coffee is a stimulant that might make your lung function better when you are having an attack. Don't drink more than 12 ounces at a time, as coffee can dehydrate

you. Interestingly, coffee is somewhat similar in chemical structure to the asthma drug Theopylline.

- **Eucalyptus:** Essential oil of eucalyptus, used in a steam or direct inhalation, is well-known to open airways. Rub a few drops of oil between your hands and breathe in deeply. Alternatively, a few drops in some steaming water will be good respiratory therapy.

- **Honey:** Honey was used in the 19th century to treat asthmatic attacks. Breathe deeply from a jar of honey and you should see improvement in a few minutes. To decrease the frequency of attacks, stir one teaspoon of honey in a twelve ounce glass of water and drink it three times daily.

- **Turmeric:** Take one teaspoon of turmeric powder in 6-8 ounces of warm water three times a day.

- **Licorice and Ginger:** Mix licorice and ginger (1/2 teaspoon of each) in a cup of water. Warning: Licorice can raise your blood pressure.

- **Black Pepper, Onion, and Honey:** Drink ¼ cup of onion juice with a tablespoon of honey, after adding 1/8 tablespoon of black pepper.

- **Mustard Oil Rub:** Mix mustard oil with camphor and rub it on your chest and back. There are claims that it gives instant relief in some cases.

- **Gingko Biloba leaf extract:** Thought to decrease hypersensitivity in the lungs; not for people who are taking aspirin or ibuprofen daily, or anticoagulants like Coumadin.

- **Vitamin D:** Some asthmatics have been diagnosed with Vitamin D deficiency.

- **Lobelia:** Native Americans actually smoked this herb as a treatment for asthma. Instead of smoking, try mixing tincture of lobelia with tincture of cayenne in a 3:1 ratio. Put 1 milliliter (about 20 drops) of this mixture in water at the start of an attack and repeat every thirty minutes or so.

With a number of these substances, further research is necessary to corroborate the amount of effect that they have on severe asthma, so take standard medications if your peak flow reading is 60% or less than normal.

Don't underestimate the effect of your diet on your condition. Asthmatics should:

- Replace animal proteins with plant proteins.
- Increase intake of Omega-3 fatty acids
- Eliminate milk and other dairy products.
- Eat organically whenever possible.
- Eliminate trans-fats; use extra-virgin olive oil as your main cooking oil.
- Always stay well-hydrated; more fluids will make your lung secretions less viscous.

Finally, various breathing methods, such as taught in Yoga classes, are thought to help promote well-being and control the panic response seen in asthmatic attacks. Acupuncture is thought by some to have some promise as well in treating the condition.

Anaphylactic reactions

In a small percentage of people, a response to an allergen may affect more than just a local area. Severe allergic reactions involve various organ systems and can be quite dangerous.

Anaphylactic reactions were first identified when researchers tried to protect dogs against a certain poison by desensitizing them with small doses. Instead of being protected, many of the dogs died suddenly the second time they got the poison. They were killed by their own immune systems going out of control.

The word used for preventative protection is "**prophylaxis**". Think of a condom, also known as a prophylactic. A condom protects you from and prevents sexually transmitted diseases. The word "**anaphylaxis**", therefore, means the opposite of protection. The dog experiment allowed scientists to understand that the same "anti-protective" (harmful) effect can occur in humans. This allergic reaction can be caused by drug exposure or pollutants, but even ordinary foods, such as peanuts, can be culprits.

Our immune system exists to protect us from infection. Unfortunately, sometimes it goes haywire and inflicts real damage. Anaphylaxis has become a timely issue because more and more people are experiencing the condition.

Why the increase? When medicines are the cause, the explanation is likely that we are simply using a lot of drugs these days. Widespread use of antibiotics and other medications are exposing us to more and more possible allergens to react against.

Why foods should be causing anaphylaxis more often, however, is more perplexing. Common allergies such as asthma, food allergies and hay fever are becoming epidemic all over the world. Pollutants and pesticides in our food might certainly be a factor. As well, it wouldn't surprise me if food allergies are being caused by the proliferation of so many genetically modified (GMO) foods in our diet. They can now produce pigs that glow in the dark by controlling their genes; A company has just received permission from the FDA to send genetically modified salmon to market. More and more genetic modifications are likely in the future.

Proven causes of anaphylaxis are:

- Drugs: dyes injected during x-rays, antibiotics like Penicillin, anesthetics, aspirin and ibuprofen, and even some heart and blood pressure medicines.
- Foods: Nuts, fruit, seafood.
- Insects stings: Bees and Yellow Jacket Wasps, especially.
- Latex: Rubber gloves made of latex, especially in healthcare workers.
- Exercise: Often after eating (yes, you can actually be allergic to exercise).
- Idiopathic: This word means "of unknown cause"; a substantial percentage of cases.

It's important to recognize the signs and symptoms of anaphylaxis because the faster you treat it, the less likely it will be life-threatening. You will see:

- Rashes: Often at places not associated with the actual exposure. For example, an all-over rash in someone with a bee sting on the arm.
- Swelling: Can be generalized, but sometimes isolated to the airways or throat.
- Breathing difficulty: Wheezing is common, as in asthmatics.
- GI symptoms: Diarrhea, nausea and vomiting, or abdominal pain.
- Loss of consciousness: The patient may appear to have fainted.
- Paresthesias: Strange sensations on the lips or oral cavity, especially with food allergies.
- Shock: Blood pressure drops, respiratory failure leading to coma and death.

Fainting is not the same thing as anaphylactic shock. You can tell the difference in several ways. Someone who has fainted is usually pale in color, but anaphylactic shock will often present with the patient somewhat flushed. The pulse in anaphylaxis is fast, but a person who has fainted will have a slow heart rate. Most people who have just fainted will rarely have breathing problems and rashes, but these will be very common signs and symptoms in an anaphylactic reaction.

In food allergies, victims may notice the effects occur very rapidly; indeed, their life may be in danger within a few minutes. Sometimes, the reaction occurs somewhat later. People who have had a serious anaphylactic reaction should be observed overnight, as there is, on occasion, a second wave of symptoms. This can happen several hours after the exposure. Some reactions are mild and probably not anaphylactic, but a history of mild symptoms is not a guarantee that every reaction will be that way.

Why does our immune system go awry during anaphylactic events? Anaphylaxis happens when the body makes an antibody called immunoglobulin E (IgE for short) in response to exposure to an allergen. IgE sticks to cells which then release substances that affect blood vessels and air passages.

The first time you're exposed is called the "**sensitization**". Usually, nothing exciting happens with the first exposure. The second time you are exposed to that allergen, however, these substances throw your immune system into overdrive. Your blood pressure can drop and generalized swelling (also called "edema" can occur. In severe cases, the airways can tighten and arteries can spasm. Respiratory difficulty and cardiac effects ensure, sometimes leading to shock and even death.

A major player in this cascade is "histamine"

Histamine, when released in this situation, triggers an inflammatory response. Medications which counteract these ill effects are known, therefore, as "**antihistamines**".

These drugs may be helpful in mild allergic reactions. In tablet form, antihistamines like Diphenhydramine (Benadryl) take about an hour to get into the bloodstream properly. In an anaphylactic reaction, this isn't fast enough to save lives. If it's all you have, chew the pill to get it into your system more quickly.

Other antihistamines like Claritin (loratidine) come in wafers that melt on your tongue, and get into your system more quickly; they are options, but probably too weak for a severe reaction. It's important to know that the same cells with IgE antibodies release other substances which may cause ill effects, and antihistamines do not protect you against these.

As such, we look to another medicine that IS more effective: Adrenaline, known in the U.S. as Epinephrine. Adrenaline (Epinephrine) is a hormone that is produced in small organs near your kidneys called the "adrenal" glands. This substance activates the well-known "flight or fight" response.

Epinephrine makes your heart pump faster, widens the air passages so you can breathe, and raises your blood pressure. The hormone works successfully against all of the effects of anaphylaxis. Therefore, it should be part of your medical supplies if you are going to responsible for the medical well-being of your family or group in any long-term disaster scenario.

Unfortunately, Adrenaline (Epinephrine) comes as an injectable. Inhalers have been tried in the past, but have disadvantages. Anaphylactic reactions cause difficulty breathing. If you can't inhale, you won't get much benefit from an inhaler.

The "**Epi-Pen**" is the most popular of the various commercially available kits to combat anaphylaxis. It's important to learn how to use the Epi-Pen properly:

- Remove the EpiPen from its case.
- Hold it firmly in your fist.
- Remove the cap (some have two caps).
- Have the patient sit or lie down.
- Hold the thigh muscle still.
- Press the end firmly against the thigh in a perpendicular fashion; it should click.
- Hold for 10 seconds.
- Massage the injection site.
- Dispose of the needle safely.

You can cause more harm than good if you fail to follow the above instructions. Adrenaline (Epinephrine) can constrict the blood vessels if injected into a finger by mistake, and prevent adequate circulation to the digit. In rare cases, gangrene can set in. Also, remember that the Epi-Pen won't help you if you don't carry it with you or don't have it readily accessible. Any allergic members of your family or group should always have it in their possession.

Since it's a liquid, Adrenaline (Epinephrine) will not stay effective forever, like some pills or capsules might. Be sure to follow the storage instructions. Although you don't want to store it someplace that's hot, the Epi-Pen shouldn't be kept in any situation where it could freeze, which will damage its effectiveness significantly.

If the solution changes color, it may be losing potency. It can do that without changing color also, so use with caution if expired. Adrenaline (Epinephrine) must be protected from light and usually comes in a brown container. Make sure you know exactly where it is in your medical kit.

You will have limited quantities of this drug in collapse situations, so when do you break into those precious supplies? An easily remembered formula is the **Rule of D's**:

- Definite reaction: Your patient is obviously having a major reaction, such as a large rash or difficult breathing.
- Danger: Any worsening of a reaction after a few minutes.
- Deterioration: Use the Epi-Pen before the condition becomes life-threatening. When in doubt, use it.

An imminent danger is probably likely only if your patient has difficulty breathing or has lost consciousness. Inhalation of stomach acid into the lungs or respiratory failure is a major cause of death in these cases. Know your CPR.

If you are ever in doubt, go ahead and give the injection. The earlier you use it, the faster a person will resolve the anaphylaxis. One injection is enough to save a life, but have more than one handy, just in case. This is especially pertinent when you are away from your retreat or base camp.

Some people may not be able to take Adrenaline (Epinephrine) due to chronic heart conditions or high blood pressure. Make sure that your people consult with their healthcare providers now. You have to determine that it wouldn't be dangerous for them to receive the drug.

In a collapse, you'll be exposed to a lot of strange things and you never know when you might be allergic to one of them. Stockpile the appropriate drugs, especially if you have family members with histories of reactions. If you learn the signs and symptoms of anaphylaxis and act quickly, you'll stay out of trouble.

POISON IVY, OAK, AND SUMAC

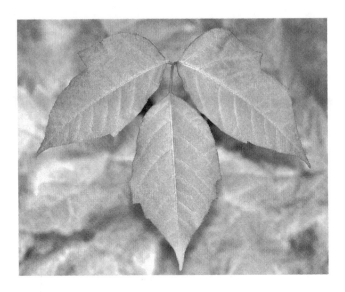

Poison Ivy

Unless you live in Alaska or Hawaii, a mountaintop, or the middle of the desert, the outdoors will have a population of poison ivy, poison oak, and/ or poison sumac. Once exposed to one or the other, 85% of the population will develop antibodies against it that will generate an itchy rash of varying degrees of severity. Winter does not eliminate the possibility of a reaction, as you can react against even the dormant vines or shrubs.

The old saying goes: "Leaves of three, let it be". Although it is true that poison ivy comes in "leaves of three", so do many other plants. Familiarize yourself with what it looks like.

Poison ivy and poison oak are very similar, with the same chemical irritant. Poison ivy leaves may be pointier, with poison oak often looking more like, well, oak leaves. One or both is present just about everywhere in the continental United States.

Poison Sumac is a shrub or small tree, growing up to nearly 30 feet in height in parts of the Eastern United States. Each leaf has 7–13 pointy leaflets. Although poison sumac has the same irritant present in poison ivy and poison oak, it is far more powerful. Simply inhaling smoke from burning poison sumac has been reported to cause death by suffocation.

All of these plants contain toxic oil that causes a reaction after the first sensitizing exposure. The oil is in just about every part of the plant: The vines, leaves, and roots. The best prevention is not touching the plant and getting the toxin on your skin. If you can't avoid exposure, here is advice before you head out into the woods:

- Long pants, long-sleeved shirts, work gloves, and boots are imperative if you're doing work in areas known to have poison plants.
- Some recommend an over-the-counter lotion called Ivy Block as a preventative. Apply it like you would a sunblock to likely areas of exposure. Theoretically, it will prevent the oil from being absorbed by your skin.

Unfortunately, many times people don't identify the exposure before it's too late. The rash takes from several hours to several days to become apparent, and will appear as red itchy lumps that tend to be patchy. Sometimes the rash appears almost linear. Itching can be prolonged and severe.

The resin or oil from the plant that causes the reaction will remain active even on your clothes, so thorough laundering will be required. Routine body washing with soap will not be useful after 30 minutes of exposure, as your system will already be producing antibodies. Hot water seems to help the oil absorb into the skin, so use only cold water early on. After all the irritant has absorbed, however, hot water baths are actually recommended by some to relieve itching.

Cleansers that remove resin or oil such as Fels-Naptha soap or Tecnu Poison Oak and Ivy Cleanser are more effective than regular detergent and can be used even several hours after exposure. Rubbing alcohol is another reasonable option and easily carried as hand sanitizers or prep pads, but is very drying to the skin.

The good news is that, even if you choose not to treat the rash, it will go away by itself over 2-3 weeks. Even though it is temporary, it could be so itchy as to make you absolutely miserable. Diphenhydramine (Benadryl) at 25-50 mg dosages 4 times a day will be helpful in relieving the itching. It's important to know that the 50mg dosage will make you drowsy. Unfortunately, calamine lotion, an old standby, and hydrocortisone cream will probably not be very effective.

Severe rashes have been treated with the prescription Medrol dose pack, (a type of steroid known as Prednisone). Prednisone is a strong anti-inflammatory drug and will be more effective in preventing the inflammatory reaction that your antibodies will cause.

Some astringent solutions such as Domeboro have been reported to give relief from the itching. The active ingredient is aluminum acetate, which is similar to the aluminum chlorohydrate in many antiperspirants.

There are several alternative treatments for poison ivy, oak and sumac:

- Cleansing the irritated area with apple cider vinegar.
- Essential oils mixed with Aloe Vera gel, such as tea tree, lemon, lavender, peppermint, geranium, and chamomile.
- Baking soda paste
- Epsom salt baths.
- Jewelweed (mash and apply)
- Chamomile tea bag compresses

For those who prefer drinking their tea, passion flower, skullcap, and chamomile are all thought to be soothing.

RADIATION SICKNESS

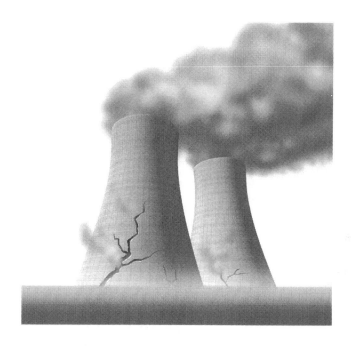

Some of the most common Doomsday scenarios involve atomic weapons and the decimation of the population from thermal blasts and radiation. Although populated areas have experienced nuclear blasts only twice, (Hiroshima and Nagasaki in 1945), nuclear events have occurred from time to time since then.

In an atomic bomb explosion, radiation is just one of the possible causes of casualties; thermal blast and kinetic energy damage near the blast will cause deaths and injuries close to ground zero. Radiation, however, can have devastating effects far from an actual detonation.

Our utilization of nuclear reactors for power places us at risk for radiation exposure when they malfunction or are damaged. Examples include the "meltdowns" at Chernobyl (1986) and Fukushima (2011). A **meltdown** (technically known as a "core melt accident") happens when reactor heat increases beyond safe levels, causing a nuclear element to exceed its melting point.

Meltdowns usually occur as a result of failure of the nuclear plant coolant system. This failure can occur as a result of damage caused by natural disasters, such as earthquakes or tsunamis. They can, however, also be caused by human error or terrorist attack. Regardless of the cause, the melted radioactive elements are released into the atmosphere; this has serious implications for populations living both near and far from the event.

Radiation released into the atmosphere is known as "fallout". **Fallout** is the particulate matter (dust) that is thrown into the air by a nuclear explosion. This dust can travel hundreds (if not thousands) of miles on the prevailing winds, coating fields, livestock, and people with radioactive material.

The higher the fallout goes into the atmosphere, the farther it will travel downwind. This material contains substances that are hazardous if inhaled or ingested, like Radioiodine, Cesium and Strontium. Even worse, fallout is absorbed by the animals and plants that make up our food supply. In large enough amounts, it is hazardous to our health.

A nuclear power plant meltdown is usually less damaging that a nuclear blast, as the radiation doesn't make it as high up in the sky as, let's say, a mushroom cloud from an atomic bomb. The worst effects will be felt by those in the area of the reactors. Lighter particles, like radioactive iodine, will travel the farthest, and are the main concern for those far from the actual explosion or meltdown. The level of radiation in an area depends on the distance that it has to travel from the meltdown, and the time it took for the radiation to arrive.

The medical effects of exposure are collectively known as "**radiation sickness**" or "Acute Radiation Syndrome". A certain amount of radiation exposure is tolerable over time, but your goal is to shelter your group as much as possible.

To accomplish this goal, we should first clarify what the different terms for measuring the quantities of radiation mean. Scientists use terms such as RADS, REMS, SIEVERTS, BECQUERELS or CURIES to describe radiation amounts. Different terms are used when describing the amount of radiation being given off by a source, the total amount of radiation that is actually absorbed by a human or animal, or the chance that a living thing will suffer health damage from exposure:

BECQUERELS/CURIES – these terms describe the amount of radiation that, say, a hunk of uranium gives off into the environment. Named after scientists who were the first to work with (and die from) radioactivity.

RADS – the amount of the radiation in the environment that is actually absorbed by a living thing.

REMS/SIEVERTS – the measurement of the risks of health damage from the radiation absorbed.

This is somewhat confusing, so, for our purposes, let's use RADS. A RAD (Radiation Absorbed Dose) measures the amount of radiation energy transferred to some mass of material, typically humans.

An acute radiation dose (one received over a short period of time) is most likely to cause damage. Below is a list of the effects on humans corresponding to the amount of radiation absorbed. For comparison, assume that you absorb about 0.6 RADs per year from natural or household sources. These are the effects of different degrees of acute radiation exposure on humans:

- **30-70 RADS:** Mild headache or nausea within several hours of exposure. Full recovery is expected.
- **70-150 RADS:** Mild nausea and vomiting in a third of patients. Decreased wound healing and increased susceptibility to infection. Full recovery is expected.
- **150-300 RADS:** Moderate nausea and vomiting in a majority of patients. Fatigue and weakness in half of patients. Infection and/or bleeding may occur due to a weakened immune system. Medical care will be required for some, especially those with burns or wounds. Occasional deaths at 300 RADS exposure may occur.
- **300-500 RADS:** Moderate nausea and vomiting, fatigue, and weakness in most patients. Diarrheal stools, dehydration, loss of appetite, skin breakdown, and infection will be common. Hair

loss is visible in most over time. At high end of exposure, expect a 50% death rate. is expected.

- **Over 500 RADS:**   Spontaneous bleeding, fever, anorexia, stomach and intestinal ulcers, bloody diarrhea, dehydration, low blood pressure, infections, and hair loss is anticipated in almost all patients. Death rates approach 100%.

The effects related to exposure may occur over time, and symptoms are often not immediate. Hair loss, for example, will appear at 10-14 days. Deaths may occur weeks after the exposure.

In the early going, your goal is to prevent exposures of over 100 RADS. A radiation dosimeter will be useful to gauge radiation levels and is widely available for purchase. This item will give you an idea of your likelihood of developing radiation sickness.

There are three basic ways of decreasing the total dose of radiation:

1. **Limit the time unprotected.** Radiation absorbed is dependent on the length of exposure. Leave areas where high levels are detected and you are without adequate shelter. The activity of radioactive particles decreases over time. After 24 hours, levels usually drop to 1/10 of their previous value or less.
2. **Increase the distance from the radiation.** Radiation disperses over distance and the effects will be decreased. To make an analogy, you have less chance of drowning the farther away you are from deep water.
3. **Shield people to decrease radiation where they are.** Shielding will decrease exposure exponentially, so it is important to know how to construct a shelter that will provide a barrier between your people and the source. A dense material will give better protection that a light material.

Barrier effectiveness is measured as "**halving thickness**". This is the thickness of a particular shield material that will reduce gamma radiation (the most dangerous kind) by one half. When you multiply the halving thickness, you multiply your protection.

For example, the halving thickness of concrete is 2.4 inches or 6 centimeters. A barrier of 2.4 inches of concrete will drop exposure to one half. Doubling the thickness of the barrier drops it to one fourth (1/2 x 1/2) and tripling it will drop it to one eighth (1/2 x 1/2 x 1/2) the exposure, etc. Ten halving thicknesses will drop the total radiation exposure to 1/1024.

Here are the halving thicknesses of some common materials:

Lead:	0.4 inches or 1 centimeter
Steel:	1 inch or 2.5 centimeters
Concrete:	2.4 inches or 6 centimeters
Soil (packed):	3.6 inches or 9 centimeters
Water:	7.2 inches or 18 centimeters
Wood:	11 inches or 30 centimeters

To take an example, let's assume you are in a concrete bunker (2.4 inches halving thickness). You would need it to be 24 inches thick to drop your radiation exposure to 1/1024 of the outside environment.

Emergency treatment of radiation sickness involves dealing with the symptoms. Antibiotics may be helpful to treat infections, fluids for dehydration, and drugs like Zofran (Ondansetron) to treat nausea. In severely ill patients, stem cell transplants and multiple transfusions are indicated but will not be options in an austere setting. This underscores the importance of an adequate shelter.

There is protection available against some of the long term effects of radiation, however. Potassium Iodide (known by the chemical symbol KI) is a 130 mg tablet that prevents radioactive Iodine from damaging the specific organ that it targets, the thyroid gland. **Radioactive Iodine** is the most common component in fallout that is not in the immediate area of the nuclear event.

Taking KI 30 minutes to 24 hours prior to a radiation exposure will prevent the eventual epidemic of thyroid cancer that will result if no treatment is given. Radiation from the 1986 Chernobyl disaster has accounted for more than 4,000 cases of thyroid cancer so far, mostly in children and adolescents. More are expected in the coming years.

Although there is a small amount of KI in ordinary iodized salt, not enough is present to confer any protection by ingesting it. It would take 250 teaspoons of household iodized salt to equal one Potassium Iodide tablet!

If radiation exposure is expected, take the KI tablet once a day for 7-10 days, or longer if prolonged or multiple exposures are expected. Children should take 1/2 doses. It is also recommended to consider 1/2 tablet for large dogs, and 1/4 tablet for small dogs and cats. The largest commercial retailer for KI tablets is KI4U.com.

Don't depend on supplies of the drug to be available after a nuclear event. Even the federal government will have little KI in reserve to give to the general population. In recent power plant meltdowns, there was little or no Potassium Iodide to be found anywhere for purchase. If you have a limited supply, it is important to know that children are the most likely to develop thyroid cancer after an exposure and should be treated first.

If you find yourself without a supply, consider this alternative: 2% tincture of Iodine solution (brand name Betadine). "Paint" 8 ml of Betadine on the abdomen or forearm 2-12 hours prior to a radiation exposure and re-apply daily. Enough should be absorbed through the skin to give protection against radioactive Iodine in fallout.

Apply 4 ml. on children 3 and older (but under 150 lbs. or 70 kg.). Toddlers should have 2ml painted on, and infants 1 ml. This strategy should also work on animals. If you don't have a way to measure in ml, remember that a standard teaspoon is about 5 milliliters. Discontinue the daily treatment after 3 days or when Radioiodine levels have fallen to safer levels.

Be aware that those who are allergic to seafood will probably be allergic to Iodine. Adverse reactions may also occur if you take medications such as diuretics and Lithium.. It is also important to note that you cannot drink Betadine, as it is poisonous if ingested.

Although many in the preparedness community don't view a nuclear event as the most likely disaster scenario, it's important to learn about ALL the possible issues that may impact your family in uncertain times.

BIOLOGICAL WARFARE

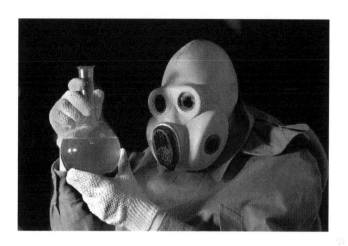

The preparedness community is concerned about the possibility of various calamities. Economic collapse, solar storms, global warming, and civil unrest are just a few. There is one scenario, however, that few consider as a possible cause of a long-term survival situation: biological warfare.

Biological warfare is the term given to the use of infectious agents such as bacteria, viruses, fungi or their by-products to wreak death and havoc among a specific population. As a result, the user achieves control over an area or a segment of the population by weakening the ability to resist. Biological weapons don't necessarily have to kill humans: unleashing a horde of locusts to destroy crops or agents that kill livestock can be just as effective.

This type of weapon has been used since ancient times, and even appears in the bible as part of the plagues visited upon Pharaoh by a wrathful God. Medieval accounts of Bubonic plague-ridden corpses catapulted into besieged cities abound; this method was used as late at 1710, when the Russians attacked the Swedish city of Reval (present day Tallinn) in this manner.

The Western hemisphere was changed forever by inadvertent introduction of smallpox into the Native American population, killing 90% in some areas and opening vast swaths of land for European colonization. In addition, purposeful biological warfare occurred against

Native Americans when the British presented a large "gift" of infected blankets as a "peace" offering during Pontiac's War in the mid-1700s.

As time progressed, new methods and infectious agents (Anthrax) were used in certain situations during World War I. As a result, use of biological weapons was banned by the Geneva Protocol in 1925, but research and production was still carried out by both sides during World War II. Research into the use of Anthrax by the United Kingdom left their laboratory area in Scotland contaminated for the next five decades.

In 1972, the storage, production, and transport of biological warfare agents was banned by the Biological Weapons Convention (BWC). Despite this, there are a number of violations that have been documented in the former Soviet Union and Iraq, and various others suspected. As of 2011, 165 countries have signed the BWC pact.

The perfect biological weapon would have these characteristics:

- Be infectious and contagious in a large percentage of those exposed.
- Cause severe long-term debilitation or death of the infected organism.
- Have few available antidotes, preventives or cures.
- Be easily deliverable to the area or population targeted.
- Have low likelihood of causing damage to those using the agent.

The concerns about "accidents" affecting the aggressor have most countries reluctant to use such weapons in normal tactical situations. During the largest such accident in 1979, a Russian lab released anthrax into the surrounding area, killing 42 people, infecting sheep over 200 miles away, and causing the immediate area to be off-limits even today.

Some candidates for use as biological agents include Anthrax, Smallpox, Viral hemorrhagic Fevers (Ebola, etc.), and Pneumonic Plague.

Anthrax can be contracted in several ways, by skin contact, inhalation, and gastrointestinal infection. More common in livestock than people, **Anthrax** is not an ideal "weapon of mass destruction" in that no person-to-person contagion occurs, except in skin cases (the least lethal form). A "cloud" of Anthrax would be necessary to affect a large population, although large numbers of infected livestock could result in an epidemic of the disease in humans.

The bacterium exists as spores which, in the right environment, release toxins that cause a flu-like syndrome which eventually destroys cells in lymph nodes, spreading to the lungs and blood, and may be highly lethal. Although Penicillin, Doxycycline, and Ciprofloxacin (Fish-Pen, Bird-Biotic, and Fish-Flox, respectively) are effective against this bacteria as a preventative or for early treatment, full-blown inhalation Anthrax may be difficult to survive; the toxins released by the spores remain even if the spores are killed.

Inhalation Anthrax can progress to shock and death in many cases; luckily, not everyone exposed will get symptoms. Because of higher risk of exposure, certain individuals, such as livestock workers, are often offered a vaccine against the disease.

"Pneumonic" is one of three types of **Plague** and, by far, the most contagious, easily spread by coughing bacteria into the air. It is caused by a bacterium known as Yersinia Pestis, usually found on rodents and other small animals in their fleas. Also starting off as a flu-like syndrome, it quickly develops into pneumonia with fever, weakness, shortness of breath, and cough (often with blood).

Pneumonic plague is different from Bubonic plague in that the patient will not have the classic swellings in the groin or armpit (called "Buboes"). Unlike inhalation Anthrax, which may take weeks to develop symptoms, patients with **Pneumonic Plague** may be dead in 2-4 days if not treated early.

Tetracycline (veterinary equivalent: Fish-Cycline), Doxycycline (Bird-Biotic) and Ciprofloxacin (Fish-Flox), and IV Gentamycin are effective treatments for victims of Plague. Oxygen is often used to support the sick individual, and protective masks are imperative for those who are caring for them.

There are several types of viral fevers associated with different organisms that normally infect rodents. **Hemorrhagic Fevers** like **Ebola** start off with fever, diarrhea, and weakness, but progress to more serious problems relating to internal and external hemorrhaging. Patients may bleed from eyes, ears, nose, mouth, or rectum and may have bruising on the skin from subcutaneous bleeding.

Normal antivirals don't seem to cure this disease, and death rates may be as high as 90%. The illness is spread by bodily fluids and other contact, so masks and gloves, again, are extremely important for health care workers.

Smallpox is another viral illness that is highly contagious and was responsible for the decimation of the Native American population. Related to the chickenpox virus, it differs in that all the blisters develop at the same time, rather than their being at different points of developing and healing. Contact with these blisters causes the disease to be contagious. Fever and fatigue accompany the illness. Although rare in developed countries now, it was prevalent in the past and FEMA stockpiles Smallpox vaccines in enough quantity to vaccinate every U.S. citizen. No curative treatment is currently available, and complications can lead to shock and death.

By-products released by microbes and plants walk the fine line between biological weapons and chemical weapons. Toxin released by the bacteria that causes botulism causes paralysis of muscles, and is used in small quantities as the cosmetic agent Botox. Ingredients in castor beans contain Ricin, a potent toxin that causes respiratory and circulatory failure. 3 mg. of ricin is potent enough to kill an average-sized adult if inhaled.

A classic example of old-time survivalism that may be useful is the "**gas mask**". A gas mask is placed over the face to protect the wearer from inhaling airborne pollutants and toxic gases. It forms a sealed cover over the nose and mouth with filters that allow breathing. Oftentimes, it will also cover the eyes or the entire face. Although cumbersome, it is superior to the surgical mask as a barrier. The user is still vulnerable to chemicals that can penetrate the skin, unless they are wearing a protective suit as well.

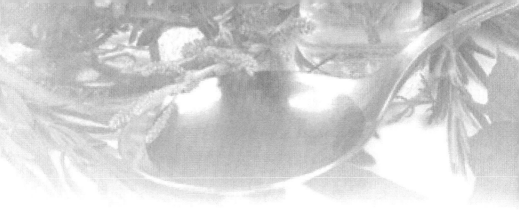

SECTION 6

✚ ✚ ✚

INJURIES

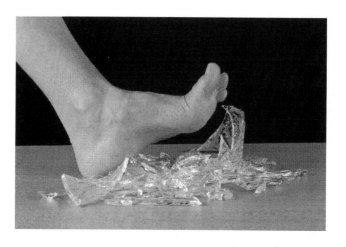

In a collapse situation, the performance of tasks like chopping wood, cooking food, etc. will likely lead to a number of soft tissue injuries (those that do not involve bony structures). From a simple cut to a severe burn, any damage to skin is akin to a chink in your body's protective armor.

Your skin is a considered an organ, indeed, the largest organ in the body, and serves as a barrier against infection and loss of fluids. When this barrier is weakened by a laceration or burn, your health is in jeopardy. Rapid and effective treatment of these injuries will prevent them from becoming life-threatening.

Being the rugged individualists that they are, some in the preparedness or homesteading community may be likely to shrug off minor injuries as inconsequential. This couldn't be farther from the truth. Any minor injury has the potential to cause trouble down the road. As a healthcare provider during troubled times, you must monitor the healing process of every wound.

Each wound is different and must be evaluated separately. If not present at the time the wound is incurred, the medic should begin by asking the simple question: "What happened"? A look around at the site of the accident will give you an idea of what type of debris you might find in the wound and the likelihood of infection. Always assume a wound is dirty initially.

Other questions to ask are whether the victim has chronic medical problems, like diabetes, and whether they are allergic to any medications. You might be surprised to find that (even close) friends may have not imparted this history to you in all the time that you've known them.

The physical examination of a wound requires the following assessment: Location on the body, length, depth, and the type of tissue involved. Circulation and Nerve involvement must also be evaluated. If an extremity, have the patient show you a full range of motion, if possible, during your examination. This is especially important if the injury involves a joint.

This section will deal with various injuries, their evaluation, and treatment. With close observation, your people will have the best chance of staying out of trouble.

MINOR WOUNDS

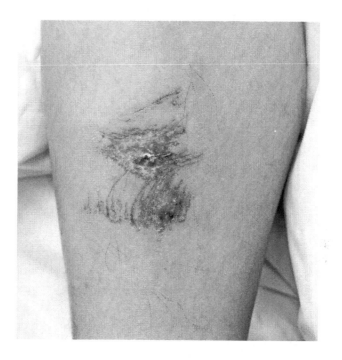

A soft tissue injury is considered minor when it fails to penetrate the deep layer of the skin, called the "**dermis**". This would include cuts, scrapes and bruises.

- **Cuts and Scratches:** These tears in the skin only penetrate the "**epidermis**" (superficial skin layer) and become infected on an infrequent basis in a healthy person.
- **Abrasions or Scrapes:** A portion of the epidermis has been scraped off. You probably have experienced plenty of these as a child.
- **Bruises or Contusions:** These result from blunt trauma and do not penetrate the skin at all. However, there is bleeding into the skin from blood vessels that have been disrupted by the impact.

All of the above minor injuries can be easily treated. Wash the wound anywhere that the epidermis has been violated. The use of an antiseptic such as Betadine (Povidone-Iodine solution), honey, or triple antibiotic ointment such as Neosporin or Bactroban will be helpful to prevent infection. Ibuprofen and Acetaminophen are useful over-the-counter drugs to treat minor pain.

Minor bleeding can be stopped with a wet styptic pencil, an item normally used for shaving cuts. The wound, if it broke the skin, should have a protective adhesive bandage (such as a Band-Aid) to prevent infection.

Applying pressure and ice (if available) wherever a bruise seems to be spreading will stop it from getting bigger. Bruises will change color over time from blackish-blue to brown to yellow. Bruises may be gravity-dependent and may descend slightly and time goes on.

The Liquid Skin bandage is an excellent way to cover a minor injury with some advantages over a regular bandage. You apply it once to the cut or scrape; it dries within a minute or so and seals the wound. It also stops minor bleeding, and won't fall out during baths. There are various brands (Band-Aid Liquid Bandage, New Skin, Curad, 3M No Sting liquid bandage) and many come as a convenient spray. These injuries will heal over the next 7-10 days, dependent on the amount of skin area affected.

You don't always have to travel the traditional road to treat many medical problems. If you have one of the minor injuries mentioned, why not consider natural remedies? Here's an alternative process to deal with these issues:

1. Evaluate seriousness of wound; if minor, you may continue with herbal treatment.
2. Stop minor bleeding with herbal blood clotting agents such as Cayenne Pepper powder, and compress the area with gauze. Substances that clot blood are called "hemostatic" agents. These include:
   - Essential oils- Geranium, Helichrysum, Lavender, Cypress, Myrrh, or Hyssop- Any oil applied to a gauze compress.
   - Medicinal Herbs- Cayenne pepper powder or cinnamon powder with direct application, Yarrow tincture soaked in a gauze compress.

3. After minor bleeding is stopped, the wound should be cleaned with an herbal antiseptic: Mix a few drops of oil with sterile water and wash out the wound thoroughly. Essential oils with this property include:
   - Lavender oil
   - Tea tree
   - Rosemary
   - Eucalyptus
   - Peppermint
4. Apply herbal antiseptic to the wound using the above essential oils; for example, use peppermint oil in a 50/50 mix with carrier oils such as olive or coconut oil. Other natural antiseptics include garlic, raw unprocessed honey, Echinacea, witch hazel, and St. John's Wort.
5. If needed, use natural pain relievers, such as:
   - Geranium oil
   - Helichrysum oil
   - Ginger oil
   - Rosemary oil
   - Oregano oil

   Apply 2-4 drops of a 50/50 dilution around the wound's edges.
6. Dress the wound using clean gauze. Do not wrap too tightly.
7. Change the dressing, reapply antiseptic, and observe for infection twice daily until healed.

   Infected wounds are discussed in the section on cellulitis in this book.

Some naturopaths advocate the use of activated charcoal to help wounds heal. To make a poultice:

- Mix 1-2 tablespoons of actuvated charcoal with a small amount of water to form a moist paste.
- Add Flax seed meal to help retain moisture.
- Spread the paste on gauze cut to fit the wound and fold it over.
- Apply to the injury and cover completely with plastic food wrap if available.
- Tape the poultice securely in place and leave overnight.

HEMORRHAGIC AND MAJOR WOUNDS

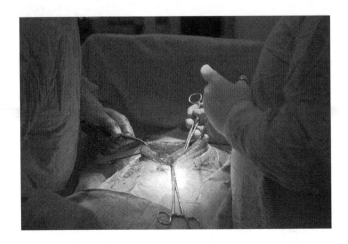

In a destabilized society, the risk of civil unrest is high. Traumatic wounds may be commonplace. Therefore, the medic for a family or group must be prepared for the worst possible injuries without the benefit of a surgeon and operating room (image above).

Cuts in the skin can be minor or catastrophic, superficial or deep, clean or infected. Most significant cuts (also called 'lacerations') penetrate both the dermis and epidermis and are associated with bleeding, sometimes major. Knowing how to manage a hemorrhagic wound quickly and effectively will be of paramount importance.

Bleeding can be venous in origin, which manifests as dark red blood, draining steadily from the wound. Bleeding can also be arterial, which is bright red (due to higher oxygen content) and comes out in spurts that correspond to the pulse of the patient. As the vein and artery usually run together, a serious cut can have both.

Once below the level of the skin, large blood vessels and nerves may be involved. Assess circulation, sensation, and the ability to move the injured area. You will notice more problems with vessel and nerve damage in deep lacerations and crush injuries.

For an extremity injury, evaluate what we call the "**Capillary Refill Time**" to test for circulation beyond the area of the wound. To do this, press the nail bed or finger/toe pad; in a person with normal circulation, this area will turn white when you release pressure and then return to a normal color within 2 seconds. If it takes longer or the fingertips are blue, you may have a person who has damaged a blood vessel. If motor function or sensation is decreased (test by lightly pricking with a safety pin beyond the level of the wound), there may be nerve damage.

Evaluating blood loss is an important aspect of dealing with wounds. An average size human adult has about 10 pints of blood. The effect on the body caused by blood loss varies with the amount of blood loss incurred:

- 1.5 pints (0.75 liters) or less: little or no effect; you can donate a pint of whole blood, for example, as often as every 8 weeks.
- 1.5-3.5 pints (0.75-1.5 liters): rapid heartbeat and respirations. The skin becomes cool and may appear pale. The patient is usually very agitated. If you are not accustomed to the sight of blood, you might be also. Even a small amount of blood on the floor or on the patient may make an inexperienced medic queasy.
- 3.5-4 pints (1.5-2 liters): Blood pressure begins to drop; the patient may appear confused. Heartbeat is usually very rapid.
- Over 4 pints (more than 2 liters): Patient is now very pale, and may be unconscious. After a period of time with continued blood loss, the blood pressure drops further, the heart rate and respirations decrease, and the patient is in serious danger.

When you encounter a person with a bleeding wound, the first course of action is to stop the hemorrhage. Oftentimes, direct pressure on the bleeding area might stop bleeding all by itself. Bleeding in an extremity may be slowed by elevating the limb above the level of the heart.

The medic should always have nitrile gloves in his or her pack; this will prevent the wound from contamination by a "dirty" hand. Try to avoid touching the palm or finger portions of the gloves as you put them on. If there are no gloves, grab a bandanna or other cloth barrier and press it into the wound.

Additionally, pressing on the "**pressure point**" for the area injured may help slow bleeding.

Pressure points are locations where major arteries come close enough to the skin to be compressed manually. Pressing on this area will slow down bleeding further down the track of the blood vessel.

Using pressure points, we can make a "map" of specific areas to concentrate your efforts to decrease bleeding. For example, there is a large blood vessel behind each knee known as the Popliteal Artery. If you have a bleeding wound in the lower leg, say your calf, applying pressure on the back of the knee will help stop the hemorrhage. A diagram of some major pressure points is below:

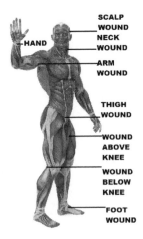

If this fails to stop the bleeding, it may be appropriate to use a tourniquet. The military uses a CAT (Combat Application Tourniquet) tourniquet, which is simple to use and could be even be placed with one hand. This is especially useful if the bleeding victim is you. Tourniquets must be placed tightly; arterial bleeding requires more pressure than simple venous bleeding to stop.

The placement of a tourniquet to a wound must be made judiciously. The tourniquet stops bleeding from the open blood vessel, but it also stops circulation in nearby intact blood vessels as well. It is important to note that the tourniquet, once placed, should be loosened every ten minutes or so, to allow blood flow to uninjured areas and to determine whether the bleeding has stopped due to the natural clotting process.

HEMORRHAGIC AND MAJOR WOUNDS

Tourniquets are painful if they are in place for too long, and prolonged use could actually cause your patient to lose a limb due to lack of circulation. As well, your body may build up toxins in the extremity; these become concentrated and rush into your body core when you release the tourniquet. It takes less than an hour or two with a tourniquet in place to cause this problem.

Once you are comfortable that major bleeding has abated, release pressure from the tourniquet while leaving it within easy reach. Flush the wound aggressively with sterile water or a 1:10 Betadine solution. This procedure is known as "**irrigation**". You may have heard of cleaning wounds with alcohol or hydrogen peroxide; this method is acceptable for a first cleaning if you have nothing else but not for later wound care (see the section on soft tissue wound care).

Packing the wound with bandages is not just for sopping up blood; bandages are useful to apply pressure. More than one bandage may be required to keep the wound from bleeding further. It's important to make sure that you put the most pressure where the bleeding was occurring in the wound. If the blood was coming from the top of a large wound, start packing there. Again, keep compressing the wound.

Now, cover the whole area with a dry dressing for further protection. The Israeli army developed an excellent bandage which is easy to use and is found almost everywhere survival gear is sold. The advantage of the Israel battle dressing is that it applies pressure on the bleeding area for you. Don't forget that bandages get dirty and should be changed often. Twice a day is a minimum until it has healed.

The above process of stopping hemorrhage and dressing a wound will also work for traumatic injuries such as knife wounds and gunshot wounds. You have probably heard that you should not remove a knife because it can cause the hemorrhage to worsen. This will give you time to get the patient to the hospital, but what if there are no hospitals? You will have to transport your victim to your base camp and prepare to remove the knife. It can't stay in there for months while you're waiting for society to re-stabilize. Have plenty of gauze and clotting agents available.

Bullet wounds are the opposite, in that the bullet is usually removed if at all possible when modern medical care is available. In you do not have the luxury of transferring the patient to a trauma center, you will want to avoid digging for a hard-to-find bullet. Even though there are instruments made for this purpose, manipulation could cause further contamination and bleeding.

For a historical example, take the case of President James Garfield. In 1881, President Garfield was shot by an assassin. In their rush to remove the bullet, 12 different physicians placed their (ungloved) hands in the wound. The wound, which would not have been mortal in all probability, became infected. As a result, the president died after a month in agony. In austere settings, think twice before removing a projectile that isn't clearly visible and easily reached.

Commercial Hemostatic Agents

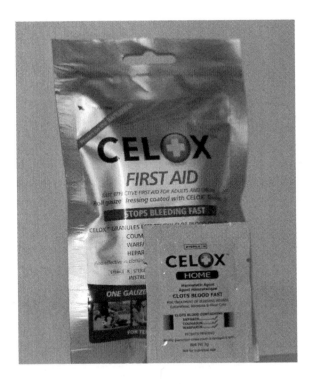

In studies of casualties in the recent wars, 50% of those killed in action died of blood loss. 25% died within the first "golden" hour after being wounded. A victim's chance of survival diminishes significantly after 1 hour without care, with a threefold increase in mortality for every 30 minutes without care thereafter.

Therefore, the question we must pose is, to paraphrase Hamlet, "To bleed or NOT to bleed". Ever since there have been traumatic injuries, we have been concerned with deaths due to hemorrhage. The Egyptians mixed wax, barley, and grease to apply to a bleeding wound. The Chinese and Greeks used herbs like bayberry, stinging nettle, yarrow, and others for the same purpose. Native Americans would apply scrapings from the inside of fresh animal hides mixed with hot sand and downy feathers. These treatments would sometimes be successful, sometimes not.

The control of major hemorrhage may be the territory of the trauma surgeon, but what if you find yourself without access to modern medical care? In the last decade or so, there have been major advancements in hemostasis (stopping blood loss). Knowledge of their appropriate use in an emergency will increase the injured patient's chance of survival.

Although there are various types of hemostatic agents on the market for medical storage, the two most popular are Quikclot and Celox. They are two different substances that are both available in a powder or powder-impregnated gauze.

Quikclot originally contained a volcanic mineral known as zeolite, which effectively clotted bleeding wounds but also caused a reaction that caused some serious burns. As a result, the main ingredient was replaced with another substance that does not burn when it comes in contact with blood.

The current generation of Quikclot is made from Kaolin, the same stuff you find in the anti-diarrheal product Kaopectate. It is so common that it is said to be what makes Georgia clay red. It does not contain animal, human, or botanical components.

Contact between kaolin and blood immediately initiates the clotting process by activating Factor XII, a major player in the clotting process. The powder or impregnated gauze is applied and pressure placed for several minutes. Quikclot is FDA-approved and widely available; the gauze dressing is easier to deal with than the powder, but can be expensive.

Quikclot has a shelf life of 3 years or so, less if the packages are left out in the sun.

One negative with Quikclot is that it does not absorb into the body and, some believe, can be difficult to remove from the wound. This was certainly true of previous generations but it is claimed to no longer be as big an issue, especially if you use the gauze dressing.. If more than one dressing is required, don't remove the first one: Place the second gauze on top. Use an irrigation syringe to flush the wound after the gauze is finally removed.

In a study published in the The Journal of Trauma, Injury, Infection, and Critical Care, (Volume 68, Number 2, February 2010), the kaolin gauze was found to be as safe as standard surgical gauze.

Celox is the other popular hemostatic agent, and it is composed of chitosan, an organic material processed from shrimp shells. As such, those allergic to seafood could possibly have a reaction to Celox. This "powder" product is actually made up of high surface area flakes. When these tiny flakes come in contact with blood, they bond with it and form a clot that appears as a gel. Like Quikclot, it also comes in impregnated gauze dressings, which are, again, relatively expensive.

Celox will cause effective clotting even in those on anti-coagulants like Heparin, Warfarin or Coumadin without further depleting clotting factors. Chitosan, being an organic material, is gradually broken down by the body's natural enzymes into other substances normally found there. Like Quikclot, Celox is FDA-approved.

Studies by the U.S. government compare Celox favorably to other hemostatic agents.

Both Quikclot and Celox gauze dressings have been tested by the U.S. and U.K. military and have been put to good use in Iraq and Afghanistan. Although effective, you shouldn't use these items as a first line of treatment in a bleeding patient. Pressure, elevation of a bleeding extremity above the heart, gauze packing and tourniquets should be your strategy here. If these measures fail, however, you have an effective extra step towards stopping that hemorrhage.

SOFT TISSUE WOUND CARE

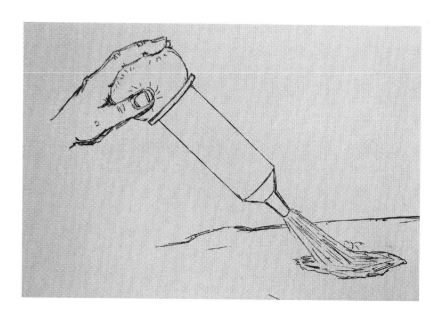

Irrigating the wound

Once you have stopped the bleeding and applied your dressing, you are in safer territory than you were. In an austere setting, however, you must follow the status of the wound until full recovery in your role as medic. Continued wound care is your responsibility.

An open wound can heal by two methods:

Primary Intention (Closure): The wound is closed in some way, such as with sutures or staples. This results in a smaller scar, but carries the risk of inadvertently sequestering bacteria deep in the wound.

Secondary Intention (Granulation): Leaving a wound open causes the formation of "**granulation tissue**". Granulation tissue is rapidly growing early scar tissue that is rich in blood vessels. It fills in spaces where the wound edges are not together. After a period of time, it turns into mature scar tissue. This scar is larger than if the wound were closed by primary intention, but decreases the risk of infection if properly cared for.

Often, it is safest to allow a wound to heal on its own rather than suture or staple it closed. Wound dressings must be changed regularly (at least twice a day or whenever the bandage is saturated with blood, fluids, etc.) in order to give the best chance for quick healing. When you change a dressing, it is important to clean the wound area with drinkable water or an antiseptic solution such as dilute Betadine (povidone-iodine). Use 1 part Betadine to 10 parts water.

Remember the old saying, "The solution to pollution is dilution". Using a bulb or irrigation syringe (60-100 ml) will provide pressure to the flow of water and wash out old clots and dirt. Lightly scrub any open wound with diluted Betadine or sterilized water. You may notice some (usually slight) bleeding. This is a sign of tissue that is forming new blood vessels and not necessarily a bad sign. Apply pressure with a clean bandage until it stops.

Interestingly, most studies find that sterilized (drinkable) water is just as good as a concentrated antiseptic solution for wound healing (sometimes better). Although it is acceptable to perform a first cleaning with Betadine or Hydrogen Peroxide, later cleaning should definitely not use these concentrated products. New cells are trying to grow, and they do this best in a moist environment. Concentrated antiseptics dry out these fragile new cells and make slow down healing.

An alternative antiseptic solution that is easy to make using common storage supplies is **Dakin's Solution.** First used during WWI, Dakin's solution is used to disinfect wounds on the skin, such as pressure sores in bedridden patients. It is inexpensive to put together, dissolves dead cells, and uses the following:

- Sodium hypochlorite solution (regular strength household bleach).
- Sodium bicarbonate (baking soda)
- Boiled tap water

To make Dakin's solution, take 4 cups of sterilized water and add ½ teaspoon of baking soda. Then, add a certain amount of bleach to reach the strength that you'll need. 3 teaspoons will act as a mild antiseptic effect (plenty for clean wounds that are healing) and 3 tablespoons will give you a stronger effect for infected wounds. You can use a full 3 fluid ounces (about 100 milliliters) for a full strength solution to treat the worst infections. Do not take Dakin's solution internally and watch for allergic reactions in the form or rashes or other irritation. Store in darkness at room temperature and make a new batch every few days, as it loses potency relatively quickly. Do not freeze or heat up the solution.

To assure rapid healing of open wounds, we use a type of dressing method known as "**wet-to-dry**". Apply a bandage directly to an open wound which has been soaked in sterilized water and wrung out. In this fashion, we prevent the drying out of new cells by keeping them in a moist environment.. On top of the bandage which touches the healing wound, you will place a dry bandage and some type of tape to secure it in place. Thus, you have a "wet-to-dry" dressing.

It may also be a good idea to apply some triple antibiotic ointment around a healing wound to prevent infection from bacteria on the skin. Raw honey, lavender oil, and tea tree oil are some natural alternatives.

As time goes on, you might see some blackish material on the wound edges. This is non-viable material and should be removed. It might just scrub out, or you might need to take your scissors or scalpel and trim off the dead tissue. This is called "**debridement**" and removes material that is no longer part of the healing process.

WOUND CLOSURE

When a laceration occurs, our body's natural armor is breached and bacteria get a free ride to the rest of our body. Once there, our health is in real danger. Therefore, it only makes common sense that we want to close that breach.

There is always some controversy as to whether to close a wound. A laceration may be closed either by sutures, tapes, staples or medical "superglues" such as Derma-Bond. When and why would you choose to close a wound, and what method should you use? After rendering first aid, which includes removal of any foreign objects, hemostasis (stopping the bleeding), irrigation, and antiseptic application, you will have to determine the answer.

Tapes, Glues, and Staples

There are several methods available to close a laceration. It makes common sense to use the simplest and least invasive method that will do the job. The easiest to use are "**Steri-Strips**" and butterfly closures. These are adhesive bandages which adhere on each side of the wound to pull it together. They don't require puncturing the skin and will fall off on their own, in time. Even duct tape can be used to make a butterfly closure.

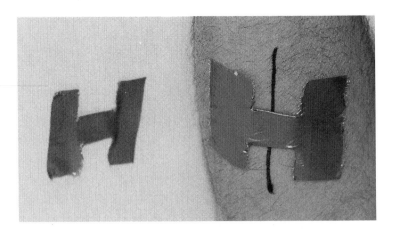

improvised butterfly closure with duct tape

The second least invasive method is Cyanoacrylate, special "glue" sold as **Derma-Bond** or Liquiseal. This is medical- grade adhesive that is made specifically for use on the skin. Simply approximate the skin and run a thin line of glue down the laceration. Hold in place until dry. It will naturally peel off as the skin heals.

Some have recommended (the much less expensive) household "**Super-Glue**" for wound closure. This preparation is slightly different chemically, and is not made for use on the skin. It may cause skin irritation in some, and burn-like reactions have been reported.

If it's all you have, however, you may choose to use it. You can test super-glue for allergic reactions by placing a small amount on the inside of your forearm and observe for a rash over the next 24 hours.

Another closure method is the use of **skin staplers**. They work by "pinching" the skin together and should be removed in about 7 days. You will require two toothed tweezers (also called "Adson's Forceps") to evert the skin edges and approximate them for the person doing the stapling. As such, stapling is best done if you have an assistant. Interestingly, the most skilled person is the one holding the tweezers, not the person stapling.

Staples are best removed with a specific instrument known as a staple remover. Stapling equipment is widely available, but probably not as cost-effective as other methods.

Sutures are your most invasive method of wound or laceration closure. As it can be done by a single person, it is the one that requires the most skill. Before you choose to close a wound by suturing, make sure you ask yourself why you can't use a less invasive method instead.

Keep it simple. Use the other methods first, and save your precious suture/staple supplies for those special cases that really need them. In a long-term survival situation, it's unlikely you'll ever be able to replenish those items.

All About Sutures

I am asked to teach suturing more than any other first aid procedure, even though it really isn't FIRST aid at all. Suturing is best done by someone with experience, and you don't get that kind of experience in your typical first responder course. Survival medical training teaches you to stabilize and transfer the patient to modern facilities. But what if there is no modern care available? You'll need to obtain the knowledge to be able to function effectively; that means learning how to suture. You must also understand when a wound should be closed and, more importantly, when it shouldn't.

Human skin has probably been sutured ever since we learned to make needles from bone and antler 30,000 years ago. The first documentation of suturing was from the Egyptians 5,000 years ago, and actual stitches have been found in mummies more than 3,000 years old. The Greeks and Romans, as well as various native cultures, also worked with sutures.

Using needles of bone, ivory and copper, they would use various natural materials such as hemp, flax, cotton, silk, hair and animal sinew to put wounds together. The classical era physician Galen, in the 2nd century A.D., was well known for stitching together the severed tendons and ligaments of gladiators, sometimes restoring function to a damaged extremity. He was one of the first to distinguish between a "clean" and a "dirty" wound.

In primitive cultures, ingenious ways were developed to close wounds. In some tropical rain forests, the natives would collect army ant soldiers whenever there was a wound to close. They would place the jaws of the ant on the skin, the ant would bite the skin closed, and then they would twist its body off! The head stayed on, with the jaws shut and the skin closed. Native Americans would pull off agave cactus needles along with a strip of the plant material attached, and use that as suture.

Suture technology didn't really advance much until the late 19th century, when the concept of sterilization of needles and suture material came into fashion. By this time, suture material was either "chromic catgut" (actually made from the intestinal lining of sheep and cows) or silk. Both of these materials are still available today in one form or another.

Suture "string" is either absorbable or non-absorbable. Catgut, for example, will dissolve in the body over the course of several weeks. Absorbable sutures are used for internal body work or areas such as the inside of the cheek or the vagina.

Silk is non-absorbable, and is used on the skin (where it can be eventually removed) or anywhere internally that you are willing to have the suture material stay forever. Around 1930, synthetic materials made their debut in the form of Nylon and polypropylene (Prolene). These are non-absorbables that are also available to this day and are, essentially, like fishing line. Since that time, various different manufactured types of suture material have reached the market, both absorbable (such as polyglycolic acid or Vicryl) and non-absorbable.

Suture material comes in various thicknesses: 0, 2-0, 3-0, 4-0, 5-0 and 6-0 are most commonly used on humans. The higher the number, the thinner the thread will be. This is not dissimilar to buckshot; 00 is thicker than 000 (2-0 vs. 3-0). 0-Nylon, for example, is thickest of the above, with 6-0 Nylon being very fine for use in delicate cosmetic work on, for example, the face. The heavier suture has more strength, but the finer suture leaves less of a scar.

Needles have progressed, also. Needles can be straight, curved, or various other shapes. Originally, needles were "eyed" and separate from the string. You threaded the needle and began your stitching, which caused two lengths of suture to go through the wound. This process caused some trauma to the tissues sutured, and so this type of needle is called a "traumatic" needle.

In 1920, a process called "swaging" was developed, which allowed the back end of the needle to be attached to the string. The diameter of the string was slightly thinner than the needle and only one single length of suture was passed through the tissue; this type of needle was named "atraumatic". Some swaged needles are built to "pop-off" with a quick tug after placing each stitch. This may be handy, but it is incredibly wasteful of suture material; therefore, I can only discourage its use unless you have unlimited supplies.

Needles are also categorized based on the point. The two most common needle points are "tapered" and "cutting", although there are various others. One is round and "tapers" smoothly to a point, like a sharpened pencil does. "Cutting" needles are triangular and have a sharp "cutting" edge on the inside curve of the needle. Cutting needles are used in dense tissue, such as skin.

When To Close A Wound/ When To Leave A Wound Open

Now that we are acquainted with sutures, we must ask ourselves the following question: What am I trying to accomplish by stitching this wound closed? Your goals are simple. You close wounds to repair the defect in your body's armor, to eliminate "dead space", and to promote healing. A well-approximated wound also has less scarring.

Unfortunately, here is where it gets complicated. Closing a wound that should be left open can do a lot more harm than good, and could possibly put your patient's life at risk. Take the case of a young woman injured in a "zipline" accident: She was taken to the local emergency room, where 22 staples were needed to close a large laceration. Unfortunately, the wound had dangerous bacteria in it, causing a serious infection which spread throughout her body. She eventually required multiple amputations. We learn from this an important lesson: Namely, that the decision to close a wound is not automatic but involves several considerations.

The most important consideration is whether you are dealing with a clean or a dirty wound. Most wounds you will encounter in a wilderness or collapse setting will be dirty. If you try to close a dirty wound, you have sequestered bacteria and dirt into your body. Within a short period of time, the infected wound will become red, swollen, and hot. An abscess may form, and pus will accumulate inside.

The infection may spread to your bloodstream and, when it does, you have caused a life-threatening situation. Leaving the wound open will allow you to clean the inside frequently and observe the healing process. It also allows inflammatory fluid to drain out of the body. Wounds that are left open heal by a process called "**granulation**"; that is, from the inside out. The scar isn't as pretty, but it's the safest option in most cases.

Other considerations when deciding whether or not to close a wound are whether it is a simple laceration (straight thin cut on the skin) or whether it is an avulsion (areas of skin torn out, hanging flaps). If the edges of the skin are so far apart that they cannot be stitched together without undue pressure, the wound should be left open. If the wound has been open for more than 8 hours, it should be left open; bacteria have already had a good chance to colonize the injury.

IF you're certain the wound is clean, you should close it if it is long, deep or gapes open loosely. Also, cuts over moving parts, such as the knee joint, will be more likely to require stitches. Remember that you should close deep wounds (except bites) in layers, to prevent any un-approximated "dead space" from occurring. Dead spaces are pockets of bacteria-laden air in a closed wound that may lead to a major infection.

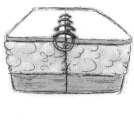

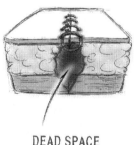

DEAD SPACE

If you are unsure, you can choose to wait 72 hours before closing a wound to make sure that no signs of infection develop. This is referred to as "delayed closure". Some wounds can be partially closed, allowing a small open space to avoid the accumulation of inflammatory fluid. Drains, consisting of thin lengths of latex, nitrile, or even gauze, might be placed into the wound for this purpose. Of course, you should place a dressing over the exposed area.

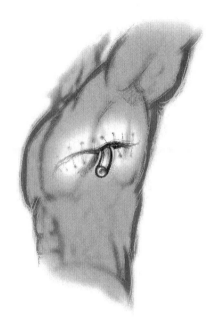

PENROSE DRAIN IN PLACE

Many injuries that require closure also should be treated with antibiotics to decrease the chance of infection. Natural remedies such as garlic or honey may be useful in an austere setting.

Deep layer sutures are never removed, so try to use absorbable material such as chromic catgut or Vicryl if possible. If you must use non-absorbables such as Silk, Nylon or Prolene, the body will wall off the sutures and may form a nodule known as a "**granuloma**". This may be disconcerting, but has little effect on a patient's health.

Sutures on the skin should be removed in 7 days (5 days if on the face); if over a joint, 14-21 days. Stitches placed over a joint, such as the knee, should be placed close together. In other areas, ½ inch or so between sutures is acceptable. It is alright to allow space for drainage of inflammatory fluid from the wound to occur. Always be certain to keep the wound clean as previously described.

LOCAL ANESTHESIA AND NERVE BLOCKS

When a person is injured and a wound must be sutured, the area will be sensitive and difficult to repair without causing significant discomfort to a person already in pain. As such, I am often asked about the use of Lidocaine (brand name Xylocaine), and other injectable local anesthetics for the purpose of preparing an injured area for suturing.

Lidocaine may be placed around the actual wound superficially (local infiltration) or may be directed to "block" a specific nerve that serves the area to be repaired. This procedure is known as a nerve block. Each nerve block is intended to numb a portion of the course of a nerve as it travels through the body, in an effort to numb the injured area.

Relatively small and superficial lacerations are best anesthetized by injecting the subcutaneous tissues with the numbing agent. The procedure is described in the next section on how to suture skin.

In other circumstances, specific nerve blocks are more appropriate. As each area of the body and wound is different, the corresponding nerve block is different as well; let's take the example of a hand injury. In this case, these situations would include:

- o Multiple lacerations to the hand or fingers
- o Injuries with multiple embedded foreign objects and debris
- o Large lacerations
- o Burns where extensive removal of dead tissue (debridement) is required
- o Poisonous bites that involve the removal of significant foreign material, such as a stingray spine
- o Areas that are sensitive or calloused (e.g., the palm of the hand)

There are various injectable local anesthetics on the market, such as Procaine (Novocain), Bupivacaine (Marcaine), and Mepivacaine (Carbocaine). Lidocaine (Xylocaine) is, however, the most widely used these days, due to the rapidity and effectiveness of its anesthetic action.

Lidocaine also comes in the form of an ointment, jelly, patch, and aerosol spray. Injecting the drug gives, of course, a much stronger effect.

You can obtain 1% or 2% Lidocaine; the more concentrated dosage is useful for longer procedures.

You can expect full effect about 10 minutes after administration, and the effect should last 1-2 hours. Epinephrine 1.200,000-1,000,000 has been used in conjunction with lidocaine to help decrease bleeding and prolong the effect further.

This combination should NOT be used in areas with limited circulation, such as the fingers or earlobes. The epinephrine could constrict the blood vessels excessively and cause lack of blood flow to the tissues (also called "**ischemia**").

Before you consider the use of local anesthetic, you should be aware of your patient's medical history. Some, such as those with liver disease, cardiac disease, or the elderly, should receive less quantities of the drug or none at all.

Of course, you'll need some equipment: Sterile towels and gauze will create a sterile field in which to work. You'll need an antiseptic such as Betadine, at least one 6cc or 10cc syringe, and a thin gauge needle (25 or 27 gauge will do fine). You can decrease the "sting" of the injection by warming the local anesthetic somewhat and/or adding 1cc of sodium bicarbonate solution to 10cc of medication.

Using an alcohol wipe on the end of the bottle, fill a small syringe with air. Inject the air into the bottle, and the pressure will cause the local anesthetic to fill the syringe. Place an injection at a 45 degree angle to the skin, and then inject enough to form a shiny raised area on each side of the laceration. This is called a "wheal". Within a few minutes, the area will be numb.

It should be noted that Lidocaine is a prescription medication and is difficult to procure. When used in subcutaneous tissue, it acts as an anesthetic; used intravenously, however, it has cardiac and other effects. An accidental injection into a blood vessel is possibly life-threatening, causing heart irregularities and seizures.

To determine if you are in a blood vessel, pull the plunger back. It will draw blood into the syringe if it's in the wrong place. If you lack Lidocaine, you can apply an ice cube to the area to be sutured until sensation decreases.

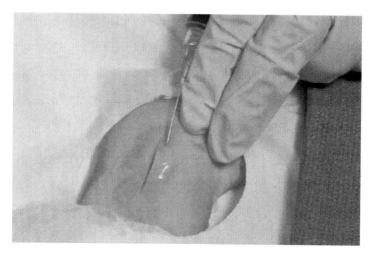

Injecting local anesthetic

Repeat until each side appears slightly swollen. You can decrease the discomfort of multiple injections by entering in an area already anesthetized by a previous injection. To see this procedure in real time, check out my YouTube video "How to Suture with Dr. Bones".

The Radial Nerve (Wrist) Block

To describe every type of nerve block would take an entire medical textbook, so let's pick a specific one and go through the procedure. We'll use the example of a laceration on the back of hand.

The nerve we want to block is the radial nerve, as it supplies sensation to that area. You can see how helpful it can be to have a book on anatomy in your medical library; it helps to know where the nerve travels in the injured area. For now, see the image below to see the nerve distribution.

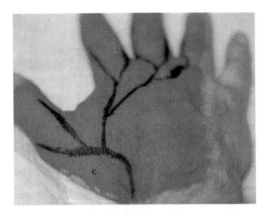

Radial Nerve Distribution

You'll start with the patient's hand in the palm-up position. Clean the entire wrist and back of the hand with Betadine. Feel the radial artery pulse; this is the one that the doctor takes your pulse with when you have a physical exam. Then feel the "radial styloid"; this is the part of the wrist that protrudes slightly below the thumb area (see image below).

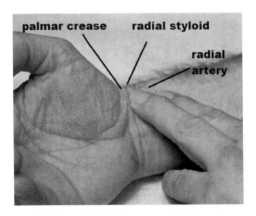

Radial Artery Pulse

Insert your needle between the radial artery and the styloid near the crease of the palm, and inject 2-3cc of the anesthetic (see image below). Always pull back the plunger before you inject to make sure you haven't entered a blood vessel. Blood in the syringe should warn you to start over.

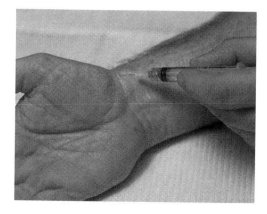

Next, you will turn the hand over. Using the same insertion site, inject another 5cc or so of Lidocaine along the back of the wrist to about the midpoint area. Use a longer needle than the one in the image below if you can; this will decrease the numbers of injections you'll have to do.

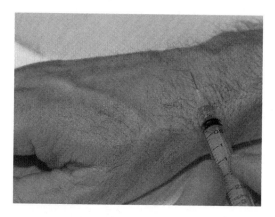

Finally, wait 10 minutes and then test the area for anesthetic effect by lightly touching the area to be sutured with a needle.

Complications of injecting local anesthesia include:

- **Nerve injury** – a sign of this is severe pain during the injection.
- **Vascular injury** – excessive constriction leading to insufficient circulation. This is usually seen with Lidocaine in combination with epinephrine.

- **Hematoma** – blood accumulating under the skin due to puncture of a blood vessel
- **Lidocaine toxicity** – accidental injection of anesthetic directly into a blood vessel

Lidocaine toxicity presents with lightheadedness, visual changes, numbness (often in the tongue), metallic taste, and ringing in the ears. Severe cases can progress to unconsciousness and convulsions. In rare instances, a patient could develop heart arrhythmias, respiratory arrest, and even go into a coma.

The Digital (finger) block

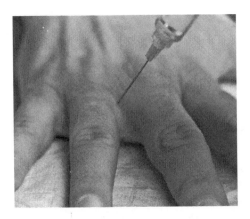

Injecting The Finger Base

The procedure to give anesthesia to a finger is relatively simple. Due to circulation issues, always use plain Lidocaine 1 or 2% WITHOUT epinephrine.

Place the hand pronated on the sterile field (use more Betadine than I did in the photos). With your small gauge needle and a Lidocaine syringe, place a small amount of local anesthesia on either side of the base of the finger, raising a wheal (a slight swelling) just under the skin. This will make any later injections less painful.

After waiting a minute or so, insert the needle in the wheal and forward toward the base of the finger bone. Begin injecting the local anesthesia. Repeat on each side of the injured finger. 1-2 ml, injected as you slowly withdraw the needle, on each side should be sufficient. Too much may cause compression of blood vessels.

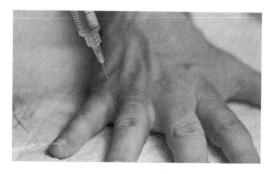

Injecting the other side

An alternative to this approach, or perhaps an addition for more complete anesthesia, is the "transthecal" finger block. The benefit is that this approach may numb the finger with a single injection, if done correctly.

To perform this type of block, turn the hand palm up, and follow the tendon of the finger down to the level of the first palmar crease line. Inserting the needle at a 45 degree angle, go down to the tendon and inject 2 ml of plain Lidocaine. If you notice resistance you are too close to the tendon and should pull back a little. Some suggest rubbing the area afterwards to distribute the medication.

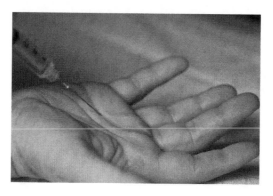

Transthecal Injection

Wait about 10 minutes or so before assessing for completeness of anesthesia. This may be done by lightly pricking with a safety pin or applying slight pressure to the area.

After any work on the finger injury, immobilize it with a finger splint or the "buddy method" of using an adjacent finger for support. Cover with a generous wrapping.

Some important things to know:

- Don't inject any area that is clearly infected (red, swollen, warm to the touch).
- Use small gauge needles to avoid hitting blood vessels and causing bleeding.
- Don't inject into any visible veins.
- Pull back on the needle before you inject anesthesia; if you see blood in the syringe, abort and try again.
- Avoid Epinephrine on fingers and toes.
- No more than 2 ml on each side of a finger block.
- If the injection is extremely painful, you may be hitting the nerve with the needle; abort and try again.

Finally, it's important to remember that, while we have the luxury of modern medical care, injuries and wounds should be treated by medical professionals. There are doctors with a lot of experience performing nerve blocks; take advantage of their expertise while they're still there for you.

HOW TO SUTURE SKIN

Suturing is best done by someone with experience, but you don't get that kind of experience in your typical first responder course. You'll need to obtain the know-how to be able to function effectively, and that means knowing how to close a wound. Here's a practice session that will give you an introduction to a brand new skill: Suturing.

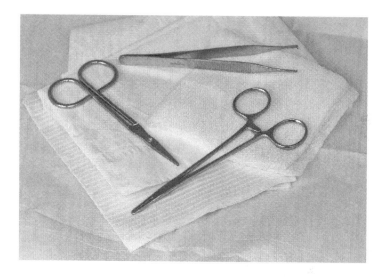

First, you need some supplies. Suture kits are available commercially at various online sites, and are comprised of the following items: A needle holder, a toothed forceps (looks like tweezers), gauze pads, suture scissors, and a sterile drape to isolate the area being repaired. Some type of antiseptic solution such as Betadine (Povidone-Iodine) or Hibiclens (Chlorhexidine) will be needed and, of course, don't forget gloves. Some people are allergic to latex, so consider nitrile products.

A good all-purpose suture material for skin would be monofilament Nylon, which is permanent and must be removed later. Other permanent materials include Prolene, Silk, and Ethibond are also used for skin closure. There are other suture materials that are absorbable, such as Catgut and polyglycolic acid (PGA); these are best used on deeper layers and do not have to be removed. These disappear after anywhere from

3 to 12 weeks. Although you can suture deep layers with non-absorbable materials like Nylon, your body's immune system will wall off each one. This is significant, mostly, from a cosmetic standpoint.

Suture material comes in various thicknesses: 0, 2-0, 3-0, 4-0, 5-0 and 6-0 are most commonly used on humans. 0-Silk, for example, is thickest, with 6-0 Silk being very fine for use in delicate cosmetic work on, for example, the face. The heavier suture has more strength, but the finer suture leaves less of a scar. For purposes of practice, try 2-0 or 3-0.

Of course, you'll need something to stitch together. I have used pig's feet, chicken breast, orange peel, and even grape skin (for delicate work) as a medical student and none are exactly like living human skin. The skin of a pig's foot is probably the closest thing you'll find to the real thing.

For the following, refer to the figures below and/or access my YouTube video called: HOW TO SUTURE WITH DR. BONES. This video goes through the entire process in real time with narration.

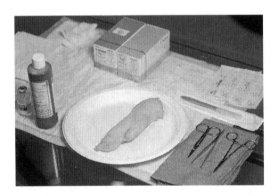

Place your pig's foot on a level surface after defrosting it and washing it thoroughly. Put your gloves on. In a real wound, you would have irrigated the area well with an antiseptic to eliminate any debris from inside the wound. You will then paint the area to be sutured (this is called the "skin prep") with a Betadine 2% solution or other antiseptic. Alcohol may be used if nothing else is available.

Next, you will isolate the "prepped" area by placing a sterile drape. The drape will usually be "fenestrated", which means it has an opening in the middle to expose the area to be sutured. Taken together, we refer to this the "surgical" or "sterile field". Although you are suturing a (deceased, I hope) pig's foot, I'll describe the process as if you are working with living tissue.

Assuming your patient is conscious, you would want to numb the area with 1% or 2% Lidocaine solution (prescription). Use an alcohol wipe on the end of the bottle, then fill a small syringe with air. Inject the air into the bottle, and the local anesthetic will fill the syringe. Place an injection at a 45 degree angle to the skin, and then inject enough to form a raised area on each side of the laceration (see figure below). Within a few minutes, the area will be numb.

It should be noted that Lidocaine is a prescription medication and is difficult to procure. When used in subcutaneous tissue, it acts as an anesthetic; used intravenously, however, it has cardiac and other effects. An accidental injection into a blood vessel is possibly life-threatening, causing heart irregularities and seizures. To determine if you are in a blood vessel, pull the plunger back. This is called "**aspiration**". Aspirating will draw blood into the syringe if it's in the wrong place. If you lack Lidocaine, you can apply an ice cube to the area to be sutured until sensation decreases.

Now, open your suture package and use your needle holder instrument to grasp the needle therein. Remove it and the attached "string" from the package. Adjust the curved needle on the needle holder so that it is perpendicular to the line of the instrument. If you are holding the needle holder in your right hand, the sharp end of the needle should point to your left. The sharp end of the needle should point to the right for left-handers. For the best command of the suture, the needle should be held at the midpoint of the curve (see figure below).

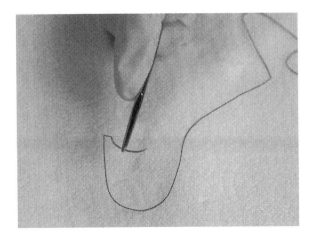

Now take your forceps (tweezers) and grasp the edge of the laceration near where you wish to place the stitch. Insert the suture needle at a 90 degree angle to the skin and drive it through that side of the laceration with a twist of the wrist. (see figure below). The needle should enter the skin no closer than a quarter inch from the edge of the laceration, or about the width of the head of your needle driver.

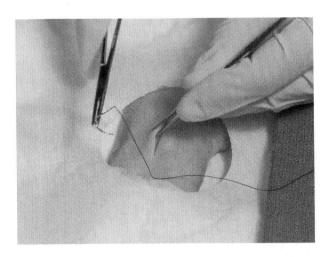

Release the needle and re-clamp it on the inside of the wound and pull it through. Replace the needle on the needle holder and, going from the inside of the wound, drive the needle with a twist of the wrist through the skin on the other side of the laceration. Pull the string through, leaving a 1-2 inch length for knot-tying (see figure below).

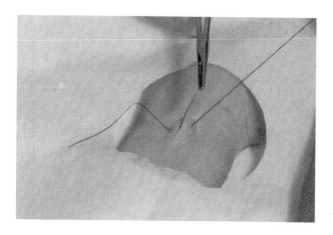

There are various ways to tie your knot, but the method that saves the most suture material (this book is meant for collapse situations, after all), is the Instrument Tie. This method uses multiple stitches, and is useful for those learning the procedure, as one bad stitch will not compromise the closure. Placing the needle holder over the wound, wrap the long end of the string twice over and around the end of the needle holder (see figure below). This will form what is known as a "Surgeon's Knot".

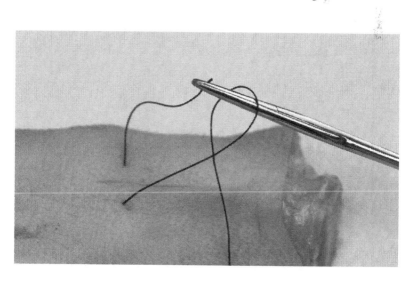

Open the needle holder end slightly and carefully grab the very end of the 2-3 inch length (see figure above), then clamp and pull it through the loops tightly to form a knot (see figure below). Repeat this knot 4 or 5 times per stitch. 1 loop is fine for every knot beyond the first.

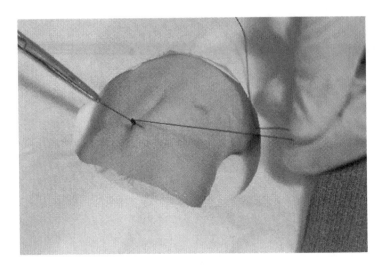

Finally, grasp the two ends and cut the remaining suture material ¼ inch from the knot with your suture scissors. Place each subsequent suture about ½ inch apart from the previous one (see below).

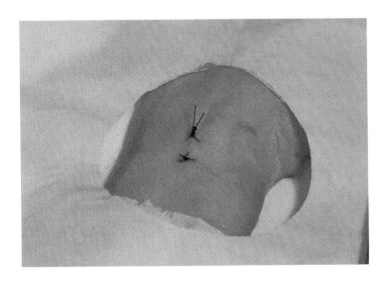

It's important to tighten your knots only enough to close the wound. Excessive pressure from a knot that is too tight will prevent healing in the area of the suture. You can easily identify sutures that are too tight: They will cause an indentation in the skin where the string is. To finish your suture job, paint it once again with Betadine solution and cover with gauze and tape. Monitor the progress of the wound closely.

To be successful in treating lacerations or other soft tissue injuries, you must be able to:

1. Decide when it is better to close a wound than leave it open.
2. Correctly place the sutures when they are indicated.
3. Provide close follow-up of the treated injury to assure complete healing, whether you have chosen to close it or leave it open.

If you can absorb this knowledge and implement it, you will have learned an important skill.

HOW TO STAPLE SKIN

Staples vs. Sutures

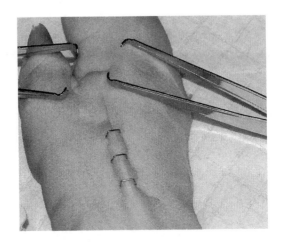

The two invasive methods of closing a wound are suturing and stapling. Both expend medical supplies that are unlikely to be renewable in a power-down situation, so conserve these vital items by using less invasive steri-strips, butterfly closures or surgical glues if possible. At one point or another, however, the medic will come across an injury that must be closed with sutures or staples.

For many minor wounds, suturing is the standard method of closure. Staples, however, are an acceptable alternative for skin wounds. According to scientific studies, the wounds that are best served by staple closure seem to be scalp lacerations (heal faster); the worst, injuries over joints (higher incidence of infection).

Straight-line lacerations are closed faster with staples than with sutures, which make them useful in mass casualty incidents or in circumstances where quick action must be taken. Sutures are going to be difficult to place quickly, especially by the medic who was not formally trained. If adequate wound cleaning did not occur before staple placement, however, the risk of infection is high. The staples may have to be removed, thorough irrigation performed, and the staples replaced.

For survival purposes, staples are used only on the skin, whereas sutures may be used in deeper layers. There are staple guns for internal organs, but these procedures require special training and will have low success rates in grid-down situations.

After thoroughly irrigating the area with an antiseptic to get rid of debris, you are ready to begin. Staples are best executed if you have an assistant that can hold the skin edges together for you. As this usually requires two hands, it will be awkward for you to staple and approximate the skin at the same time. The assistant, by the way, is the skilled labor on this team. Little technical skill is actually required in placing the staple.

On the other hand, suturing can be performed by one person and requires a bit of skill to achieve a cosmetic result. The trade-off is the fact that suturing is a much slower process than stapling. Also, there is the possibility that you might stick yourself with the suture needle during the procedure.

Both sutures and staples have a place in your medical storage. Get enough of each to deal with the various injuries you're likely to see in an austere setting.

How to Staple Skin

After thoroughly cleaning a wound and applying antiseptic to "prep" the surgical field, you are ready to use your skin stapler. You can access my YouTube video "How to Staple Skin with Dr. Bones" and follow along.

Your assistant will need two Adson's or "rat-tooth" forceps to hold the skin for you.

Most staplers are held in the hand the same way you would hold, say, a garden hose nozzle. Stand in a position so that you have an overhead view of the laceration to be closed. You can access my YouTube video "How to Staple Skin with Dr. Bones" to get an idea.

Your assistant then grabs the edges of the skin closest to you with the two forceps. Then, he/she will evert the edges (turn them inside out) SLIGHTLY and hold them together.

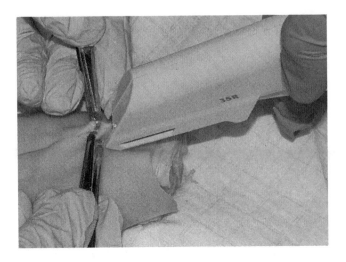

Placing the Staple

Hold your stapler at a 90 degree angle to the edges and press downward on the skin. The firmer you press, the deeper the staple. The line of the laceration should be right in the middle of the line of the stapler.

Press the "trigger" of your stapler to embed the staple and then release (completely) and retract. Check the staple placement and remove any that are not appropriately executed.

To remove staples, you will need an instrument known as a "staple remover". This instrument is similar to office staple removers of bygone days. It looks vaguely like a small scissors, but with no sharp edges.

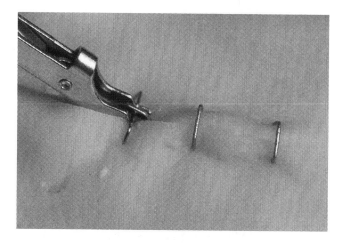

Removing the Staple

Place the lower "blade" of the staple remover between the healed skin and the staple. There will be two prongs on the lower blade and one on the upper. When the two prongs are under the staple, press the handles together; the top prong will press on the staple in such a fashion that the staple is removed. Lift the staple remover and dispose of the staple safely. Repeat until all staples are removed.

BLISTERS, SPLINTERS, AND FISHHOOKS

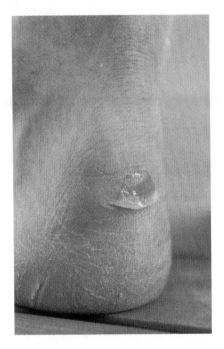

Typical broken blister

Foot Care

Anyone who has done any hiking or has bought the wrong pair of shoes has experienced a friction blister. For a relatively small soft tissue injury, it can certainly cause more than its share of problems. More than one hike has come to a screeching halt because the terrain was more than the foot wear could handle. Never underestimate the importance of a properly-fitted pair of shoes.

Even if you're an adult, your shoe size may change. Shoe size changes as you age, after a pregnancy or even during the course of the day. You should always try new shoes on after a day of walking, when your feet are a little larger than other times. Most of us have one foot that's larger than the other, so make sure your boots fit both feet (especially the larger one).

Each part of your foot should be comfortable in your new boots:

- The ball of your foot should fit the widest part of the shoe without issue.
- There should be about 1/2 inch or so from the end of your toes to the end of your shoe.
- The upper part of the shoe should be flexible enough to not cause discomfort on your instep.
- Your heel should not slip up and down when you walk.

Other considerations are important: Soles should be thick Vibram or other sturdy material. High-cut boots will help prevent ankle sprains by giving more support and will protect against the occasional snake bite.

Don't buy shoes that are too tight and expect them to stretch. They might, but you'll go through a lot of discomfort to get them there. You might be used to buying shoes online, but you really should walk in a shoe first for a while before making any purchase decisions. Your feet are shaped differently than the next guy's, so different brands of boot might be better for different people.

Heavier boots, such as those with steel toes, are great if you're chopping wood (you get to keep all ten of your toes) but are heavy. Remember that an extra pound of weight in your boot is like 5 extra pounds of weight on your back. Getting soft, flexible uppers will help. In wet climates, waterproof materials like Gore-Tex are a good investment.

A special note: Unless you can count "shoemaker" as one of your survival skills, buy a spare pair or two now while they're still available. Break them in.

Another factor in keeping your feet healthy is your socks. Most people hike in the same pair of socks all day, even in the heat of summer.

Sweaty feet are unhappy feet; Wetness increases friction and gives you blisters.

Change your socks often and have replacement pairs as a standard item in your backpack. Consider the use of a lighter, second pair of socks (sock liners) under the thicker hiking socks you use for additional protection. Use foot powders, like Gold Bond, or even corn starch to help your feet stay dry.

Blisters

If a blister is just starting, it will look like a tender red area where the friction is. Cover it with moleskin or Spenco Second Skin before it gets worse. These items are inexpensive and can be lifesavers. If you don't have any on hand, you can make use of gauze or a Band-Aid or even duct tape. The important thing here is to add padding to remove the friction from the blister.

Most people are eager to pop their blisters, but this shouldn't be done with small ones, as this could lead to infection. An intact blister serves as a sterile dressing. Large blisters are different, however, as they pop by themselves easily, allowing bacteria into damaged skin. Follow this process:

- Clean the area with disinfectant. Alcohol or iodine is especially useful.
- Take a needle and sterilize with alcohol or heat it till it is red hot.
- Pierce the side of the blister. This allows the fluid to drain. This will ease some discomfort and also will allow healing to begin.
- Preserve loose skin unless it is especially irritating.
- Cover the blister to offer protection and apply antibiotic cream if possible.
- Take some moleskin or Spenco Second Skin and cut a hole in the middle a little bigger than the blister.
- Place the moleskin on so that the blister is in the middle of where the hole is.
- Cover with a gauze pad or other bandage.
- Rest if you can.

If you absolutely must keep walking, make sure that your bandage has stopped the friction to the area. Remember, bandages frequently come off, so check it from time to time to make sure it's still on. Change the bandage frequently to maintain cleanliness.

Home Remedies for Blisters:

- Apply a cold compress to the blister by soaking a cloth in salt water.

- Apply a 10 percent tannic acid solution to the blister two or three times a day.
- Apply a few drops of Listerine antiseptic to a broken blister to disinfect the wound. Garlic oil is also very useful for this purpose.
- Place some aloe vera, vitamin E oil or zinc oxide ointment on the blister.
- Witch hazel on the blister three times a day helps with pain and is also a drying agent.
- Tea tree oil will help prevent infection.
- Apply lavender oil to help regenerate skin several times a day.

If you don't treat the blister and keep friction on it, there's a chance that it may turn into a foot ulcer. Diabetics need to be especially careful, because they're more susceptible to foot problems due to poor circulation and nerve damage. A foot ulcer is an open sore, and can become increasingly deep and even affect tendons, nerves, and bone. Infections are common. This is why prevention is so important when it comes to blisters.

Splinters

Being out in the woods or working with wood not uncommonly leaves a person with a splinter or two to deal with. You can remove a splinter by simply cutting the skin over it until the end can be grasped with a small forceps or tweezers. You'll need as fine an instrument as you can get to make this easy. Also, a magnifying glass is very useful in this circumstance..

If you can see the entire length of the splinter, use a scalpel (#11 or #15 blade) and cut the epidermis. You want to cut superficially and just enough to expose the tip of the wooden fragment. Then, take your tweezers and grasp the end of the splinter and pull it out along the angle that it entered the skin. Don't forget to wash the area thoroughly before and after the procedure.

It's unlikely that a major infection will come from simply having a splinter, with the exception of those that have been under the skin for more than 2-3 days. Redness or swelling in the area will become apparent if an infection is brewing. You might consider antibiotics in this circumstance to avoid having problems later.

Fishhooks

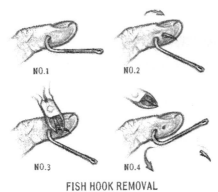

NO.1   NO.2

NO.3   NO.4

FISH HOOK REMOVAL

Even if you're an accomplished fisherman, you will eventually wind up with a fishhook embedded in you somewhere, probably your hand. Since the hook probably has worm guts on it, start off by cleaning the area thoroughly with an antiseptic.

Your hook probably has a barbed end. If you can't easily slide it out, the barb is probably the issue. Press down on the skin over where the barb is and then attempt to remove the hook along the curve of the shank.

If this doesn't work, you may have to advance the fishhook further along the skin until the barbed end comes out again. At this point, you can take a wire cutter and separate the barbed end from the shank. Then, pull the shank out from whence it came. Wash the area again and cover with a bandage. Observe carefully over time for signs of infection.

NAILBED INJURIES

Mild injuries can sometimes be detrimental to the effective function of a member of your survival group. Although perhaps not as life-threatening as a gunshot wound or a fractured thighbone, nail bed injuries are common; they will be more so when we are required to perform carpentry jobs or other duties that we may not be performing on a daily basis now.

Your fingernails and toenails are made up of protein and a tough substance called keratin, and are similar to the claws of animals. When we refer to issues involving nails, we refer to it as "ungual" (from the latin word for claw: unguis).

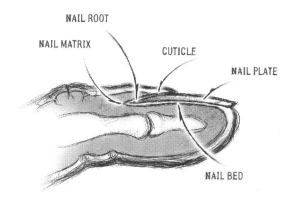

NAIL ROOT
NAIL MATRIX
CUTICLE
NAIL PLATE
NAIL BED

NAIL ANATOMY

The nail consists of several parts:

- **The nail plate (body):** this is the hard covering of the end of your finger or toe; what you normally consider to be the nail.
- **The nail bed:** the skin directly under the nail plate. Made up of dermis and epidermis just like the rest of your skin, the superficial epidermis moves along with the nail plate as it grows. Vertical grooves attach the superficial epidermis to the deep dermis. In older people, the nail plate thins out and you can see the grooves if you look closely. Like all skin, blood vessels and nerves run through the nail bed.

- **The nail matrix:** the portion or root at the base of the nail under the cuticle that produces new cells for the nail plate. You can see a portion of the matrix in the light half-moon (the "lunula") visible at the base of the nail plate. This determines the shape and thickness of the nail; a curved matrix produces a curved nail, a flat one produces a flat nail.

In a nail "**avulsion**", the nail plate is ripped away by some form of trauma. The nail may be partially or completely off, lifted up off the nail bed. Ordinarily, depending on the type of trauma, an x-ray would be performed to rule out a fracture of the digit; you won't have this available if modern medical care is not available, but you can do this:

- Numb the area by providing a digital block (discussed earlier in this book).
- Clean the nail bed thoroughly with saline solution, if available, and irrigate out any debris. Paint with Betadine (2% Povidone-Iodine solution).
- Cover the exposed (and very sensitive) nail bed with a non-adherent (telfa) dressing. Some add petroleum jelly as a covering. Change frequently. Avoid ordinary gauze, as it will stick tenaciously and be painful to remove.
- If the nail plate is hanging on by a thread, remove it by separating it from the skin folds by using a small surgical clamp. You can consider placing the avulsed nail plate on the nail bed as a protective covering; it is dead tissue but may be the most comfortable option. Avoid scraping off loose edges, as it may affect the nail bed's ability to heal.
- If the nail bed is lacerated, suture (if clean) with the thinnest gauge absorbable suture available (6-0 Vicryl is good). Be sure to remove any nail plate tissue over the laceration so the suture repair will be complete.
- Place a fingertip dressing. Some will immobilize the digit with a finger splint to protect it from further damage.
- Begin a course of antibiotics if the nail bed is contaminated with debris, etc.

In some crush injuries, such as striking the nail plate with a hammer, a bruise (also called an "**ecchymosis**") or a collection of blood may form underneath (a "**hematoma**"). A bruise will be painful, but the pain should subside within an hour or two. A hematoma, however, will continue to be painful even several hours after the event. A bruise will likely appear brownish or blue, but a hematoma may appear a deep blue-black.

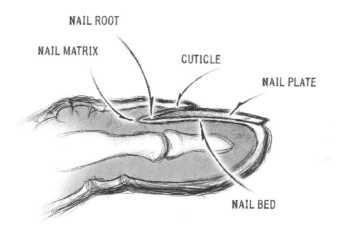

NAIL ANATOMY

For a bruised nail, little needs to be done other than given oral pain relief, such as Ibuprofen. For a significant hematoma, however, some suggest a further procedure called "**trephination**". In this instance, a very fine drill (or a hot 18 gauge needle or paper clip) is used to make a hole in the nail plate. This must be large enough to relieve pressure from the blood that has collected under the nail. It should not be too painful if you don't go too far in.

This procedure should not be performed unless absolutely necessary, as the pain will eventually decrease over time by itself. If you go too deep through the nail, you may further injure the nail bed. The finger must be kept dry, splinted and bandaged for a minimum of 48 hours afterwards.

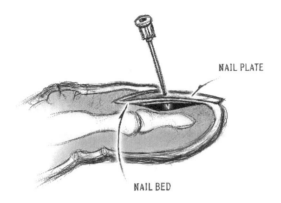

NAIL PLATE

NAIL BED

NAIL TREPHINATION

It's important to know that damage to the base of the nail (the germinal matrix) may be difficult to completely repair, and that future nail growth may be deformed in some way. In situations where modern medical care is available, a hand surgeon is often called in to give the injury the best chance to heal appropriately. Even then, a higher incidence of issues such as "ingrown" nails may occur. A completely torn-off nail will take 4-5 months to grow back.

BURN INJURIES

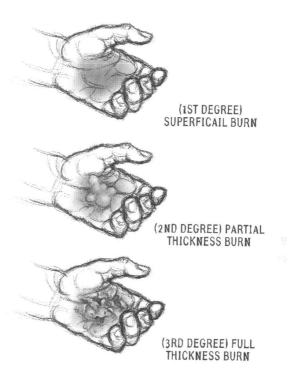

(1ST DEGREE)
SUPERFICAIL BURN

(2ND DEGREE) PARTIAL
THICKNESS BURN

(3RD DEGREE) FULL
THICKNESS BURN

BURN CATEGORIES

If we find ourselves off the power grid, we will be cooking out in the open more frequently. The potential for significant burn injuries will rise exponentially, especially if the survival group includes small children; naturally curious, they may get too close to our campfires. A working knowledge of burns and their treatment will be a standard skill for every group's medical provider.

The severity of the burn injury depends on the percentage of the total body surface that is burned, and on the degree (depth) of the burn injury. Although assessing the surface percentage is helpful to burn units in major hospitals, this practice will likely be of limited helpfulness in a collapse.

Before we discuss the different degrees of burn you might encounter, preventative measures should be put forth. Most burns you'll see will be due to too much exposure to the sun. To avoid sunburn:

- Do not sunbathe (a tan is NOT healthy).
- Avoid peak sun hours (say, 11am-4pm).
- Wear long pants and sleeves, hats, and sunglasses.
- Spend some time in the shade.

If you cannot avoid extended exposure to sunlight, be certain to apply a sunblock. They should be applied prior to going outside and frequently throughout the day. Even water resistant/proof sunscreens should be reapplied every 1-2 hours. Most people fail to put enough on their skin; be generous in your application.

By the way, a sunblock and a sunscreen are not the same thing. Sunblocks contain tiny particles that "block" and **reflect** UV light. A sunscreen contains substances that **absorb** UV light, thus preventing it from penetrating the skin. Many commercial products contain both.

The SPF (Sun Protection Factor) rating system was developed in 1962 to measure the capacity of a product to block UV radiation. It measures the length of time your skin will be protected from burning.

A SPF (sun protection factor) of at least 15 is recommended. It takes about 20 minutes without sunscreen for your skin to turn red. A product that is SPF 15 should delay burning by a factor of 15, or about 5 hours or so. Higher SPF ratings give more protection, and might be beneficial to those with fair skin.

Besides the sun, injuries will most likely be related to cooking, especially by campfire. Using hand protection will prevent many of these burns, as will careful supervision of children near any cooking area. Now, let's concentrate on learning to identify burns by their degree:

First Degree Burns

These burns will be very common, such as simple sunburn. The injury will appear red, warm and dry, and will be painful to the touch. These burns frequently affect large areas of the torso; immersion in a cool bath is a good idea or at least running cool water over the injury.

Placing a cool moist cloth or Spenco Second Skin on the area will give some relief, as will common anti-inflammatory medicines such as Ibuprofen. Aloe Vera or Zinc Oxide cream is also an effective treatment.

Usually, the discomfort improves after 24 hours or so, as only the superficial skin layer, the epidermis, is affected. Avoid tight clothing and try to wear light fabrics, such as cotton.

Second-Degree Burns

These burns are deeper, going partially through the skin, and will be seen to be moist and have blisters with reddened bases. The area will have a tendency to weep clear or whitish fluid. The area will appear slightly swollen, so remove rings and bracelets.

To treat second degrees burns:

- Run cool water over the injury for 10-15 minutes (avoid ice).
- Apply moist skin dressings such as Spenco Second skin.
- Give oral pain relief such as Ibuprofen.
- Apply anesthetic ointment such as Benzocaine.
- Use Silver Sulfadiazine (Silvadene) creams to help prevent infection.
- Consider antibiotic ointment if slow to heal.
- Lance only large blisters
- Avoid removing burned skin.

A personal aside: I had a significant second degree burn as a child (they called it "sun poisoning" back then) and my little brother thought it was a good idea to peel off some skin. He ended up with a 10 inch x 2 inch strip of skin in his hands. Don't peel off skin from a second degree burn.

Third-Degree Burns

The worst type of burn injury; it involves the full thickness of skin and possibly deeper structures such as subcutaneous fat and muscle. It may appear charred, or be white in color. The burn may appear indented if significant tissue has been lost.

Third-degree burns will cause dehydration, so giving fluids is essential to keep the patient stable. Spenco Second Skin is, again, useful, as a burn wound cover, for protection purposes.

Celox combat gauze, when wet, forms a gel-like dressing that may provide a helpful barrier. Silver Sulfadiazine (Silvadene) cream is helpful in preventing infections in third degree burns. You might see fourth, fifth and sixth degree burns described in some other medical resource books. They would be treated the same as third degree burns in a long-term survival scenario.

Any burn this severe that is larger than, say, an inch or so in diameter, usually requires a skin graft to heal completely. Unfortunately, the capacity for such restorative surgery is unlikely to be available. A person with third-degree burns over more than 10% of the body surface could be go into shock, and is in a life-threatening situation.

When a person gets burned, it's of paramount importance to remove the heat source immediately. Run cool water over any degree of burn for at least 10-15 minutes as soon as possible after the injury. Cool water is preferable to ice as it is less traumatic to the already damaged tissue. Again, be certain to remove rings or jewelry, as swelling is commonly seen in these kinds of injuries.

Natural Burn Remedies

It's important to realize that our traditional medicine resources may not be available some day and a successful medic will ensure that everyone will have some knowledge regarding alternate burn treatments. Various plants will have properties that will allow you to improve burn healing, even if no modern medical supplies are available. Although of limited use for severe burns, many first and second degree burns will respond to their effects.

The first remedy is **Aloe Vera**. Studies have shown that Aloe Vera helps new skin cells form and speeds healing. This would be an excellent option for first or second degree burns. If you have an aloe plant, cut off a leaf, open it up and either scoop out the gel or rub the open leaf directly on the burned area. Reapply 4-6 times daily, with or without a bandage covering. Simplicity and fast relief are the key benefits to using Aloe Vera on burns.

Many articles you can find on burn treatments commonly include **vinegar** (any type) as a treatment for burns. Vinegar works as an astringent and antiseptic and helps to prevent infections. The best way to use vinegar on smaller sized burns is to make a compress with 1/2 vinegar and 1/2 cool water and cover the burn until the compress feels warm, then re-soak the compress and reapply. There is no limit to how many times you can apply the vinegar soaks.

A similar method is adding vinegar to a cool bath. Start with tepid water and let the water cool off while the patient is soaking. If the burn is on the central body area, use a cotton t-shirt soaked in vinegar and then wring it out. This treatment is especially useful as help your patient sleep.

Another "cooling off" treatment for burns is the **Witch Hazel** compress. Use the extract of the bark, which decreases inflammation and soothes a 1st degree burn. Soak a compress in full strength Witch Hazel and apply to the burned area. Reapply as frequently as desired.

Elder flower and **comfrey leaf** "decoctions" are also an excellent remedy for burns. For those unfamiliar with the term **decoction**, it is an extraction of the crushed herbs produced by boiling. Using lower water temperatures produces a tea instead. The decoctions of these plants can also be used for compresses just like the Witch Hazel. However, they can also be freshly crushed and rehydrated and then applied directly to the burned area with a sterile gauze cover. We refer to this as a "**poultice**".

Black tea leaves have tannic acid that helps draw heat from a burn. There are several ways to implement the black tea treatment:

- Put 2-3 tea bags in cool water for a few minutes and use the water with compresses or just apply the liquid to the burned area.
- Make a concoction of 3 or 4 tea bags, 2 cups fresh mint leaves and 4 cups of boiling water. Then strain the liquid into a jar and allow

it to cool. To use, dab the mixture on burned skin with a cotton ball or washcloth.

- If your patient has to be mobile, make a stay-in-place poultice out of 2 or 3 wet tea bags. Simply place cool wet tea bags directly on the burn and wrap them with a piece of gauze and some tape to hold them in place.

Both **milk** and **yogurt** have also been found to help cool and hydrate the skin after a burn. Wrap whole-milk, full-fat yogurt, inside gauze or cheesecloth and use as a compress. Replace the compress as the yogurt warms on the skin. Whole milk compresses can be used the same way.

Another method of application for large burn injuries is a yogurt "spa treatment" which involves spreading yogurt all over the burn then bathing with cool water after 15 minutes.

Yet another home remedy is the **baking soda** bath. Add 1/4 cup baking soda to a warm bath and soak for at least 15 minutes or longer if needed until the water cools off.

There are two essential oils that can be used on 1st or 2nd degree burns: **Lavender** and **tea tree** oils. They help with pain due to stinging and promote tissue healing. Mix tea tree oil with a small amount of water, or lavender can be used full strength; apply all over the burned area. A loose covering of gauze over the oil may be helpful when used for 2nd degree burns.

It is important to know that butter or lard, commonly used for burns in the past, will hold in the heat and are not to be used in the treatment of your patient.

You can also make a poultice of marigold (**calendula**) petals pounded with small amounts of olive or wheat germ oil; this can be spread lightly over the burned area and covered by loose gauze or a sterile covering. Marigold is a common ingredient in skin medications, and it has been proven to have anti-inflammatory and antibacterial effects.

An **oatmeal** bath may be used to reduce itching related to healing, Crumble 1-2 cups of raw oats and add them to a lukewarm bath as the tub is filling and soak 15-20 minutes. Then, air dry so that a thin coating of oatmeal remains on your skin. You can do this as often as needed to reduce itching.

A time proven remedy related to Ancient Indian healing arts has been used for many centuries to treat even severe burns. Here are the steps to make **cotton-ash paste**:

- Take a large piece of cotton wool; or any kind of pure white cotton fabric and burn it into ashes in a Dutch oven.
- Use the ASH of the burned cotton and mix with olive oil or any kind of cooking oil available
- Mix this into a thick paste and spread the black paste on the burned skin
- Cover it with ordinary plastic cling wrap and perhaps some gauze to hold it all in place.
- Add new paste every day for a week or so, depending on the severity of the burn.

One of the best natural remedies that is useful in treating the burn patient is honey. **Honey** is best to use in its raw unprocessed state because of its antibacterial activity and hydrating properties. Honey has an acidic pH that is inhospitable to bacteria. Therefore, it will help prevent and even treat infections in many wounds. It can be used in 1st, 2nd and, if no other medical care is available, as a last resort for 3rd degree burns.

This is how to use the honey method:

- Immediately after the first 15 minute cooling-down treatment, apply a generous amount of honey in a thick layer all over the burned area
- Cover the honey with cling wrap plastic or waterproof dressings. Use tape to hold the dressing in place.
- If the dressing begins to fill up with fluid oozing out of the wound, change the dressing. The worse the burn, the more frequently the dressing will need to be changed. Repeat for 7-10 days.
- Do not remove or wash off the honey for the first 20 days (or earlier if healing is complete). Add more honey often and fill up any deeper areas as needed. Always have a thick layer of honey

THE SURVIVAL MEDICINE HANDBOOK

extending over the edges of the burn. You do not want any air getting to the burned skin until healing is completed. This will cut down the infection rate.

- Change the dressing at least three times a day regardless of the amount of oozing fluid.

Treating burns without a medical system available will require intense care and close observation. Severe fluid losses lead to dangerous consequences for these patients, so always be certain that you do everything possible to keep them well hydrated. The damage to the skin caused by burns leaves those injured to the mercy of many pathogens, so watch for fevers or other signs of infection.

ANIMAL BITES

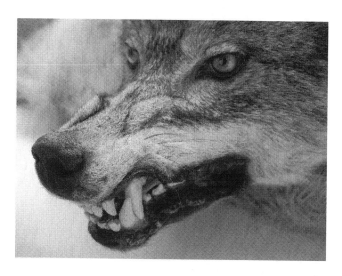

Most people have, at some time of their life, run afoul of an ornery dog or cat. Most animal bites will be puncture wounds; these will be relatively small but have the potential to cause dangerous infections. In the United States, there are millions of animal bites every year. Most animal bites affect the hands (in adults) and the face, head, and neck (in children).

Domestic pets, such as cats, dogs, and small rodents are the culprits in the grand majority of cases. Dog bites, the most common, are usually more superficial than cat bites, as their teeth are relatively dull compared to felines. Despite this, their jaws are powerful and can inflict crush injuries to soft tissues. Cats' teeth are thin and sharp, and puncture wounds tend to be deeper. Both can lead to infection if ignored, but cat bites inject bacteria into deeper tissues and seem to become contaminated more often.

Besides the trauma associated with the actual bite, various animals carry disease which can be transmitted to humans. Here are just a few diseases and the animals involved:

- Rabies: Viral disease spread by raccoons, skunks, bats, opossums, and canines.
- Plague: Bacterial disease associated with rats and fleas.

- Tuberculosis: Bacterial disease associated with deer, elk, and bison.
- Brucella: Bacterial disease associated with bison, deer, and other animals.
- Hantavirus: Viral disease caused by mice.
- Baylisascaris (raccoon roundworm): Parasitic disease associated with raccoons.
- Histoplasma: Fungal disease associated with bat excrement (guano).
- Tularemia: Bacterial disease associated with wildlife especially rodents, rabbits, and hares.

In addition, it is possible to develop tetanus from any animal bite. Tetanus is a potentially fatal infection of the muscles and nervous system caused by the bacteria Clostridia Tetani. It is discussed elsewhere in this book.

Those at highest risk from the above list of illnesses are the following:

- Those over 50 years of age
- Diabetics
- People with liver disease
- Those with weakened immune systems (transplant, chemotherapy, HIV/AIDS patients)
- People who take steroids
- Those with poor circulation
- People who have had their spleen removed

Whenever a person has been bitten, the first and most important action is to put on gloves and clean the wound thoroughly with soap and water. Flushing the wound with an irrigation syringe will help remove dirt and bacteria-containing saliva.

Benzalkonium Chloride (BZK) is the best antiseptic to use in treating animal bites, because it has some effect against the Rabies virus. Be sure to control any bleeding with direct pressure (for more information, see the section on hemorrhagic wounds).

Any animal bite should be considered a "dirty" wound and should not be taped, sutured, or stapled shut. If the bite is on the hand, any rings or bracelets should be taken off; if swelling occurs, they may be very difficult to remove afterwards

Frequent cleansing is the best treatment for a recovering bite wound. Apply antibiotic ointment to the area and be sure to watch for signs of infection. You may see redness, swelling or oozing. In many instance, the site might feel unusually warm to the touch.

Oral antibiotics may be appropriate treatment (especially after a cat bite): Clindamycin (veterinary equivalent: Fish-Cin) 300mg orally every 6 hours and Ciprofloxacin (Fish-Flox) 500 mg every 12 hours in combination would be a good choice, but Azithromycin and Ampicillin-Sulbactam are also options. A tetanus shot is indicated in those who haven't been vaccinated in the last five years.

Children who suffer animal bites may develop a form of Post-traumatic Stress Syndrome (discussed later in this book) from the experience and may require counseling.

Rabies is a dangerous but, luckily, uncommon disease that can be transmitted by an animal bite.

The grand majority of cases are found in underdeveloped countries. In the United Kingdom, rabies is almost unheard of, although there has been a report or two of infection from bat bites in 2012.

Although the classic example is the rabid dog, cat bites are the most common cause among domesticated animals. Wildlife, however, accounts for the grand majority of cases in the United States. Raccoons, opossums, skunks, coyotes, and bats are the most common vectors. It is estimated that 40,000 persons in the United States receive a rabies prevention treatment after exposure every year.

In the United States, there has never been a rabies case transmitted to humans by the following animals:

- domestic cattle
- squirrels
- rabbits
- rats
- sheep
- horses

A person with rabies is usually symptom-free for a time which varies in each case (average 30 days or so). The patient will begin to complain of fatigue, fever, headache, loss of appetite, and fatigue. The site of the bite wound may be itchy or numb. A few days later, evidence of nerve damage appears in the form of irritability, disorientation, hallucination, seizures, and eventually, paralysis. The victim may go into a coma or suffer cardiac or respiratory arrest.

Once a person develops the disease, it is usually fatal.

Vaccinations are available to prevent the disease. Regardless of your general opinion regarding them, it might be something to consider (especially if you work with animals as an occupation).

It is important to remember that humans are animals, and you might see bites from this source as well. Approximately 10-15% of human bites become infected, due to the fact that there are over 100 million bacteria per milliliter in saliva.

Although it would be extraordinarily rare to get rabies as a result of a human bite, transmission of hepatitis, tetanus, herpes, syphilis, and even HIV if possible. Treat as you would any contaminated wound. Be especially certain not to close puncture wounds from bites, as they would likely become infected if you do.

SNAKE BITES

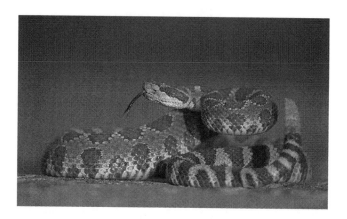

In a grid-down scenario, you will find yourself out in the woods a lot more frequently, gathering firewood, hunting, and foraging for edible wild plants. As such, we will likely encounter a snake or two. Most snakes aren't poisonous, but even non-venomous snake bites have potential for infection.

Poison is, perhaps, the wrong word to use here; venoms and poisons are not the same thing. Poisons are absorbed by the skin or digestive system, but venoms must enter the tissues or blood directly. Therefore, it is usually not dangerous to drink snake venom unless you have, say, a cut in your mouth (don't try it, though).

North America has two kinds of venomous snakes: The pit vipers (rattlesnakes, water moccasins) and Elapids (coral snakes). One or more of these snakes can be found almost everywhere in the continental U.S. A member of another viper family, the common adder, is the only venomous snake in Britain, but it and other adders are common throughout Europe (except for Ireland, thanks to St. Patrick).

These snakes generally have hollow fangs through which they deliver venom. Snakes are most active during the warmer months and, therefore, most bite injuries are seen then. Not every bite from a venomous snake transfers its poison to the victim; 25-30% of these bites will show no ill effects. This probably has to do with the duration of time the snake has its fangs in its victim.

An ounce of prevention, they say, is worth a pound of cure. Be sure to wear good solid high-top boots and long pants when hiking in the wilderness. Treading heavily creates ground vibrations and noise, which will often cause snakes to hit the road. Snakes have no outer ear, so they "hear" ground vibrations better than those in the air caused by, for instance, shouting.

Many snakes are active at night, especially in warm weather. Some activities of daily survival, such as gathering firewood, are inadvisable without a good light source. In the wilderness, it's important to look where you're putting your hands and feet. Be especially careful around areas where snakes might like to hide, such as hollow logs, under rocks, or in old shelters. Wearing heavy gloves would be a reasonable precaution.

A snake doesn't always slither away after it bites you. It's likely that it still has more venom that it can inject, so move out of its territory or abolish the threat in any way you can. Killing the snake, however, may not render it harmless: it can reflexively bite for a period of time, even if its head has been severed from its body.

Snake bites that cause a burning pain immediately are likely to have venom in them. Swelling at the site may begin as soon as five minutes afterwards, and may travel up the affected area. Pit viper bites tend to cause bruising and blisters at the site of the wound. Numbness may be noted in the area bitten, or perhaps on the lips or face. Some victims describe a metallic or other strange taste in their mouths.

With pit vipers, bruising is not uncommon and a serious bite might start to cause spontaneous bleeding from the nose or gums. Coral snake bites, however, will cause mental and nerve issues such as twitching, confusion and slurred speech. Later, nerve damage may cause difficulty with swallowing and breathing, followed by total paralysis.

Coral snakes appear very similar to their look-alike, the non-venomous king snake. They both have red, yellow and black bands and are commonly confused with each other. The old saying goes: "red touches yellow, kill a fellow; red touches black, venom it lacks". This adage only applies to coral snakes in North America, however.

Coral snakes are not as aggressive as pit vipers and will prefer fleeing to attacking. Once they bite you, however, they tend to hold on; Pit vipers prefer to bite and let go quickly. Unlike coral snakes, pit vipers may not relinquish their territory to you, so prepare to possibly be bitten again.

The treatment for a venomous snake bite is "Anti-venin", an animal or human serum with antibodies capable of neutralizing a specific biological toxin. This product will probably be unavailable in a long-term survival situation.

The following strategy, therefore, will be useful:

- Keep the victim calm. Stress increases blood flow, thereby endangering the patient by speeding the venom into the system.
- Stop all movement of the injured extremity. Movement will move the venom into the circulation faster, so do your best to keep the limb still.
- Clean the wound thoroughly to remove any venom that isn't deep in the wound, and
- Remove rings and bracelets from an affected extremity. Swelling is likely to occur.
- Position the extremity below the level of the heart; this also slows the transport of venom.
- Wrap with compression bandages as you would an orthopedic injury, but continue it further up the limb than usual. Bandaging begins two to four inches above the bite (towards the heart), winding around and moving up, then back down over the bite and past it towards the hand or foot.
- Keep the wrapping about as tight as when dressing a sprained ankle. If it is too tight, the patient will reflexively move the limb, and move the venom around.
- Do not use tourniquets, which will do more harm than good.
- Draw a circle, if possible, around the affected area. As time progresses, you will see improvement or worsening at the site more clearly. This is a useful strategy to follow any local reaction or infection.

The limb should then be rested, and perhaps immobilized with a splint or sling. The less movement there is, the better. Keep the patient on bed rest, with the bite site lower than the heart for 24-48 hours. This strategy also works for bites from venomous lizards, like Gila monsters.

It is no longer recommended to make an incision and try to suck out the venom with your mouth. If done more than 3 minutes after the actual bite, it would remove perhaps 1/1000 of the venom and could cause damage or infection to the bitten area. A Sawyer Extractor (a syringe with a suction cup) is more modern, but is also fairly ineffective in eliminating more than a small amount of the venom. These methods fail, mostly, due to the speed at which the venom is absorbed.

Interestingly, snake bites cause less infections than bites from, say, cats, dogs, or humans. As such, antibiotics are used less often in these cases.

INSECT BITES AND STINGS

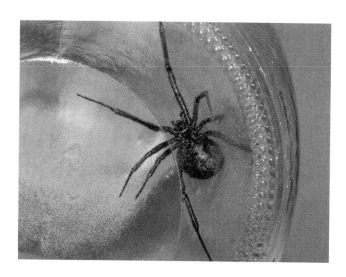

Southern Black Widow Spider

In a survival scenario, you will see a million insects for every snake; so many, indeed, that you can expect to regularly get bitten by them. Insect bites usually cause pain with local redness, itching, and swelling but are rarely life-threatening.

The exceptions are black widow spiders, brown recluse spiders, and various caterpillars and scorpions. Many of these bites can inject toxins that could cause serious damage. Of course, we are talking about the bite itself, not disease that may be passed on by the insect. We will discuss that subject in the section on mosquito-borne illness.

Bee/Wasp Stings

Stinging insects can be annoyances, but for up to 3% of the population, they can be life-threatening. In the United States, 40-50 deaths a year are caused by hypersensitivity reactions.

For most victims, the offender will be a bee, wasp or hornet. A bee will leave its stinger in the victim, but wasps take their stingers with them and can sting again. Even though you won't get stung again by the same bee, they send out a scent that informs nearby bees that an attack is underway. This is especially true with Africanized bees, which are more aggressive than native bees. As such, you should leave the area whether the culprit was a bee, wasp or hornet.

The best way to reduce any reaction to bee venom is to remove the bee stinger as quickly as possible. Pull it out with tweezers or, if possible, scrape it out with your fingernail. The venom sac of a bee should not be manipulated as it will inject more irritant into the victim. The longer bee stingers are allowed to remain in the body, the higher chance for a severe reaction.

Most bee and wasp stings heal with little or no treatment. For those that experience only local reactions, the following actions will be sufficient:

- Clean the area thoroughly.
- Remove the stinger if visible.
- Place cold packs and anesthetic ointments to relieve discomfort and local swelling.
- Control itching and redness with oral antihistamines such as Benadryl or Claritin.
- Give Acetaminophen or ibuprofen to reduce discomfort.
- Apply antibiotic ointments to prevent infection.

Topical essential oils may be applied (after removing the stinger) with beneficial effect. Use Lavadin, helichrysum, tea tree or peppermint oil, applying 1 or 2 drops to the affected area, 3 times a day. A baking soda paste (baking soda mixed with a small amount of water) may be useful when applied to a sting wound.

Although most of these injuries are relatively minor, there are quite a few people who are allergic to the toxins in the stings. Some are so allergic that they will have what is called an "**anaphylactic reaction**". Instead of just local symptoms like rashes and itching, they will experience dizziness, difficulty breathing and/or faintness. Severe swelling is seen in some, which can be life-threatening if it closes the person's airways.

Those experiencing an anaphylactic reaction will require treatment with epinephrine as well as antihistamines. People who are aware that they are highly allergic to stings should carry antihistamines and epinephrine on their person whenever they go outside.

Epinephrine is available in a pre-measured dose cartridge known as the **Epi-Pen** (there is a pediatric version, as well). The Epi-pen is a prescription medication, but few doctors would begrudge a request for one. Make sure to make them aware that you will be outside and may be exposed to possible causes of anaphylaxis. As a matter of fact, it may be wise to have several Epi-Pens in your possession. See the section on allergic reactions for a more in-depth discussion.

Spider bites

Although large spiders, such as tarantulas, cause painful bites, most spider bites don't even break the skin. In temperate climates, two spiders are to be especially feared: The **black widow** and the **brown recluse**.

The black widow spider is about ½ inch long and is active mostly at night. They rarely invade your home, but can be found in outbuildings like barns and garages. Southern black widows have a red hourglass pattern on their backs, but other sub-species may not. Although its bite has very potent venom damaging to the nervous system, the effects on each individual are quite variable.

A black widow bite will appear red and raised and you may see 2 small puncture marks at the site of the wound. Severe pain at the site is usually the first symptom soon after the bite. Following this, you might see:

- Muscle cramps
- Abdominal pain
- Weakness
- Shakiness
- Nausea and vomiting
- Fainting
- Chest pain
- Difficulty breathing
- Disorientation

Each person will present with a variable combination and degree of the above symptoms. The very young and the elderly are more seriously affected than most. In you exam, you can expect rises in both heart rate and blood pressure.

The **brown recluse** spider is, well, brown, and has legs about an inch long. Unlike most spiders, it only has 6 eyes instead of 8, but they are so small it is difficult to identify them from this characteristic.

Victims of brown recluse bites report them to be painless at first, but then may experience these symptoms:

- Itching
- Pain, sometimes severe, after several hours
- Fever
- Nausea and vomiting
- Blisters

The venom of the brown recluse is thought to be more potent than a rattlesnake's, although much less is injected in its bite. Substances in the venom disrupt soft tissue, which leads to local breakdown of blood vessels, skin, and fat. This process, seen in severe cases, leads to "**necrosis**", or death of tissues immediately surrounding the bite. Areas affected may be extensive.

Once bitten, the human body activates its immune response as a result, and can go haywire, destroying red blood cells and kidney tissue, and hampering the ability of blood to clot appropriately. These effects can lead to coma and, eventually death. Almost all deaths from brown recluse bites are recorded in children.

The treatment for spider bites includes:

- Washing the area of the bite thoroughly
- Applying ice to painful and swollen areas
- Pain medications such as acetaminophen/Tylenol
- Enforcing bed rest

- Warm baths for those with muscle cramps (black widow bites only; stay away from applying heat to the area with brown recluse bites)
- Antibiotics to prevent secondary bacterial infection

Home remedies include making a paste out of baking soda or aspirin and applying it to the wound. The same method, using olive oil and turmeric in combination, is a time-honored tradition. Dried basil has also been suggested; crush between your fingers until it becomes a fine dust, then apply to the bite. One naturopath uses Echinacea and Vitamin C to speed the healing process. Be aware that these methods may be variable in their effect from patient to patient.

There are various devices and kits available that purport to remove venom from bite wounds. Unfortunately, these suction devices are generally ineffective in removing venom from wounds. Tourniquets are also not recommended and may be dangerous. Although antidotes known as "antivenins" (discussed in the section on snakebite) exist and may be life-saving for venomous spider and scorpion stings, these will be scarce in the aftermath of a major disaster. Luckily, most cases that are not severe will subside over the course of a few days, but the sickest patients will be nearly untreatable without the antivenin.

Scorpion Stings

Most scorpions are harmless; in the United States, only the **bark scorpion** of the Southwest desert has toxins that can cause severe symptoms. In other areas of the world, however, a scorpion sting may be lethal. In the U.S., 17,000 scorpion stings were treated in emergency rooms in 2009.

Some scorpions may reach several inches long; they have eight legs and pincers, and inject venom through their "tail". They are most commonly active at night. Interestingly, scorpion exoskeletons somewhat fluorescent under ultraviolet light; you can find them most easily at night by using a "black light".

The nervous system is most often affected from a scorpion sting. Children are most at risk for major complications. Symptoms you may see in victims of scorpion stings may include:

- Pain, numbness, and/or tingling in the area of the sting
- Sweating
- Weakness
- Increased saliva output
- Restlessness or twitching
- Irritability
- Difficulty swallowing
- Rapid breathing and heart rate

When you have diagnosed a scorpion sting, do the following:

- Wash the area with soap and water.
- Remove jewelry from affected limb (swelling may occur)
- Apply cold compresses to decrease pain.
- Give an antihistamine, such as diphenhydramine (Benadryl)
- If done quickly, this may slow the venom's spread.
- Keep your patient calm to slow down the spread of venom.
- Limit food intake if throat is swollen.
- Give pain relievers such as Ibuprofen or Acetaminophen, but avoid narcotics, as they may suppress breathing.
- Don't cut in the wound or use suction to attempt to remove venom.

Although not likely available in an austere environment, an antivenin is now available that eliminates symptoms in children (the group most severely affected) after four hours.

Fire Ant Stings and Bites

Fire ants are about ¼ inch in length and can be red or black. If their nest is disturbed, it triggers a mass attack of, sometimes, thousands of colony members. The ants bite with their jaws and have a rear-end stinger that they can use multiple times. Hypersensitivity to fire ants causes about 80 deaths a year in the Southeastern U.S.

If you are attacked by fire ants, do the following:

- Brush them away with your hands (although it may be difficult if they have clamped their jaws into you).
- Move away from the mound.
- Remove clothes if they may have gotten inside them.
- Elevate the bitten extremity to reduce swelling.
- Place a cool compress on the area.
- Take antihistamines such as diphenhydramine (Benadryl) or apply hydrocortisone cream.
- If a blister develops, don't pop it. It will usually not get infected if it stays intact.
- If a blister pops, wash with soap and water.
- Consider antibiotics, such as Amoxicillin, if the wounds appear to worsen with time.

Bedbugs

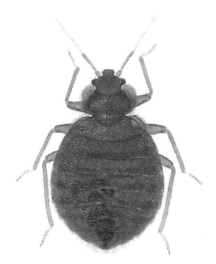

Of all the creepy-crawlies that raise an alarm in a household, few are worse than bed bugs. Although poor standards of living and unsanitary conditions have been associated with bed bug infestations, even the cleanest house in the most developed country can harbor these parasites.

Bed bugs were once so common that every house in many urban areas was thought to harbor them in the early 20th century; they declined with the advent of modern pesticides like DDT, but a resurgence of these creatures has been noted in North America, Europe, and even Australia over the last decade or so. Cities such as New York and London have seen 5 times as many cases reported over the last few years. This may have to do with the restriction of DDT-like pesticide. On the other hand, the general over-use of pesticides may be leading to resistance.

The common bed bug (Cimex Lectularius) is a small wingless insect that is thought to have originated in caves where both bats and humans made their homes. Ancient Greeks, such as Aristotle, mention them in their writings. They were such a serious issue during WWII that Zyklon, a Hydrogen Cyanide gas infamously used in Nazi concentration camps, was implemented by both sides to get rid of infestations.

There are a number of species of bed bug that are found in differing climates. Unlike lice, bed bugs are not always species-specific (exclusive to humans). For example, Cimex hemipterus, a bed bug found in tropical regions, infests poultry and bats as well as humans.

Adult bed bugs are light to medium brown and have oval, flat bodies about 4mm long (slightly more after eating). Juveniles are called "nymphs" and are lighter in color, almost translucent. There are several nymph stages before adulthood; to progress to adulthood, a meal of blood (yours!) is necessary.

Bed bugs, which are mostly (but not exclusively) active at night, bite the exposed skin of sleeping humans to feed on their blood; they then retreat to hiding places in seams of mattresses, linens, and furniture. Their bites are usually painless, but later on, itchy raised welts on the skin may develop. The severity of the response varies from person to person.

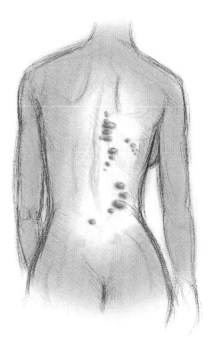

BEDBUG BITE PATTERN

Bed bugs can make you miserable and have been known to harbor other disease-causing organisms, but there have not been, as yet, cases of illness specifically caused by them. This is in contrast to body lice or fleas, which has been associated with outbreaks of Typhus, Relapsing fever, and even Plague.

Strangely, bed bugs don't like to live in your clothes, like body lice, or on your skin or hair, like fleas. They apparently don't care much for heat, and prefer to spend more time in your backpack or luggage than your underarm.

Many confuse the bites of bed bugs with mosquitos or fleas. Most flea bites will appear around the ankles, while bed bugs will bite any area of skin exposed during the night. Flea bites often have a characteristic central red spot. Bed bug bites may resemble mosquito bites; bed bugs, however, tend to bite multiple times in a straight line. This has been referred as the classic "breakfast, lunch, and dinner" pattern.

The most common treatment for bed bug bites is hydrocortisone cream to treat inflammation and the use of diphenhydramine (Benadryl) for allergic symptoms and itching. The cure, however, is to eradicate the bed bug from your shelter or camp; that's a little harder to do.

First, find their nests: Look at every seam in your mattress, linens, backpacks, and furniture. Bed bugs will also hide in joints in the wooden parts of headboards and baseboards. You will usually find bed bug "families" of various ages, along with brown fecal markings and, perhaps, even small amounts of dried blood.

Most people, once bed bugs are identified, will immediately want to treat with chemicals. Pesticides in the pyrethroid family and Malathion have been found to be effective. Propoxur, an insecticide, is highly toxic to bed bugs as well, but is not approved for indoor use in the U.S. due to health risks.

If you use chemicals, be sure you cover all areas on the bed, including the frame and slats. Expect several treatments to be required to eliminate the infestation; repeat at least once about 10 days after the initial treatment.

Those concerned with the over-use of pesticides or with lack of availability, as in a long term survival situation, could consider using natural predators, but this is highly impractical, as the bed bug predator list consists of everything else you don't want in your shelter: ants, spiders, cockroaches, and mites.

One reasonable option is the use of bedding covers. These are impervious sheets or padding that, essentially, trap bed bugs inside your mattress until they starve. If they can't reach you to get a meal of blood, they will eventually die out. This method (known as "encasing") is the least risky, as it doesn't involve the use of chemicals.

If you have electricity, make sure to place all bedding and clothes in a hot dryer for, say, an hour. Usually, washing clothes alone will not kill bed bugs although hot, soapy water over 125 degrees Fahrenheit may work. This strategy, by the way, includes your backpack when you return from a trip out of town or an extended foraging patrol. Extreme cold is also considered an effective treatment. If you live far enough north, 4 or 5 days of temperatures approaching 0 degrees Fahrenheit should kill them.

If you have access to a working vacuum, use it on flooring and upholstery. A stiff brush is helpful to scrub mattress seams before vacuuming.

Natural remedies to treat bed bugs include dusting seams with diatomaceous earth; the bugs consume it and it tears up their insides. Many people swear by tea tree oil and rubbing alcohol as well. Here's a time-honored herbal bedbug treatment:

- 1 Cup Water
- Lavender essential oil (10 drops)
- Rosemary essential oil (10 drops)
- Eucalyptus essential oil (10 drops)
- Clove bud essential oil (optional)
- Place in a fine mist spray bottle
- Shake well before using

As bed bugs can live for months without a meal, it's important to maintain long-term diligence in identifying these pests wherever you hang your hat during rough times. These bugs may not end your life, but they can certainly affect the quality of it. Educate your loved ones to be aware of the environment and look for dangerous insects (and, of course, snakes) whenever they are doing outside work.

Others

Some insect bites are not dangerous due to toxins, but can cause infectious disease. Ticks can transfer Lyme disease and mosquitos can transfer Malaria, for example. The best way to prevent these is by wearing protective clothing whenever you go outside, and having insect repellant (DEET) in good amount in your storage. Both tick and mosquito bites are dealt with in other sections of this book.

Citronella, commonly used as an insect repellant in candles, can be found naturally in some plants. The citronella plant is hardy and grows anywhere there are periods of warm weather. It is distasteful to a number of pests. Consider it for your medicinal garden.

HEAD INJURIES

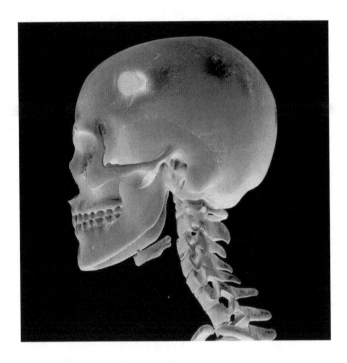

Head injuries can be soft tissue injuries (brain, scalp, blood vessels) or bony injuries (skull, facial bones), so I've placed this section between soft tissue and orthopedic problems. Damage is usually caused by direct impact, such as a laceration in the scalp or a fracture of the part of the skull that contains the brain (also called the "**cranium**").

An "open" head injury means that the skull has been penetrated with possible exposure of the brain tissue. If the skull is not fractured, it is referred to as a "closed" injury.

Damage can also be caused by the rebound of the brain against the inside walls of the skull; this may cause tearing of the blood vessels in the brain, which can result in a hemorrhage. There may be no obvious penetrating wound in this case; the original trauma may even have occurred at a site other than the head. An example of this would be the violent shaking of an infant.

Anyone with a traumatic injury to the head must always be observed closely, as symptoms from bleeding and swelling may take time to develop.

The brain requires blood and oxygen to function normally. An injury which causes bleeding or swelling inside the skull will increase the intracranial pressure. This causes the heart to work harder to get blood and oxygen into the brain. Blood accumulation (known as a "hematoma") could occur within the brain tissue, itself, or from between the layers of tissue covering the brain.

Without adequate circulation, brain function ceases. Pressure that is high enough could actually cause a portion of the brain to push downward through the base of the skull. This is known as a **"brain herniation"** and, without modern medical care, will almost invariably lead to death.

Most head injuries result in only a laceration to the scalp and a swelling at the site of impact. Cuts on the scalp or face will tend to bleed, as there are many small blood vessels that travel through this area. This bleeding, although significant, does not have to signify internal damage; most cases can be treated as any other laceration. There are a number of signs and symptoms, however, which might identify those patients that are more seriously affected. They include:

- Loss of Consciousness
- Convulsions (Seizures)
- Worsening Headache
- Nausea and Vomiting
- Bruising (around eyes and ears)
- Bleeding from Ears and Nose
- Confusion/Apathy/Drowsiness
- One Pupil More Dilated than the Other
- Indentation of the Skull

A person with trauma to the head may be knocked unconsciousness for a period of time or may remain completely alert. If consciousness is NOT lost, the patient may experience a headache and could require treatment for superficial injuries. After a period of observation, a head injury without loss of consciousness is most likely not serious unless one of the other signs and symptoms from the above list are noted.

Loss of consciousness for a very brief time (say, 2 minutes or so) will merit close observation for the next 48 hours. A head injury of this type is called a "**concussion**". This patient will usually awaken somewhat "foggy", and may be unclear as to how the injury occurred or the events shortly before. It will be important to be certain that the patient has regained normal motor function. In other words, make sure they can move all their extremities with normal range and strength. Even so, rest is prescribed for the remainder of the day, so that they may be closely watched.

When your patient is asleep, it will be appropriate to awaken them every 2-3 hours, to make sure that they are easily aroused and have developed none of the danger signals listed above. In most cases, a concussion causes no permanent damage unless there are multiple episodes of head trauma over time, as in the case of boxers or other athletes.

If the period of unconsciousness is over 10 minutes in length, you must suspect the possibility of significant injury. Vital signs such as pulse, respiration rate, and blood pressure should be monitored closely. The patient's head should be immobilized, and attention should be given to the neck and spine, in case they are also damaged. Verify that the airway is clear, and remove any possible obstructions. In a collapse, this person is in a life-threatening situation that will have few curative options if consciousness is not regained.

Other signs of a significant injury to this area are the appearance of bruising behind the ears or around the eyes (the "**raccoon**" **sign**) despite the impact not occurring in that area. This could indicate a fracture with internal bleeding. Bleeding from the ear itself or nose without direct trauma to those areas is another indication. The fluid may be clear and not bloody; this may represent spinal fluid leakage.

In addition, intracranial bleeding may cause pressure that compresses nerves that lead to the pupils. In this case, you will notice that your unconscious patient has one pupil more dilated than the other.

A **stroke**, (also known as a **cerebrovascular accident** or CVA), is damage to the brain caused by lack of blood supply. This could occur in a head injury due to a blockage of blood to a portion of the brain. This blockage could be due to a clot, a hemorrhage, or anything else that compromises the circulation in the area. Whatever functions are associated with the part of the brain affected will be lost or impaired. This might include the inability to speak, blindness, or loss of normal comprehension. Symptoms, such as paralysis or weakness, are often on one side of the body and/or face. The stroke is usually heralded by a sudden severe headache.

Strokes may also occur due to other reasons as well, such as uncontrolled high blood pressure. Although it may not be difficult to diagnose a major CVA in an austere setting, few options will exist for treating it. Blood thinners might help a stroke caused by a clot, but worsen a stroke caused by hemorrhage. It could be difficult to tell which is which without advanced testing.

Keep the victim on bed rest; sometimes, they may recover partial function after a period of time. If they do, most improvement will happen in the first few days.

Trauma to the head may have negligible consequences, or it could have life-threatening consequences. In some circumstances, there may be little that you, the medic, can do in a long-term survival situation.

SPRAINS AND STRAINS

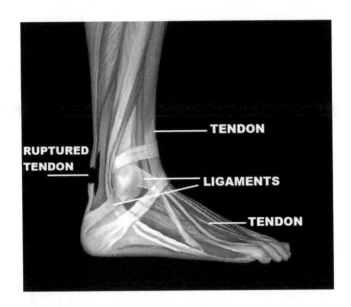

Bones, joints, muscles and tendons give the body support and locomotion, and there is no substitute for having all your parts in good working order. The amount of work these structures will be called upon to do after a disaster will be greatly increased. Off the grid, there will be additional strain put on the body. Therefore, the medic will expect to see more injuries; it is important to know how to identify and treat these problems.

Prior to a collapse, it is recommended to have whatever surgical repairs of any orthopedic faults you happen to have. Knees, shoulders, ankles and other joints are commonly damaged due to long-term abuse, and it pays to "tune" these up while modern surgical care is still available. Many surgeries these days are done through very small incisions, and most can be done as an outpatient.

Many people have heard of ligaments, tendons, sprains, and strains but have little idea of what they really are. Therefore, let's define some anatomical terms:

- **Joint:** the physical point of connection between two bones, usually allowing a certain range of motion. For example, the knee or elbow joint.

- **Ligament:** The fibrous tissue that connects one bone to another, oftentimes across a joint.
- **Tendon:** Tissue that extends from muscle to connect to bone.
- **Sprain:** An injury where a ligament is excessively stretched by forcing a joint beyond its normal range of motion.
- **Strain:** When the muscle or its connection to the bone (tendon) is partially torn as a result of an injury.
- **Rupture:** A complete tear through a ligament or muscle.

Sprains

Our joints are truly marvels of engineering. They help provide mobility and locomotion and sometimes bear an incredible amount of stress without mishap. They are moving parts, however, and moving parts wear down. In long-term survival situations, our level of physical exertion goes up a notch and the risk of injury to the joints increases as well.

You can expect the most common sprains in your group to involve the ankle, wrist, knee or finger. The most likely signs and symptoms are bruising, swelling, and pain. It's a rare individual who has never experienced this injury, in varying degrees of severity, over the course of their life.

Treatment for most sprains is relatively straightforward and follows the easy-to-remember **R.I.C.E.S.** protocol:

REST: It is important to avoid further injury by not testing the injured joint. Stop whatever actions led to the injury and you will have the best chance to recover fully. Failure to rest is a common mistake for many athletes, who will continue to stress the joint by continuing strenuous activity. As a result, the partially-healed ligament will re-injure itself and permanent damage may occur.

In a survival scenario, you may not have the luxury of rest. If not, expect chronic problems in the weakened joint.

ICE: Cold therapy decreases both swelling and pain. The earlier it is applied, the better effect it will have in speeding up the healing process. If you're in the wilderness, you might have to stick your ankle in a stream to get some cooling action, although you can keep some cold packs in your backpack that can be activated by shaking.

Cold therapy should be performed several times a day for 20-30 minutes or so each time for the first 24-48 hours. This is followed each time by applying compression.

COMPRESSION: A compression bandage is useful to decrease swelling and should be placed after each cold therapy. This will also help provide support to the joint. After applying some padding to the area, wrap an elastic "ACE" bandage, starting below the joint and working your way up beyond it. The wrap should be tight, but not uncomfortably so.

Any tingling, increased pain or numbness tells you that the wrap is too tight, and should be loosened somewhat. Additionally, an excessively tight wrap may affect the circulation, and you may notice the fingertips or toes becoming white or even blue.

ELEVATION: Elevate the sprain above the level of the heart. This will help prevent swelling at the site of the injury. Swelling is caused by fluid that pools where the inflammation is ("**edema**"), and likes to accumulate where gravity will allow. By elevating the leg, you allow the fluid to process itself back into your circulation and aid the healing process, or at least not impede it.

This also works for swollen ankles due to chronic medical problems, like high blood pressure; even pregnant women achieve relief from swollen ankles in this fashion.

STABILIZATION: Immobilizing the injury will prevent further damage. This may be accomplished by the compression bandage alone or may best be supported with a splint or a cast. if the patient is unable to place much weight on the joint, this strategy will be especially useful.

Splints may be commercially produced, such as the very useful **SAM (Structural Aluminum Malleable) splint,** or may be improvised with sticks, cloth or pillows and duct tape. Make sure the injured joint is immobile after placement of the splint.

I am often asked how to tell the difference between a sprain and a fracture. Sometimes it's quite easy, as when a straight bone is suddenly "zig-zag" in shape. Many times, it's quite difficult and hard to determine without modern diagnostic tests (which won't be available in a long-term survival situation).

You can, however, look for one or more of these signs:

- A fracture will generally have more pronounced swelling and bruising.
- A fracture is generally so painful that no traction or pressure may be placed on the injury.
- A fracture may have a deep cut in the area of the injury (This is called an "open" fracture and is particularly dangerous due to the risk of infection).
- A fracture may show motion in an area beyond the joint (if your finger suddenly has five knuckles, you probably broke it).
- A fracture may present a grating sensation when pressing upon it.

For sprains, Ibuprofen serves as an excellent anti-inflammatory and pain reliever. Natural remedies may also help. The underbark of willow, aspen and poplar trees have Salicin, a natural pain medicine.

Most sprains, (such as wrist and ankle sprains) commonly heal well over time using the R.I.C.E.S. protocol, pain relievers, and a lot of rest. Others, however, such as severe knee sprains with torn or ruptured ligaments, may heal completely only with the aid of surgical intervention.

It's important to get joint issues dealt with while we still have modern medicine to help us. If you need surgery to fix a bum knee, do it now. In uncertain times, you (and your joints) want to be in the best shape possible to face the challenges ahead.

Strains

By far, the most frequently seen strain will be to the back muscles. Strains, especially back strains, involve injury to the muscle and their tendons (which connects them to the bone). As the lower part of the back holds the majority of the body's weight, you can expect the most trouble here. Some of these injuries are preventable with some simple precaution:

- Every morning, you should perform some stretching, to increase blood flow to cold, stiff muscles and joints.
- When you lift a heavy object, such as a backpack, keep your back straight and let your legs perform the work.
- The object should be close to your body as you lift it (don't reach for it).
- For packs, keep the weight on the hips rather than the shoulders.
- If you are on rocky or unstable terrain, consider using a walking stick for balance. Remember, any weight-lifting action that you perform while being off-balance is likely to result in a strained muscle.

Ibuprofen is an excellent anti-inflammatory and pain reliever for these types of injury. For muscle injuries, prescription relaxants such as Diazepam (Valium) or Cyclobenzaprine (Flexeril) will also provide relief. If these are not available, the patient will benefit from mild massage.

A number of alternative remedies exist for the treatment of mild-moderate sprains and strains. Essential oils are considered helpful to clear up bruising. Apply 2-3 drops of oil of Helichrysum, cypress, clove, or geranium, mixed half and half with carrier oil such as coconut or olive, 3-5 times a day on the area of bruising.

To decrease swelling, apply Helichrysum oil, undiluted, to the affected area. Willow under bark or ginger tea has anti-inflammatory properties; drink with warm raw honey, several times a day.

Common herbal pain relievers for orthopedic injuries include direct application of Oil of wintergreen, helichrysum, peppermint, clove, or diluted arnica to the affected area. Blends of the above may also be used. Herbal teas that may give relief are valerian root, willow under bark, ginger, passion flower, feverfew, and turmeric. As always, drink warm with raw honey several times a day.

Some sprains and strains, (such as wrist and ankle sprains or back strains) commonly heal well over time with the above therapy. Other injuries may cause chronic pain and eventual degeneration of the joint. It will be difficult to foretell the progress of an injured joint without modern diagnostic imaging.

DISLOCATIONS

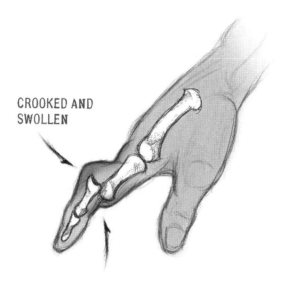

CROOKED AND
SWOLLEN

DISLOCATED FINGER

A dislocation is an injury in which a bone is pulled out of its joint by some type of trauma. Dislocations commonly occur in shoulders, fingers, and elbows, but knees, ankles and hips may also be affected. The joint involved looks visibly abnormal and is unusable. Bruising, pain, and/or numbness often accompany the injury.

If the dislocation is momentary and the bone slips back into its joint on its own, it is called a **subluxation**. Subluxations can be treated the same way that sprains are, using the R.I.C.E.S. method. It should be noted that the traditional medical definition of subluxation is somewhat different from the chiropractic one.

Of course, if there is medical care readily available, the patient should go directly to the local emergency room. General anesthesia if often used to resolve the problem. In a collapse, however, you are on your own and will probably have to correct the dislocation yourself. This is known as performing a "reduction" of the injury.

Reduction is easiest to perform soon after the dislocation, before muscles spasm and the inevitable swelling occurs. Not only does reducing the dislocation decrease the pain experienced by the victim, but it will lessen the damage to all the blood vessels and nerves that run along the line of the injury.

The faster the reduction is performed, the less likely there will be permanent damage. It should be noted that a dislocated joint may be permanently damaged. It may have a tendency to go out of place again in the future.

Expect significant pain on the part of the patient during the actual procedure, however. Some pain relievers like ibuprofen might be useful to decrease discomfort from the reduction. Muscle relaxers such as Cyclobenzaprine (Flexeril) are also helpful, but these are "by prescription only".

The use of traction will greatly aid your attempt to fix the problem. Traction is the act of pulling the dislocated bone away from the joint to give the bone room to slip back into place.

The procedure is as follows:

- Stabilize the joint that the bone was dislocated from (the shoulder, for example) by holding it firmly.
- Using a firm but slow pulling action, pull the bone away from the joint. This will make space for the bone to realign.
- Use your other hand (or preferably a helper's hands) to push the dislocated portion of the bone so that it will be in line again with the joint socket. The bone will naturally want to revert to its normal position in the joint.
- After the reduction is complete and judged successful, splint the bone as if it were a fracture (see next section).

Some dislocations, such as a dislocated finger, may take as little as 2-3 weeks to regain normal function. Others, such as hip dislocations, may take many months to heal.

FRACTURES

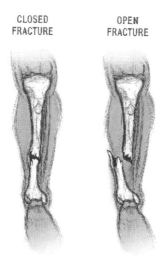

CLOSED
FRACTURE

OPEN
FRACTURE

FRACTURE TYPES

If enough force is applied, an injury to soft tissues can damage the skeletal structure underneath. When a bone is broken, it is termed a fracture. There are several types of fractures:

- **Reduced or "Stable" fracture.** In the simplest fracture, the broken ends of the bone are barely out of place.
- **Open or compound fracture.** In a compound fracture, the skin is pierced by the broken bone or there is some other penetrating trauma. The end of the bone may be above or below the level of the skin.
- **Comminuted fracture:** The bone shatters into several pieces.
- **Oblique/Transverse fracture:** the line of the broken bone may be horizontal or at an oblique angle.
- **Greenstick fracture:** One side of the bone snaps, the other remains intact. Reminiscent of the result of trying to snap live wood in two.

For our purposes, let's assume that they are all either "open" or "closed". A closed fracture is when there is a break in the bone, but the skin is intact (all of the above except the compound fracture). An open fracture is when the skin is broken.

Needless to say, there is usually more blood loss and infection associated with an open wound. The infection may be deep in the skin (**cellulitis**), the blood (**sepsis**), or the bone itself (**osteomyelitis**) and could be life threatening if not treated. If poorly managed, a closed fracture can become an open fracture.

The diagnosis of a broken bone can be simple, as when the bone is obviously deformed, or difficult, as in a minimal, "hairline" fracture. X-rays can be helpful to differentiate a small fracture from a severe sprain, but that technology won't be available in a power-down situation. There are some ways to tell, however (also discussed under sprains):

- A fracture will manifest with severe pain and inability to use the bone (for example. The patient cannot put any weight whatsoever on a broken ankle). Someone with a sprain can probably put some weight, albeit painfully, on the area.
- More pronounced swelling and bruising will likely be present on a fracture than a sprain.
- A grinding sensation may be felt when broken ends of a bone rub together.
- A deep cut in the area of the injury is a likely sign of an open fracture.
- Motion of the bone in an area where there is no joint is another dead giveaway that there is a fracture. If you notice that your injured finger appears to have 5 knuckles, you're probably dealing with a fracture.

Dealing with a fractured bone involves first evaluating the injured area for the above signs and symptoms. Use your bandage or EMT scissors to cut away the clothing over the injury. This will prevent further injury that may occur if the patient was made to remove their own clothing. First, check the site for bleeding and the presence of an open wound; if present, stop the bleeding before proceeding further.

Fractures may cause damage to the patient's circulation in the limb affected, so it is important to check the area beyond the level of the injury for changes in coloration (white or blue instead of normal skin color) and for strong and steady pulses. Usually, normal color returns to skin in the fingertips within 2 seconds of applying pressure and then releasing. This is known as the "Capillary Refill Time" and is discussed in the section of this book on triage.

To find out what a strong pulse feels like, place two fingers on the side of your neck until you feel your neck arteries pulsing. You will do this same action on, say, the wrist, if the patient has broken their arm. Lightly prick the patient in the same area with a safety pin to make sure they have normal sensation. If not, the nerve has been injured.

If the bone has not deformed the extremity, a simple splint will immobilize the fracture, prevent further injury to soft tissues and promote appropriate healing. Oftentimes, however, the bone will be obviously bent or otherwise deformed, and the fracture must be "reduced" as we discussed with dislocations. Although this will be painful, normal healing and complete recovery will not occur until the two ends of the broken bone are realigned to their original position.

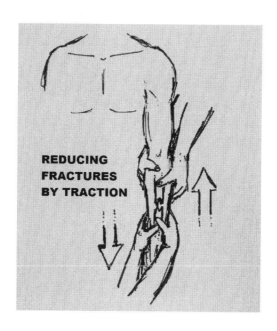

REDUCING
FRACTURES
BY TRACTION

Reducing a deformity is best performed with 2 persons and a sedated patient. One supports and provides traction on the side closest to the torso, and the other exerts steady traction on the area beyond the fracture. Often, some form of traction is needed to keep the broken ends of the bone in place. There are risks to this procedure; nerves and blood vessels can be damaged, but normal healing will not occur in a deformed limb.

Splint the extremity in place immediately after performing the reduction. In an open fracture, thorough washing of the wound is absolutely necessary to prevent internal infection. Infection will invariably occur in a dirty wound, even if the reduction is successful. Therefore, antibiotics are important to prevent complications such as osteomyelitis. Always check the pulses and capillary refill time after the reduction is performed; this will assure adequate circulation beyond the level of the injury.

It is very important to immobilize the fractured bone in such a fashion that it is allowed to heal. When you are responsible for the complete healing of the broken bone, remember that the splint should immobilize it in a position that it normally would assume in routine function.

- For legs: The leg should be straight, with a slight bend at the knee.
- For arms: The elbow should be flexed at a 90 degree angle to the upper arm.
- For ankles: The ankle should be at a 90 degree angle to the leg.
- For wrist: The wrist should be straight or slightly extended upward.
- For fingers: The fingers should be slightly flexed, as if holding a glass of water.

As previously mentioned, splints can be commercially produced (e.g., SAM splints), or may be improvised, using straight sticks with bandannas or T-shirt strips to immobilize the area. Another option is to fold a pillow around the injury and duct tape it in place.

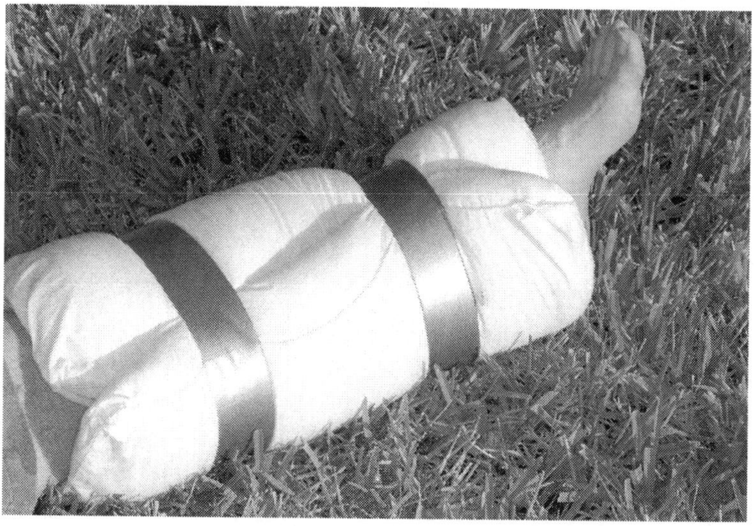

Pillow Splint

For most fractures, you will want to consider the placement of a cast to enforce immobilization. Casting material using plaster of paris or fiberglass is easy to obtain and lasts a long time. It's a useful addition to any medical storage.

When placing a cast, you will first start with a liner of cotton known as a "stockinette". Then, you will need rolls of padding to form a barrier between the skin and the cast. Rolls of plaster of Paris or fiberglass are then immersed in water for 20 seconds or so. Wring out the excess water (keep the end of the roll between your fingers or it will stick and be difficult to find).

Then, you will begin to slowly roll the casting material around the area of the fracture, smoothing it out as you go along. Advance one half of the thickness of the roll as you go from beyond the fracture towards the torso. You will want perhaps three layers of casting material on the area, more in places where there is a bony prominence, such as the wrist.

Each fracture is casted somewhat differently: Stockinettes, padding, and casting rolls are available in different widths and lengths appropriate to the particular fracture. For comfort and cleanliness, plastic wrap is helpful to cover the cast during bathing. A wet cast is a smelly cast.

Although oscillating saws are used today to remove casts, they require the availability of electricity. There are still special heavy-duty shears available for the purpose, although some effort is needed to perform the removal.

To review: Your goal is to immobilize the fracture in a position of function. Use padding under the splint or cast as possible to keep the injured area stable and protected. Most fractures require 6-8 weeks to form a "callous"; this is newly formed tissue that will reunite the broken ends of the bone. Larger bones or more complicated injuries take longer. If not well-realigned, the function of the affected extremity will be permanently compromised. References to books devoted to the subject are listed at the end of this volume.

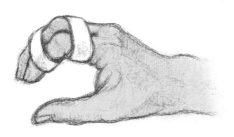

FRACTURED FINGER BUDDY

Fingers and toes may be splinted by taping them to an adjoining digit. This is called the "buddy method". There are small manufactured splints that will also do the job. Neck injuries may be particularly serious, and an investment should be made in purchasing a good neck "collar".

Rib Fractures and Pneumothorax

Rib fractures are commonly treated by firmly taping the affected area, as it is the motion of breathing that causes the pain associated with the injury. Although reduction is usually not necessary, taping the area may help provide pain relief.

Rib fractures become more serious if the fracture punctures a lung, causing a condition known as a "pneumothorax". Air from the puncture enters the chest cavity, which compresses the lung and collapses the organ.

Although a person with a rib fracture will complain of pain with breathing, a person with a pneumothorax will have signs of bluish skin coloration (this is called "**cyanosis**"), distended neck veins, and signs of shock. If you use a stethoscope, you will hear the sounds familiarly associated with Rice Krispies cereal when you listen to the lungs, or perhaps no breath sounds at all from the affected area.

If, and only if, the pneumothorax has become life-threatening (known as a "**tension pneumothorax**"), should you act. Lung decompression can't be taken lightly, and should only be attempted if it's clear the patient will die without action taken on their behalf.

This is what you do: Clean the area of the chest above the third rib midway between the top of the shoulder and the nipple. Using a sharp object no wider than a pencil, poke a hole ABOVE the rib (the blood vessels travel below the rib) deep enough to hear air pass through. A large gauge (14g or larger) spinal needle will be large and long enough to do the job, so consider purchasing this from a medical supply store.

You goal is to provide a way for the air to continue to escape from the incision you made, but not to go back in. Take a square of saran wrap or a plastic bag and firmly tape it above the skin incision on three sides only. This will serve as a valve, and allow air to escape, while allowing the lung to re-inflate. It should be noted that there are lung decompression kits that are available commercially.

Inflammatory or bloody fluid is likely to accumulate in many lung wounds. You will have to rig a drainage system to prevent too much fluid from preventing adequate air passage. A rubber tube connected to a jar placed below the patient may perform this duty by using gravity. It will not, however, be as efficient as the electric suction systems available at your local hospital. It's important to realize that this type of wound will be difficult to recover from. If modern medical care is not available, expect the worst.

AMPUTATION

In rare circumstances, damage to a limb may be so extensive that it cannot be saved. Amputation is the surgical removal of all or part of an extremity. This procedure is performed on arms, legs, hands, feet, fingers, or toes. Amputation of a part of the leg is the most common amputation surgery.

An amputation, in a survival situation, is a procedure of last resort. In many cases, your patient will not survive it. At least 25% of American civil war soldiers undergoing the procedure lost their lives due to complications. The closer to the body that the amputation was performed, the higher the death rate will be. It's unlikely there will be much improvement in survival in future times of trouble.

There are various reasons that an amputation may be necessary. The most common is poor circulation because of damage to blood vessels. Without reasonable blood flow, tissue may not get enough oxygen to remain viable. Infection and gangrene (discussed in the section on frostbite) may set in.

Below are some reasons that an amputation may be indicated:

- Extensive injury from trauma or burns.
- Cancerous tumors
- Serious infection that does not get better with antibiotics
- Severe frostbite
- Gangrene

Several methods are used to identify where to cut and how much to remove:

- Checking where an extremity loses a pulse.
- Areas when a limb loses normal temperature.
- Looking for areas of reddened skin (infection) or blackened skin (gangrene)
- Checking where the extremity is no longer sensitive to touch.
- Identifying areas where the bone has been crushed beyond repair.

AMPUTATION

Basic measures to increase the chances of a successful amputation are:

- Sedate the patient as much as possible.
- Clean the damaged area with Betadine or other antiseptics before the procedure.
- Use sterile gloves in a sterile field
- Remove debris and bits of shattered bone.
- Tie off bleeding blood vessels.
- Preserve an adequate amount of living tissue to cover the exposed end of the bone.
- Shorten and smooth the bone enough to decrease irritation to the covering soft tissue.
- Stitch remaining muscle to the bone lining (also known as the "**periosteum**"). This is difficult without special equipment.
- Before closing completely, place a drain (discussed earlier in this book) to allow blood and inflammatory fluid to leave the surgical site.
- Adequately close the wound with sutures or staples.
- Change dressings regularly.
- Observe for infection. Start a course of antibiotics.

Amputation is a procedure I hope you will never have to consider. In severe injuries, however, it may be life-saving.

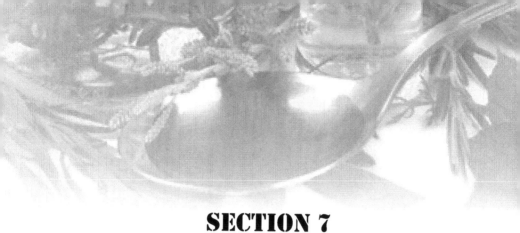

SECTION 7

✚ ✚ ✚

CHRONIC MEDICAL PROBLEMS

As a caregiver in a long-term survival scenario, you cannot expect that everyone under your care will start off in perfect health. It is likely that one or more members of your family or group will have a longstanding medical issue that cannot be ignored.

The amount and diversity of chronic medical issues may test the medic's fund of knowledge. You will be challenged to formulate strategies for power-down situations that you know are inferior to those available in modern times. Despite this, you must take action to be ready for difficult times or your patient may suffer the consequences.

You would probably be surprised at how many of your friends have chronic illnesses or conditions that you are unaware of. Even those you may have known for decades may not make it a habit of discussing their medical issues with you. As the person responsible for their medical well-being in a collapse, however, it is your duty to obtain full histories from everyone in your party. Without obtaining this information, you will be less effective in your role.

Thyroid malfunction, diabetes, and heart disease are just some of the issues; these illnesses require medications that will not be manufactured in times of trouble. We must, therefore, think "outside the box" to formulate a medical strategy for these patients that does not include modern technology.

Its goes without saying that medical conditions that are poorly controlled now could be completely out of control in a collapse situation. The most important way to preserve your family's health will be to have any chronic conditions appropriately treated and monitored **prior** to a catastrophe.

While you have the benefit of modern medical care (and, perhaps, medical insurance), take full advantage of any option that will tune up chronic problems. Eliminate dental issues you might have ignored, repair that defective knee joint or get corrective vision surgery. In hard times, you'll need to function at 100% efficiency. If you ignore your medical issues now, how can you expect to keep it together if things fall apart, whether it's your health or that of others?

This section will discuss some of the most common diseases that people have to deal with today. The successful caregiver will develop a plan of action that will keep those with chronic medical problems out of trouble. If we ever find ourselves on our own, having a plan in place will increase a medic's effectiveness and improve the health of the community.

THYROID DISEASE

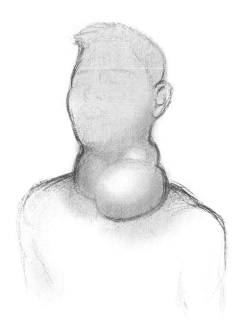

GOITER

The thyroid gland is positioned just in front of and below the Adam's apple ("also known as the laryngeal prominence") and produces hormones that help regulate your metabolism. The organ produces substances that regulate growth, energy and the body's utilization of other hormones and vitamins.

The thyroid gland is involved in maintaining a hormonal balance between itself and two other organs, the "pituitary gland" and the "hypothalamus". These two organs can be found near the base of the brain. When this balance is disturbed in some way, we experience thyroid dysfunction. Thyroid conditions usually involve the production of either too little or too much of these hormones. These malfunctions are most commonly seen in women.

A thyroid problem that might be common in an austere setting is the development of a lump on the thyroid (known as a "**goiter**"). This is the result of a deficiency of iodine in the body, and is one of the reasons why common table salt is "iodized". Potassium Iodide tablets (discussed in the section on radiation) may be a treatment option if no other source of iodine is available. It should be noted that iodine-containing drugs should not be administered to those with allergies to seafood.

A person may have a lump on the thyroid that is not associated with iodine deficiency. It can exist without causing symptoms or even disturbed thyroid hormone levels. A lump may present as a **cyst** (a mass filled with fluid) or a **nodule** (a solid mass), and usually has no major ill effect. These are considered to be "cold" tumors. Some thyroid tumors, however, are "hot" and produce excessive amounts of hormone. Thyroid cancer is relatively rare, even in the elderly, unless there has been exposure to radiation.

Hyperthyroidism

The excessive production of thyroid hormone is known as Hyperthyroidism. Determination of thyroid malfunction depends on certain blood tests and sometimes a scan of the gland. These modalities will be gone in a collapse, so it's important to learn what a person with elevated thyroid levels looks like. Some common signs and symptoms of this condition in adults are:

- Insomnia
- Hand tremors
- Nervousness
- Feeling excessively hot in normal or cold temperatures
- Eyes appear to be bulging out or "staring"
- Frequent bowel movements
- Losing weight despite normal or increased appetite
- Excessive sweating
- Weight loss
- Menstrual period becomes scant, or ceases altogether
- Growth and Puberty issues (children)
- Muscle Weakness, Chest Pain and Shortness of Breath (elderly)

Poorly controlled hyperthyroidism can lead to a condition known as **thyroid "storm"**, in which large levels of hormone cause major effects on the heart and brain. All the above symptoms may combine with elevated heart rate and blood pressure to endanger the patient's life.

Treatment of hyperthyroidism involves medications such as Propylthiouracil and Methimazole, which block thyroid function. These medications should be stockpiled if you're aware of a member of your group with hyperthyroidism, as they will be hard to find if modern medical care is no longer available.

Substances such as I-131 (also known as radioiodine) have been used to actually destroy the thyroid. As you can imagine, this often results in the patient producing no thyroid hormone at all. I-131 treatment is useful in severe hyperhyroidism, but is also unlikely to be available in a collapse.

Iodide is also useful in blocking the excessive production of thyroid hormone, and can be found in Kelp in good quantity. The anti-radiation medication KI (Potassium Iodide) might be an additional option in this situation. Unfortunately, the use of Iodides, while a known treatment, may actually worsen the condition in some cases.

Dietary restriction of nicotine, caffeine, alcohol and other substances that alter metabolism will be useful as well. Vitamins C and B12 are thought to have a beneficial effect on those with this condition, as does L-Carnitine. L-Carnitine is beneficial in that it may lower thyroid hormone levels without damaging the gland.

Foods that are thought to depress production of thyroid hormone include cabbage, cauliflower, broccoli, Brussels sprouts, and spinach. In addition, foods high in antioxidants are thought to reduce free radicals that might be involved in hyperthyroidism. These include blueberries, cherries, tomatoes, squash and bell peppers, among many others.

Hypothyroidism

More commonly seen than hyperthyroidism, hypothyroidism is the failure to produce enough thyroid hormone. Various causes of low thyroid levels exist, such as certain drugs or exposure to radiation. Also, the immune system sometimes misfires and targets the thyroid. The most commonly seen signs and symptoms of hypothyroidism in adults are:

- Fatigue
- Intolerance to cold
- Constipation
- Poor appetite
- Weight gain
- Dry skin
- Hair loss
- Hoarseness
- Depression
- Menstrual irregularity
- Poor Growth (Children)

If ignored, additional symptoms might appear, such as:

- Thickened skin
- Hair loss
- Vocal changes
- Swollen appearance of hands, feet, and face

It should be noted that untreated hypothyroidism in a pregnant woman may cause birth defects in the baby.

The treatment of this condition is based on the oral replacement of the missing hormone, which is called "**thyroxine**". These drugs come in a variety of dosages, and it is important to determine the appropriate dose for your patient while modern medical care is still available. The lowest dose that will maintain normal thyroid levels is indicated; too much may cause hyperthyroidism.

Once you have determined the right dosage, you may consider, in normal times, asking a physician for additional supplies or perhaps a prescription for a higher dose. This might allow you to use, say, half of the pill in the present and stockpile the other half for the uncertain future. Only do this if you intend to follow your physician's advice as to your dose. There is no benefit (but significant risk) to taking more thyroid replacement medicine that you should.

Besides standard thyroid medications such as Synthroid and Levothyroid, there are a number of other remedies that may have effect in improving hypothyroidism. A number of thyroid extracts are available which consist of desiccated and powdered pig or cow thyroid gland. The amount of thyroid hormone in these extracts may be variable; therefore, the medical establishment recommends against the use of these supplements.

Having said this, in the absence of modern medications, it is better than nothing. One strategy that may help you decide what natural supplement may be right for you is to ask your physician to monitor your thyroid levels for 2-4 weeks or so while you try it out. If your thyroid levels drop precipitously, it may have little or no effect, and you should research other options. If your thyroid levels remain normal, continue monitoring long term to determine whether the particular product might be worthwhile to stockpile.

From a dietary standpoint, you should avoid foods that depress thyroid functions. These include:

- Cauliflower
- Broccoli
- Brussels sprouts
- Spinach
- Cabbage

A number of natural supplements, such as Thyromine, are commercially available. They are combinations of various herbs that are touted as beneficial for both low and high thyroid conditions. Your experience may vary.

DIABETES

Diabetes is a common, yet devastating disease. It is characterized by high sugar (also called "glucose") levels. Uncontrolled diabetes is known to cause damage to various organs, such as the kidneys, eyes, and heart. The incidence of the disease has been increasing over time in developed countries, perhaps due to issues relating to obesity.

Diabetes is especially problematic for the survival medic in that the medications used to treat the worst cases are unlikely to be produced in a grid-down scenario. Diabetic medications, such as insulin, lose potency over time. Therefore, an alternative strategy to keep diabetics from losing complete control of their blood sugar will have to be formulated.

Type 1 Diabetes (known in the past as juvenile diabetes or insulin-dependent diabetes) results from the failure of the pancreas to produce insulin. Insulin is a hormone that controls the level of sugar in your system. The destruction of the cells in the pancreas that produce Insulin is thought to be caused by an **autoimmune** response. This means that the body's own immune system attacks parts of itself. Type 1 diabetes is often first diagnosed in childhood, but 60% of new cases are now found in those over the age of 40.

Type 2 Diabetes (known in the past as adult-onset or non-insulin dependent diabetes) is more commonly the result of the resistance of the cells in your body to the insulin produced by the pancreas. Insulin is required to move sugar (glucose) into cells; there, it is stored and later used to produce energy for the body.

In type 2 diabetes, certain cells do not respond appropriately to insulin. This is referred to as "insulin resistance". Glucose fails to enter these cells and, therefore, it accumulates in the blood. High blood sugar is known as "**hyperglycemia**".

Obesity is thought to be a major factor in Type 2 diabetes. Most people are, indeed, overweight when the diagnosis is made. Although rare in the past, more children are being found with the condition; again, this is related to the epidemic of obesity in modern societies.

Diabetes (mild or severe) may also develop in some pregnancies, even in non-diabetic women. Some believe that those that get diabetes during their pregnancies may be prone to diabetic issues later in life.

The three classic symptoms of diabetes are:

1. Excessive thirst
2. Excessive hunger
3. Frequent urination.

Uncontrolled diabetes causes eye and kidney problems, leading to blindness and renal failure. It worsens coronary artery disease, increasing the chances for heart attacks and other cardiac issues. Weight loss may occur despite the consumption of more food; the cells cannot access the glucose in the blood for energy to produce mass.

Cuts and scrapes, especially in the extremities, are slow to heal. Over time, nerve damage occurs which causes numbness, pins and needles sensations and, in the worst cases, gangrene. Many severely uncontrolled diabetics may require amputation.

As type 2 Diabetes is most often seen in older, heavier, and less active individuals, weight control and close attention to controlling the amounts of carbohydrates (which the body turns into sugars) in the diet is important. In some cases, decreasing excess weight and frequent small meals may reverse Type 2 diabetes in its entirety. Regular exercise will also decrease blood sugar levels, and improve glucose control. The most popular medication used for treatment is called Metformin, which works in various ways, including increasing the cells' sensitivity to insulin. In tablet form, it is a good candidate for medical storage.

Type 1 Diabetes is more problematic, as many with this medical problem have large swings in their sugar (glucose) levels. Insulin has been used since its formulation in 1921 to control severe diabetes. Regular monitoring of blood glucose levels and appropriate treatment with the right amount of Insulin is necessary to remain healthy.

There are two common diabetic emergencies. These are related either to very low or very high glucose levels. If a diabetic, especially Type 1, fails to eat regularly or in accordance with his Insulin therapy, he or she may develop "**hypoglycemia**". Hypoglycemia can occur very rapidly, and symptoms commonly seen are sweating, loss of coordination, confusion, and loss of consciousness.

In this case, a drink containing sugar will rapidly resolve the condition. Never give liquids to someone who is unconscious, however; the fluids could go down the respiratory passages and suffocation could occur. If the patient is not mentally alert, place some sugar granules under the tongue. This will absorb rapidly without causing the tendency to choke.

On the other hand, very high glucose levels lead to a condition called "**Diabetic Ketoacidosis**". This occurs as a result of missed Insulin doses and/or chronically under-dosed Insulin. The patient will have a characteristic "fruity" odor to his or her breath. In addition to the usual symptoms, there will be nausea, vomiting, and abdominal pain as well. This is a major emergency which could lead to coma and even death. Small amounts of clear liquids are acceptable in someone with this condition, but without Insulin, the prognosis is grave.

Insulin can be purchased without a prescription in the U.S. Needless to say, Insulin, like most liquid medications, will lose potency relatively soon after its expiration date. Due to the complexity of the manufacturing process, it is unlikely to be available in a collapse situation. What, then, can be done to maximize glucose control?

Prevention is the best way to avoid hypoglycemia and/or Diabetic Ketoacidosis. In a collapse situation, alternatives will be needed to provide a modicum of diabetic control. In hard times, the goal will be to prevent ketoacidosis. Diabetics will be unlikely to have perfect control, especially Type 1 diabetics, but it may be possible to keep their sugars low enough to prevent a major complication. Even a few months of less than optimal control may be survivable and might give you some time for society to re-stabilize.

One therapeutic option is to stockpile the highest dose of Metformin (oral diabetes medicine) in the hope that it will have some benefit to the Insulin-deprived Diabetic. It will be helpful for type 2 diabetics, but will only deal with the issue of insulin resistance. Unfortunately, it will not make the pancreas produce insulin. Metformin is not as strong a drug as Insulin, and it is uncertain what benefit it may do a pure Type 1 case.

Even if it just prevents the diabetes from going completely out of control for a time, however, it is worth a shot.

A recent study suggests that Metformin may be used along with insulin. In some diabetics, the addition of Metformin resulted in lower amounts of insulin required for control. This is of interest to the survival medic, who may have expiring insulin medications that may be made more effective by adding Metformin. More study is warranted.

Another option is to regulate diet severely and subsist on a diet almost entirely comprised of protein and fats. The key is to restrict caloric intake significantly. This will be harmful in the long run, but frequent, small, high-protein meals may give some time for a short-term societal destabilization to resolve.

Type 2 diabetics (especially obese ones) may actually improve from the increased physical exertion and dietary restrictions that will be part and parcel of a long-term survival situation. An emphasis on limiting food intake to frequent small meals will be helpful here.

HIGH BLOOD PRESSURE

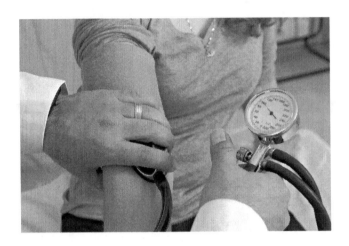

One of the most common chronic medical conditions that we will see in a collapse situation is high blood pressure (also known as "**hypertension**"). Stress associated with activities of daily survival can raise blood pressure in the short term and may worsen chronic conditions. Lack of blood pressure medications may cause complications in people who were previously under good control.

To begin with, the "**blood pressure**" is the measure of the blood flow pushing against the walls of the arteries in your body. If this pressure is elevated over time, it can cause long-term damage. Many millions of adults in the U.S. have this condition, which is often asymptomatic (no signs or symptoms). Because of this, it has been referred to as a "silent killer". Blood pressure tends to rise with increasing age and weight.

The group medic should have, as part of his equipment, a stethoscope for listening and a pressure monitor called a "sphygmomanometer" (blood pressure cuff). This is relatively inexpensive and will allow evaluation of the blood pressures of the members of the community.

Taking a Blood Pressure

To use a sphygmomanometer, place the cuff around the upper arm and fill it up with air, using the attached bulb. Place your stethoscope over an area with a pulse (usually the inside of the crook of the arm) and listen while looking at the gauge on the cuff. Some new compact blood pressure units are shaped like wristbands and are one piece. With these, it is important to have your wrist at the level of your heart when taking a reading.

When you take a blood pressure, you are listening for the pulse to register on your stethoscope. A Blood pressure is measured as systolic and diastolic pressures. "**Systolic**" refers to blood pressure when the heart beats and "**Diastolic**" refers to blood pressure when the heart is at rest. Therefore, blood pressure is written down as systolic over diastolic: for example: (systolic pressure) 120 over 80 (diastolic pressure). You will see it written in this manner: 120/80.

Wherever the gauge is when you FIRST hear the pulse is the "systolic" pressure. As the air deflates from the sphygmomanometer, the pulse will fade away. When it first appears to fade is the "diastolic" pressure. You should be concerned with numbers that are above 140/90 in the supine or sitting position.

As blood pressures tend to vary at different times of the day and under different circumstances, you would be looking for at least 3 elevated pressures in a row before making the diagnosis of high blood pressure (hypertension). Readings above 160/100 are associated with higher frequency of complications. Persistent hypertension can lead to stroke, heart attack, heart failure and chronic kidney failure. Commonly seen symptoms may include:

- Headaches
- Blurred vision
- Nausea and vomiting

Sometimes, elevated pressures can cause a blood vessel in the brain to have an "accident". **Strokes** (also known as "cerebrovascular accidents" or CVAs) are bleeding episodes or clots in the brain that can occur as a high pressure event and cause paralysis. Suspect this condition if your patient has suddenly found themselves unable to speak, control the extremities on one side of their body or move one side of their face. They will usually complain of the sudden onset of a severe headache, as well.

You will have few options other than placing the stroke victim on bed rest and observation. There is often some improvement over the first 48 hours or so. Beyond this point, further recovery may be limited.

Pregnancy-induced hypertension ("Pre-Eclampsia") is a serious late pregnancy condition that may lead to seizures ("Eclampsia") and blood clotting abnormalities. See the section on pregnancy for more information.

The first step to controlling elevated blood pressures is to return to a normal weight for your height and age. Most people who are overweight find that their pressures decrease (often back to normal) when they lose weight. Over the years, I have documented my own blood pressures and find this correlation to be completely true. Even a change of 10 pounds seem to affect my average readings.

Physical exercise and dietary control are the best way to get there. Dietary restriction of sodium is paramount in importance when it comes to decreasing pressures. Sodium is in just about everything you eat, so stop adding salt to food. Alcohol, nicotine, and perhaps, caffeine are also known to raise blood pressures, so avoiding these substances is an additional strategy. In a long-term survival situation, forced abstention may actually have a beneficial effect on overweight patients with hypertension.

The National Institute of Health recommends the DASH (Dietary Approaches to Stop Hypertension) diet. A major feature of the plan is limiting intake of sodium and it generally encourages the consumption of nuts, whole grains, fish, poultry, fruits and vegetables while lowering the consumption of red meats, sweets, and sugar. It is also rich in protein, potassium, calcium, and magnesium. Studies have found that the **DASH diet** can reduce high blood pressure within two weeks in certain cases. These are the daily guidelines of the DASH diet:

- 7 to 8 servings of grains
- 4 to 5 servings of vegetables
- 4 to 5 servings of fruit
- 2 to 3 servings of low-fat or non-fat dairy
- 2r less servings of meat, fish, or poultry
- 2 to 3 servings of fats and oils
- 4 to 5 servings per week of nuts, seeds, and dry beans

- Less than 5 servings a week of sweets

Serving Sizes

-1/2 cup cooked rice or pasta
-1 slice bread
-1 cup raw vegetables or fruit
-1/2 cup cooked vegetables or fruit
-8 oz. of milk
-1 teaspoon olive oil

Optimize your results on this diet by implementing the following tips:

- Choose foods that are low in saturated fat, cholesterol, and total fat, such as lean meat, poultry, and fish.
- Eat plenty of fruits and vegetables; aim for eight to ten servings each day.
- Include two to three servings of low-fat or fat-free dairy foods each day.
- Choose whole-grain foods, such as 100 percent whole-wheat or whole-grain bread, cereal, and pasta.
- Eat nuts, seeds, and dried beans -- four to five servings per week (one serving equals 1/3 cup or 1.5 ounces nuts, 2 tablespoons or 1/2 ounce seeds, or 1/2 cup cooked dried beans or peas).
- Go easy on added fats. Choose soft margarine, low-fat mayonnaise, light salad dressing, and unsaturated vegetable oils (such as olive, corn, canola, or safflower).
- Cut back on sweets and sugary beverages.

The above is good advice about nutrition in almost every circumstance, whether you are dealing with high blood pressure or not.

A number of medications with impressive names are available for the control of high blood pressure: ACE inhibitors, alpha blockers, angiotensin II receptor antagonists, beta blockers, calcium channel blockers, diuretics, and others. Those with hypertension will be placed on one or more of these medications until their readings are back to normal.

All of these commercially prepared products will be scarce in times of trouble, so consider asking for higher doses of your specific medication than what you need, so that you can break them in half and store some of it. Again, always take your medication in the dosage prescribed by your physician.

Natural supplements have been used to help lower blood pressure, as well. Any herb that has a sedative effect will likely also lower pressures. Valerian, Passion Flower, and Lemon Balm are some examples. Garlic and Cayenne Pepper is also well-known to have a modest lowering effect. Coenzyme Q10 has shown some promise in this field. Antioxidants like Vitamin C and fish oil may prevent free radicals from damaging artery walls. Foods rich in Potassium, like bananas, are also recommended.

Don't forget natural relaxation techniques. Meditation, Yoga, and mild massage therapy will relax your patient. Take their blood pressure after a session and see what effect it has had. You will probably be quite surprised at the results.

Any avenue you can find that will keep blood pressures within normal range will keep the people under your care healthier. Diet, mild natural sedatives, and conventional medications are all tools in the medical woodshed. Use them well.

HEART DISEASE AND CHEST PAIN

Unlike most medical books, I will not be spending a great deal of time discussing coronary artery disease, even though it is one of the leading causes of death in today's society. Why? It will be difficult in a collapse situation to do very much about heart attacks, due to the loss of all the advances that have been made to deal with coronary disease.

The loss of the power grid would throw us back into an earlier era from a medical standpoint. There will not be a cardiac intensive care unit or a cardiac bypass surgeon at your disposal. This is a shame, as the stress associated with the aftermath of a major disaster is known to have a damaging effect on the heart. We will have to accept that some folks with heart problems will do better than others in hard times.

Heart attacks, also called "**myocardial infarctions**", involve the blockage of an artery that gives oxygen to a part of the heart muscle. That portion of the heart subsequently dies, either killing the patient or leaving them so incapacitated as to be unable to function in a post-collapse scenario. This decrease in function is most likely permanent.

Does that mean that you can't or shouldn't do anything if you suspect that your patient is having a heart attack? No, there are low tech approaches; they just won't do much if there has been a lot of damage caused.

Cardio-pulmonary resuscitation (CPR) may be limited in its usefulness (it is most helpful if you have modern medical facilities the patient could benefit from). Despite this hard reality, it is still compulsory for any effective medic and is described later in this book. Additionally, you have an obligation now, before a disaster, to encourage all your group members to eat well, exercise regularly, avoid smoking, and drink alcohol only in moderation.

You would suspect a heart event if your patient experiences the following:

- "Crushing" sensation in the chest area
- Pain down the left arm
- Pain in the jaw area

- Weakness
- Fatigue
- Sweating
- Pale coloring

The main approach is to immediately give your patient a chewable adult aspirin (325 mg). This will act as a blood thinner; it aids in preventing further damage to the coronary artery and preserve oxygen flow. Aspirin works within 15 minutes to prevent the formation of blood clots in people with known coronary artery disease. One adult-strength aspirin contains 325 milligrams. The current study suggests that 325 milligrams of CHEWABLE aspirin would be preferred in the setting of a heart attack or sudden onset of "**angina**" (cardiac-related chest pain). Angina occurs when not enough oxygen reaches the heart due to clogged coronary arteries.

A natural substance (Capsaicin) found in cayenne pepper may also be helpful during a myocardial infarction. The strength of peppers are based on a measurement system called Scoville heat units (H.U.). For use during a heart attack, the H.U. should be at least 90,000. Give the conscious patient a glass of warm water mixed with 1 teaspoon of cayenne pepper. An alternative is to give 2 full droppers of cayenne pepper tincture or extract underneath their tongue. Studies at the University of Cincinnati show an 85% decrease in cardiac cell death if cayenne pepper is given. The tincture, extract or a salve can be used for an unconscious person as a possible life saving procedure.

A person suffering a heart attack will feel most comfortable lying down at a 45 degree angle. Complete rest will cause the least oxygen demand on the damaged heart. Don't forget to loosen constrictive clothing; tight clothes make a cardiac patient feel anxious and cause their heart to beat faster. This would cause more strain on an already damaged organ.

Aspirin, in small doses, is also reasonable as a preventative strategy. One baby aspirin (81 mg) daily is thought to help prevent the deposition of plaque inside the blood vessels. You might consider having all of your adults 40 and over on this treatment. Men are most likely to have coronary artery disease, as female hormones seem to protect women, at least before menopause. If your patient takes heart medications, administer them immediately.

Those in your survival community with coronary artery issues should stockpile whatever medications they take to deal with their symptoms. Angina (cardiac-related chest pain) can be treated with nitroglycerine tablets. Placed under the tongue, they will give rapid relief in most cases.

High Cholesterol

In developed countries, high cholesterol is a major cause of coronary artery disease. In an austere setting, the tests performed to follow a person's cholesterol levels will be unavailable, but you can still devise a strategy to decrease the risk of heart attack due to this problem.

Cholesterol is a fat-like substance made in the liver and other cells. It can be found in foods such as dairy products, meat, and eggs. The body needs some cholesterol in order to function properly, but the presence of too much of it negatively impacts the heart.

There is good cholesterol (HDL) and bad cholesterol (LDL). High levels of bad cholesterol cause plaque. Plaque is a deposit that forms on the inside of arterial linings, eventually forming a blockage that can lead to a heart attack. These are the different types of cholesterol which comprise "good" and "bad":

- Low density lipoproteins (LDL) or Very low density lipoproteins (VLDL): LDL and VLDL can cause buildup of plaque on the walls of arteries. The more you have of these, the greater the risk of heart disease.
- High density lipoproteins (HDL): HDL helps the body counteract bad cholesterol in the blood. The more HDL cholesterol you have, the better. If levels of HDL are low, the chance of coronary artery disease increases.
- Triglycerides: Triglycerides are another type of fat that is carried in the blood by very low density lipoproteins. Sugar, Alcohol and overly high caloric intake increase the amount of triglycerides, making your blood "fatty".

Many factors are involved in increasing "bad" cholesterol levels:

- Poor diet - Saturated fat and cholesterol in the food you eat increase cholesterol levels.
- Weight. Obesity can also increase cholesterol. Losing weight can help lower your LDL and total cholesterol levels, as well as increase HDL ("good") cholesterol.
- Inactivity: Regular exercise can lower LDL cholesterol and raise HDL cholesterol.
- Age: As we get older, cholesterol levels rise.
- Sex: Young women tend to have lower total cholesterol levels than men of similar age. After menopause, however, women's levels rise just like a man's does.
- Diabetes. Poorly controlled diabetes increases cholesterol. Heredity. Families may have multiple members with high cholesterol due to genetic factors.

Despite this, you can take action to improve the situation:

- Change your diet. If you have heart disease, limit daily intake of fatty foods to less than 200 milligrams. Staying away from saturated fats can make major changes in the amount of "bad" cholesterol in your system.
- Avoid Smoking. Smoking lowers HDL ("good") cholesterol levels. This trend is reversed when you quit.
- Be active. Exercise increases HDL cholesterol in some people. if done daily, weight, diabetes, and high blood pressure all benefit.
- Stockpile Medications. Make sure that your group or family members on medications for high cholesterol (called "statins" accumulate medications if at all possible.

Even if you stockpile medications, they will eventually run out in a long term survival situation. Don't despair, as various alternatives are available: Some of the herbal and nutritional supplements that may help include:

- Garlic: Garlic is an herb that has multiple beneficial effects on the body. It has been reported to decrease cholesterol levels in some people. Be aware that it may have health risks in those on blood thinners.

- Sugar Cane: Sugar cane contains policanisol, a substance that has been shown to lower cholesterol levels in several studies.
- Red Yeast Rice: Red yeast rice contains lovastatin, a substance founds in some prescription cholesterol medications. Its effect is still under study.
- Myrrh: The mukul myrrh tree contains a resin known as guggulipid. Indian studies seem to indicate that total and LDL cholesterol is lowered with regular use, although U.S. studies have failed to achieve the same results.
- Fenugreek, artichoke extract, yarrow, holy basil, ginger, turmeric, and rosemary all have been proposed as possible options to lower cholesterol.

In addition, dietary changes may be helpful. Increasing fiber, soy, omega-3 fatty acids and plant sterols may be options to help decrease "bad" cholesterol levels. Again, some of these may adversely affect those people who take blood thinners.

Other causes of chest pain

There are various other causes of chest pain. Injury to muscles and joints in the torso may mimic cardiac pain. In this type of pain, you will notice that the pain gets worse with movement of the affected area, or that you can elicit pain by pressing on it. Rest the patient and give them Ibuprofen or Acetaminophen for pain.

Acid reflux may also cause pain (usually burning in nature) in the chest area. This type of pain is usually improved with antacids in tablet form such as calcium carbonate (Tums, Rolaids, etc.) or liquid versions with magnesium hydroxide/aluminum hydroxide Maalox, Mylanta). Relaxation techniques such as massage in a sitting position may also help. For a further discussion about acid reflux and other gastro-intestinal issues, see the next chapter.

Chest pain is also seen in some patients with anxiety issues. This is usually accompanied by tremors, a rapid heart rate and hyperventilation.

Sedative herbs like Valerian Root, Passion Flower, and Chamomile may be helpful in this situation, as are some prescription medications such as diazepam (Valium). See the discussion of anxiety later in this book.

ULCER AND ACID REFLUX DISEASE

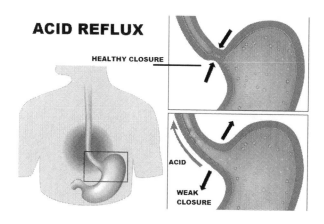

Ulcers

Chronic stress, as will be seen in a collapse scenario, can manifest itself in ways that are both emotional and physical. One of the physical effects is increased stomach acid levels.

Excessive acid can cause an inflammation of the esophagus (the tube that goes from the throat to the stomach), the stomach itself and/or the next part of the bowel, called the duodenum. The irritated lining becomes weak and an erosion is formed. This erosion is called an "**ulcer**" and can cause bleeding or even perforate the entire thickness of the lining.

The major symptom of an ulcer is a burning or gnawing discomfort in the stomach area. This pain is often described as "**heartburn**". It usually occurs in the left or mid-upper abdomen or may travel up to the breastbone. Sometimes it will be described as hunger pangs or indigestion. The discomfort that goes along with this problem is hard to ignore and will decrease work efficiency. Therefore, diagnosis and treatment are important to get your group member back to normal.

There are many causes of pain in the chest and stomach areas. Chest pain caused by coronary heart disease ("angina") is just one of the possibilities and was discussed in the last section.

To make the diagnosis of ulcer or acid reflux disease, the timing of the discomfort is important. Ulcer and acid reflux discomfort occurs soon after eating but is sometimes seen several hours after a meal. It can be differentiated from other causes of chest pain in another way: it gets better by drinking milk or taking antacids. As you can imagine, this wouldn't do much for angina.

Many ulcers and inflammation are caused by a bacterium known as Helicobacter pylori. H. pylori may be transmitted from person to person through contaminated food and water, so proper water filtration and sterilization will decrease the likelihood of this infection. Antibiotics such as Amoxicillin and Metronidazole in combination are the most effective treatment for Helicobacter pylori ulcers.

Other causes include the use of ibuprofen or aspirin, which can be an irritant to the stomach in some people. Avoidance of these drugs can prevent these ulcers and inflammatory pain. Smoking and alcohol abuse are also known causes.

Acid Reflux Disease

Acid reflux disease is caused by acid traveling up the esophagus. This is sometimes caused by a relaxation at the stomach-esophagus border, or by an out pouching of the area (called a "**hiatal hernia**"). The primary symptom is heartburn, but severe disease can cause chest pain. It is usually relieved by antacids and/or by sleeping with the upper body raised.

Your patient may benefit from avoiding certain foods. These commonly include:

- Acidic fruit (for example, oranges)
- Fatty foods
- Coffee
- Certain teas
- Onions
- Peppermint
- Chocolate

Eating smaller meals and avoiding acidic foods before bedtime is a good strategy to prevent reflux. Obese individuals seem to suffer more from this problem, so weight loss might be helpful.

Medications that commonly relieve acid reflux include calcium, magnesium, aluminum, and bismuth antacids such as Tums, Maalox, Mylanta or Pepto-Bismol, as well as other medications such as Ranitidine (Zantac), Cimetidine (Tagamet), and Omeprazole (Prilosec). These medications are available in non-prescription strength and are easy to accumulate in quantity.

Home remedies abound for acid reflux:

- Organic apple cider vinegar: Mix one tablespoon in four ounces of water, drink before each meal.
- Aloe Vera Juice: Mix one ounce in two ounces of water before a meal.
- Baking soda: Mix one tablespoon in a glass of water and drink right away when you begin to feel heartburn
- Glutamine: An amino acid that has an anti-inflammatory effect and reduces acid reflux. It can be found in milk and eggs.

It's important to remember to communicate with your patients. Many in the preparedness and homesteading community are rugged individualists. They may be unlikely to tell the medic about something they consider trivial, like heartburn. Someone that is clearly in pain, losing efficiency, or unable to sleep should always be questioned about their symptoms. It could be something that you just might be able to help them with.

SEIZURE DISORDERS

Seizures occur when the brain's electrical system misfires. Instead of sending out signals in a controlled manner, a surge of haphazard energy goes through the brain. These abnormal signals can cause involuntary muscle contractions, poor control of certain organs, and loss of consciousness. A person with chronic problems with convulsions is sometimes said to have "**epilepsy**" and may be called an "epileptic". There are several types of seizures:

Generalized Seizures may involve the entire brain. There are several types that have been identified:

- **Petit Mal seizures:** No involuntary contractions, but a temporary loss of concentration or even consciousness. Blank staring may be noticed. Strange sensations known as "auras" (smells, colors, etc.) may herald an upcoming convulsion.
- **Grand Mal seizures:** shaking and jerking with loss of consciousness, bladder control, and sometimes violent shaking and jerking. Grand mal seizures are what most people associate with epilepsy.
- **Myoclonic seizures:** Involuntary movement of the muscles without loss of consciousness (usually).
- **Partial seizures:** Also known as "Jacksonian" seizures, these are caused by abnormal signals from one part of the brain. They may involve involuntary shaking of just one limb or specific twitching behavior. The patient may notice auras prior to some partial seizures. Although vision may be temporarily impaired, there may or may not be changes in mental status.

There are various causes of convulsive disorders, such as:

- High fever (in children, mostly)
- Head injury
- Meningitis (Infection of the central nervous system)
- Stroke
- Brain tumors

- Genetic predisposition
- Idiopathic (unknown – about 50% of cases)

In a collapse situation, there won't be the sophisticated equipment such as EEGs (electroencephalograms) and Brain Scans to make the diagnosis, so we will have to watch for symptoms to identify the problem. It is important to know that one seizure does not make someone an epileptic. Multiple episodes are required to be certain. In some cases (especially childhood seizures associated with fevers), a person might even "outgrow" the condition.

In addition to auras that give some warning that an attack may be imminent, there are also triggers that sometimes cause a convulsion. A good example is a bright flashing light. Avoidance of these triggers will decrease the number of episodes.

The most important aspect of treatment when intravenous medication is no longer available will be to prevent the patient from injuring themselves during an attack. A tongue depressor with gauze taped around it and placed in the mouth was once a standard recommendation, but it was found to cause injuries to both the patient and the rescuer. Keep everything away from the patient's mouth, especially your fingers.

You shouldn't restrain the person physically, but remove nearby objects that could cause injury. An exception is if the patient is standing when the seizure starts. In this case, grab the patient and gently lower them to the floor. Placing them in the CPR "recovery" position (discussed in the CPR section of this book) will help keep their airway open.

Do not give oral fluids or medications to an epileptic after a seizure until they are fully awake and alert. If the convulsion is caused by a fever, as in children, cool them down with wet compresses. Anyone in your survival group with a convulsive disorder should work towards stockpiling their medicine. Popular drugs are Dilantin, Tegretol, Valproic Acid, and Diazepam (Valium). Emphasize the importance of extra medications in cases of natural disaster or other emergencies to your family or group members.

Natural alternatives have long been espoused to decrease the frequency and severity of convulsions. Many vitamins and herbal supplements have a sedative effect, which calms the brain's electrical energy. They may be taken as a tea (1 teaspoon of the herb in a cup of water) or as a tincture (an extract with grain alcohol). Here are some that have been reported as beneficial for prevention:

- Bacopa (*Bacopa monnieri*
- Chamomile (*Matricaria recutita*)
- Kava (*Piper methysticum*) – (too much may damage your liver)
- Valerian (*Valeriana officinalis,*
- Lemon balm (*Melissa officinalis*),
- Passionflower (*Passiflora incarnata*)
- Vitamin B12 supplements
- Vitamin E supplements

Vegetable juices may help eliminate toxins that could induce seizures. Drink a combination of carrot juice, cucumber and beet juice; if possible drink a half liter a day. Coconut oil, 3 tablespoons a day, has also been reported to decrease seizure frequency. Your experience may vary.

When a Person Collapses

Sometimes, a patient may collapse, not from a convulsion, but from simple fainting. This must be differentiated from the person who has "seized". In this circumstance, your patient should not have jerky movements as in a Grand Mal seizure or stare into space as in a petit mal seizure. A person who has had a seizure will tend to be difficult to rouse for a period of time. This is called a **"post-ictal" state** and will resolve on its own over time. If there has been a head injury, however, a concussion cannot be ruled out (discussed in the section on head trauma). Most people who have fainted will regain alertness relatively soon after the episode.

Dehydration, low blood sugar and various other medical conditions can cause fainting. Good hydration and appropriate dietary intake will prevent most episodes. If someone feels as if they are about to collapse, they should sit down and put their head down between their knees to increase blood flow to the brain. If you see someone who is fainting from a standing position, grab them and gently lower them to the ground (in this case, on their back). In normal times, of course, you would have someone call emergency medical services.

Evaluate the victim quickly. If someone has only fainted, they will be breathing and have a pulse. If this is the case, raise their legs about 12 inches off the ground and above the level of their heart/head. This will help blood flow to the brain. Assess the patient for evidence of trauma, bleeding, or seizures. If bleeding, apply direct pressure to the wound. If the person is having a convulsion, treat as previously discussed. If no pulse or breathing, begin CPR as discussed in the section later in this book.

Once a person who has fainted has been determined to be breathing normally, have a pulse, and have no bleeding injuries, tap on their shoulder and ask in a clear voice "Can you hear me?" or "Are you OK?". Loosen any obviously constricting clothing and make sure that they are getting lots of fresh air by keeping the area around them clear of crowds. If you are in an area that is hot, fan the patient or carefully carry them to a cooler area.

If you are successful in arousing the patient, ask them if they have any pre-existing medical conditions such as diabetes, heart disease or epilepsy. Stay calm and speak in a reassuring manner. Don't let them get up for a period of time, even if they say that they are fine. People oftentimes are embarrassed and want to brush off the incident, but they are still at risk for another fall.

Once the victim is awake and alert (Do they know their name? Do they know where they are? What year it is?), you may slowly have the patient sit up if they are not otherwise injured. If you are not in an austere setting, emergency medical personnel are on the way; wait until they arrive before having the patient stand up. In a survival situation, however, you will have to make a judgment as to whether and when the victim is capable to return to normal activities.

Common causes of fainting include dehydration and low blood sugar, so some oral intake may be helpful. ONLY do this if it is clear that they are completely conscious, alert, and able to function. Test their strength by having them raise their knees against the pressure of your hands. If they are weak, they should continue to rest. Close monitoring of the patient will be very important, as some internal injuries may not manifest for hours.

JOINT DISEASE

COMMON ARTHRITIS TYPES

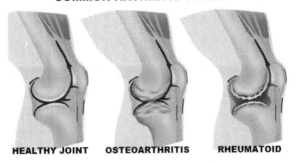

HEALTHY JOINT   OSTEOARTHRITIS   RHEUMATOID

Over the course of time, the moving parts of humans suffer wear and tear just like the moving parts of any other machine. Damage to ankles, knees, hips, and even the spine occurs chronically over the course of years. We can expect an acceleration of this process when demands on our body increase in times of trouble. The performance of activities of daily survival will, in particular, wear out our joints.

Degenerative damage to joints is called "**osteoarthritis**". Many advances in degenerative disease, such as hip replacements, may no longer be available in austere settings, so we will have to figure out other options. We will not have curative remedies, but we can still improve the quality of life of the patient.

Besides degenerative changes, inflammation of the joints (also known as "**arthritis**") can also be caused by **auto-immune** conditions. Antibodies are formed by the body that attack its own joints and sometimes cause striking deformities. Bacterial infections, some of which are sexually transmitted, also can significantly damage joint tissue. The cause must be identified and treated quickly.

Regardless of why the arthritis in the joint occurred, the signs and symptoms are frequently similar. You will see:

- Pain (mild or severe)
- Swelling
- Joint stiffness and decreased range of motion

- Reluctance to use the affected joint
- Fluid accumulation in the joint space
- Muscle weakness (with chronic arthritis)
- Fever (septic/bacterial arthritis)

Arthritis Types

Osteoarthritis

As you can imagine, Osteoarthritis is the most common form of arthritis, especially in older individuals. It can affect both larger and smaller joints of the body. Hands, feet, back, hip, and knees are most commonly affected.

The disease is acquired by daily wear and tear on the joints, although it can also be a long term effect of a previous injury. Many athletes, for example, may develop arthritis in this manner at a relatively young age. Obesity causes increased stress on joints as well and leads to osteoarthritis.

Warm compresses are useful to treat discomfort and stiffness. Non-steroidal anti-inflammatory drugs (NSAIDs) like ibuprofen or aspirin are helpful, as is Capsaicin creams or ointments. The worst cases may require oral or injectable steroids. These, however, are unlikely to be available in austere settings. Sometimes, a needle is placed to drain excess fluid from an affected joint to give relief. This is call "**arthrocentesis**" and carries with it the risk that you might introduce infection.

Rheumatoid Arthritis

Rheumatoid arthritis is the most common auto-immune disease in the world today. It is a disorder in which the body's own immune system starts to attack its own tissues. The attack is not only directed at the joint but to other parts of the body. Unlike some joint diseases, rheumatoid arthritis tends to affect the same joint on BOTH sides of the body. Women are more susceptible than men.

Rheumatoid arthritis especially affects joints in the fingers and wrists, but is also common in knees and elbows. Over time, it can lead to severe deformities in a few years if not treated. Rheumatoid arthritis occurs in younger populations than osteoarthritis, even striking children on occasion.

Other symptoms associated with rheumatoid arthritis that you might NOT see with degenerative osteoarthritis:

- Dry mouth
- Dryness, Itching or burning in the eyes
- Insomnia
- Strange sensations in the hands or feet
- Nodules under the skin
- Chest pain when taking a breath (also known as "pleurisy")

Treatments concentrate on easing the symptoms, as for osteoarthritis, but no cure exists. Medical therapy includes strong anti-inflammatory medications such as oral steroids (example: Prednisone).

Another auto-immune disorder that can cause joint disease is known as Systemic Lupus Erythematosis (SLE). Although usually diagnosed by blood testing, Lupus can be differentiated from rheumatoid arthritis due to its one-sided nature. You will also see patients with SLE experience hair loss and body rashes. Lupus is often treated with long-term oral steroids.

Even though rheumatoid arthritis cannot be cured, you can prevent the condition from worsening. Weight loss is one way to improve symptoms and prevent progression. Physical therapy to strengthen muscles and joints is thought to be helpful.

Bacterial Arthritis

Bacterial arthritis (sometimes called "septic" arthritis) is often the result of some penetrating injury that allows organisms to invade the joint space. It can also occur from within, as when someone with a blood infection (**septicemia**) or bone infection (**osteomyelitis**) has spread to a joint. Common skin bacteria, such as Streptococcus and Staphylococcus, are the usual suspects but gonorrhea, a sexually transmitted disease, can also be the cause.

Typical symptoms of a bacterial arthritis are the same as osteoarthritis, except that the patient may have a fever and may exhibit redness or warmth over the affected joint. In addition to standard treatment, antibiotics will be helpful.

Gout

Gout is another condition that destroys joints over time. It is caused by deposition of uric acid crystals in the joint, causing inflammation. Some people simply produce too much uric acid or don't eliminate it well. Obesity is a major risk factor, as is diabetes. This illness occurs primarily in men; a history of certain types of kidney stones may be associated with future episodes of gout.

The presentation of gout will appear as:

- Inflammation in one or two joints. The big toe is the classic example, but knees and ankles may also be affected.
- Warm, red, painful joints. The pain is throbbing and often severe. Even laying a sheet over it may cause pain.
- Fever.
- Episodic repeat attacks (50% of cases).

After multiple episodes, permanent damage occurs and the joint loses its range of motion. Chronic sufferers may also develop lumps called "**tophi**". Tophi are lumps below the skin, mostly around joints. They may drain chalky material from time to time.

Specialized prescription drugs are available for gout, such as Colchicine and Allopurinol. If you have a family member with gout, encourage them to stockpile extra medications; they won't be found in your standard medic's storage.

Lifestyle and dietary changes may be helpful:

- Avoid alcohol
- Reduce how many uric acid elevating foods you eat. These include: Liver, herring, sardines, anchovies, kidney, beans, peas, mushrooms, asparagus, and cauliflower. .
- Limit excessive meat intake.
- Avoid fatty foods
- Eat enough carbohydrates

Natural therapy for joint disease

From an alternative standpoint, there are several treatments for joint pain caused by arthritis.

Various glucosamine supplements are popular; glucosamine sulfate preparations have more evidence for their effectiveness than glucosamine hydrochloride. Take 1,500 milligrams once a day on a regular basis.

Glucosamine is often paired with chondroitin sulfate. 800-1,200 milligrams a day has been shown to possibly slow progression of some arthritic conditions.

Two teaspoons of lemon juice or apple cider vinegar mixed with a teaspoon of honey twice a day is a time-honored treatment. Other oral supplements reported to be effective against joint pain are:

- Turmeric powder
- Soybean Oil
- Avocado Oil
- Rose hips
- Fish Oil
- Bathua leaf juice
- Alfalfa tea

For external use:

- Use Arnica essential oil on affected areas (good for muscle aches as well)
- Apply warm vinegar to aching joints.
- Mix powdered sandalwood into a paste; it has a cooling effect when rubbed on a joint.
- Make an ointment from 2 parts olive oil and 1 part Kerosene (use extreme caution: Kerosene is flammable!).

Acupuncture, massage therapy, and physical therapy may alleviate muscle spasms associated with arthritis. Electricity delivered by a device known as a TENS unit may be helpful (if you have electricity).

KIDNEY STONES/GALL BLADDER DISEASE

The kidney and gall bladder are two organs that have the propensity in some people to develop an accumulation of crystals. These crystals form masses known as "stones". Some are large and some are as small as grains of sand, but any size can cause pain (sometimes excruciating). These issues can put group members out of commission at a time when they are most needed.

Kidney Stones

MALE

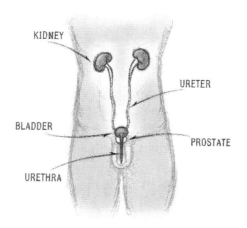

URINARY SYSTEM

Kidney stones are most commonly seen in those persons who fail to keep themselves well hydrated. Even small stones can lead to significant pain (known as "**renal colic**"), and the larger ones can cause blockages that can disrupt the function of the organ. Once you have had a kidney stone, it is likely you will get them again at one point or another. Kidney stones are usually NOT associated with infections.

Once formed in the kidney, stones usually do not cause symptoms until they begin to move down the tubes which connect the kidneys to the bladder (the "**ureters**"). When this happens, the stones can block the flow of urine. This causes swelling of the kidney affected as well as significant pain. Kidney stones as small as grains of sand may reach the bladder without incident and then cause pain as they attempt to pass through the tube that goes from the bladder to the outside (the "**urethra**").

There are several different types of kidney stones:

- **Calcium stones:** The most common, they occur more often in men than in women, usually in those 20 to 40 years old. Calcium can combine with other substances, such as oxalate, phosphate, or carbonate to form a stone.
- **Cysteine stones:** These form in people who have "cysteinuria", a condition that tends to run in families.
- **Struvite stones:** This variety is mostly found in women and can grow quite large; they can cause blockages at any point in the urinary tract. Frequent and chronic infections are a risk factor.
- **Uric acid stones:** More common in men than in women, these stones are associated with conditions such as gout.

To diagnose a kidney stone, look for pain that starts suddenly and comes and goes. Pain is commonly felt on the side of the back (the "flank"). Lightly pounding on the right and left flank at the level of the lowest rib will cause significant pain in patients with kidney stones or kidney infections. As the stone moves, so will the pain; it will travel down the abdomen and could settle in the groin or even the urethral area.

Other symptoms of renal stones can include:

- Bloody urine
- Fever and chills
- Nausea and vomiting

Some dietary changes may prevent the formation of kidney stones, especially if they are made of calcium. Avoid foods such as:

- Spinach
- Rhubarb
- Beets,

- Parsley
- Sorrel, and
- Chocolate

Also, decreasing dairy intake will restrict the amount of calcium available for stone formation. This will keep them as small as possible and, therefore, easier to pass.

Your treatment goal as medical provider is to assist the stone to pass through the system quickly. Have your patient drink at least 8 glasses of water per day to produce a large amount of urine. The flow will help move the stone along.

Some have used diuretic medications for the same purpose. Pain relievers can help control the pain of passing the stones (renal colic). For most pain, Ibuprofen will be the available treatment of choice. Stronger pain medications, if you can get them, may be necessary for severe cases.

Some of the larger stones will be chronic issues, as the high technology and surgical options used to remove these will not be available in a collapse scenario. Medications specific to the type of stone may be helpful:

- Allopurinol (prescription medicine for uric acid stones and gout).
- Antibiotics (for struvite stones).
- Sodium bicarbonate or sodium citrate (which increases the alkalinity of the urine). These drugs decrease the likelihood of formation of uric acid stones.

A good home remedy to relieve discomfort and aid passage of the stone is lemon juice, olive oil, and apple cider vinegar. With the first twinge of pain, drink a mixture of 2 ounces of lemon juice and 2 ounces of olive oil. Then, drink a large glass of water. After 1 hour, drink a mixture of 1 tablespoon of raw apple cider vinegar with 2 ounces of lemon juice in a large glass of water. Repeat this process every 1 to 2 hours until improved.

Other natural substances that may help are:

- Horsetail tea (a natural diuretic)
- Pomegranate juice

- Dandelion root tea
- Celery tea
- Basil tea

Gall Bladder Stones

GALLSTONES

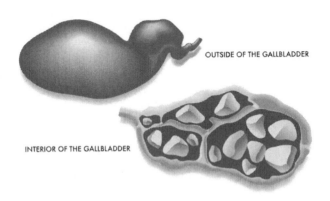

OUTSIDE OF THE GALLBLADDER

INTERIOR OF THE GALLBLADDER

The gall bladder is a sac-like organ that is attached to the liver; it stores the bile that the liver secretes. **Gallstones** are firm deposits that form inside the gallbladder and could block the passage of bile. This blockage can cause a great deal of pain and inflammation (known as "**cholecystitis**").

There are two main types of gallstones:

1. **Cholesterol stones:** The grand majority, these are not related to the actual cholesterol levels in the bloodstream.
2. **Bilirubin stones:** These occur in those people who have illnesses that destroy their red blood cells. The by-products of this destruction releases a substance called "bilirubin" into the bile and forms a stone.

Risk factors for this condition can be described as the 4 "F's":

- **FAT:** The majority of those with gallstones are overweight.
- **FEMALE:** The majority of sufferers are women.
- **FORTY:** Most people with gallstone issues are over 40 years old.

- **FERTILE:** Most women with gallstones have had children.

Additional risk factors include diabetes, liver cirrhosis (discussed in the section on hepatitis), and low blood counts ("**anemia**").

Luckily, most people with this problem don't have any symptoms. If a large stone causes a blockage, however, you may experience what is called "**biliary colic**". Symptoms of biliary colic include:

- Cramping right upper abdomen pain (constant, spreading to the back).
- Fever.
- Jaundice (yellowing of the skin and whites of the eyes).
- Discolored bowel movements (gray or grayish-white).
- Nausea and vomiting.

The classical finding on physical examination is "**Murphy's Sign**". Press with one hand just below the midline of the lowest rib on the front right. Then, ask your patient to breathe deeply. If the gallbladder is tender, the patient should complain of significant pain at the site.

Unfortunately, the main treatment for gallstones is to surgically remove the gall bladder (you can live without it and stay healthy). As surgical suites are unlikely to be available in a collapse situation, you might consider some alternative remedies. These are mostly preventative measures:

- Apple cider vinegar (mixed with apple juice)
- Chanca Piedra, (Phyllanthus niruri), a plant that is native to the Amazon; translated, the name means "Break Stones".
- Peppermint
- Turmeric
- Alfalfa
- Ginger root
- Dandelion root
- Artichoke leaves
- Beet, Carrot, Grape, Lemon juices

Sadly, it is very difficult to eliminate most of the risk factors for gall bladder disease. If you're forty, female, and have children, there is not much you can do about it. You may be able to something about being fat, however. Dietary changes to decrease intake of high-cholesterol foods may help you decrease weight and the risk of gallstones.

DERMATITIS

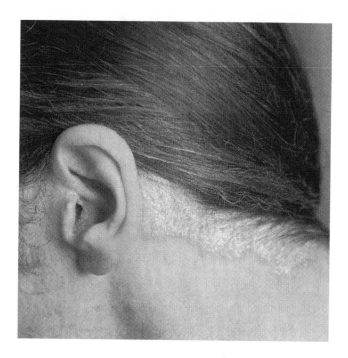

Seborrheic Dermatitis

In austere circumstances, a caregiver may consider a skin rash to be of no consequence. Symptoms associated with it, however, may cause sleep loss or irritation that make affect a group member's work efficiency. Therefore, it makes common sense to treat any condition that decreases the quality of life of a loved one.

Dermatitis simply means an inflammation of the skin. This condition may have many causes and may vary in appearance from case to case. Most types of dermatitis usually present with swollen, reddened and/or itchy skin. Continuous scratching traumatizes the irritated area and may lead to cellulitis once the skin is broken.

Some of the more common types of skin inflammation are:

- **Contact dermatitis:** Caused by allergens and chemical irritants. A good example would be poison ivy.

- **Seborrheic dermatitis**: A commonly seen condition that affects the face and scalp (common cause of dandruff).
- **Atopic Dermatitis or Eczema:** A chronic itchy rash that can be found in various areas at once and tends to be intermittent in nature. This may be accompanied by hay fever or asthma.
- **Neuro-dermatitis:** A chronic itchy skin condition localized to certain areas of the skin (as seen in a herpes virus infection known as "Shingles").
- **Stasis dermatitis:** An inflamed area caused by fluid under the skin, commonly seen on the lower legs of older individuals. Poor circulation is a major factor here.

Many of the above conditions may appear similar to the non-medical person. Indeed, some cannot be conclusively diagnosed without sending a sample of skin to a laboratory. Whatever the cause, effective treatment of symptoms will be important in a grid-down situation. Limiting trauma from repeated scratching will prevent secondary, deeper infections from developing.

Moisturizing dry skin may be one way to help decrease frequency of outbreaks of dermatitis. Bathing is a healthy habit; it may, however, dry out your skin. You can prevent this by:

- Using mild soaps: Deodorant soaps are to be avoided in patient with significant dermatitis.
- Moisturize: Apply any of a myriad of oils or creams to the skin while wet. This will seal in the moisture.
- Dry gently: Pat rather than rub dry with a towel.
- Bathe less: Sure enough, limiting the frequency and duration of baths may decrease symptoms.

Of all the types of skin conditions, you will most likely see contact dermatitis in a survival situation, as your people will be exposed to substances while scavenging that may cause reactions. Some of these include:

- Soaps, laundry soap and detergents.
- Cleaning products.
- Rubber or Latex.

- Metals, such as nickel.
- Weeds, such as poison ivy, oak or sumac.

Once you're sensitized to an allergen, future exposures will cause skin reactions. Your patient will probably experience these reactions for the rest of his or her life. The following factors seem to worsen the condition:

- Stress
- Rapid changes of temperature
- Sweating
- Harsh detergents or soaps
- Rough clothing or bedding

Avoidance is the cornerstone of prevention. Corticosteroid creams and cool moist compresses are a good start for treatment purposes. Use these only until the rash is improved. Antihistamines such as Benadryl or Claritin will help relieve itching. Of course, if the dermatitis was caused by contact with a specific irritant, avoid it if at all possible.

Scalp irritations caused by Seborrhea may be treated by shampoos that contain tar, pyrithione zinc, or ketoconazole. Scaly areas may be treated with mineral or olive oil.

Stasis dermatitis may be improved by wearing support hose. Pay careful attention to infections that may be developing. Wet dressings may soften rough areas.

Neurodermatitis caused by Shingles may be treated with anti-viral agents, such as Acyclovir, Famciclovir or Valacyclovir (Zovirax, Valtrex or Famvir, respectively).

In addition to hydrocortisone cream and wet compresses, some creams that suppress local immune response such as Pimecrolimus (Elidel) may improve atopic dermatitis. Vitamin B12 and rice bran products are both thought to be of help.

Some are proponents of light therapy. This involves exposing affected skin to controlled amounts of natural or artificial light. It may be effective in preventing recurrences of atopic dermatitis.

Other natural supplements that improve dermatitis often involve Omega-3 fatty acids, which have an anti-inflammatory effect. Used with evening primrose oil, it is thought to be especially effective. Chamomile cream is considered to be as potent as a mild hydrocortisone. Calendula has skin-soothing properties and may protect against contact dermatitis. Be aware, however, that it may trigger an allergic reaction on broken skin.

VARICOSE VEINS

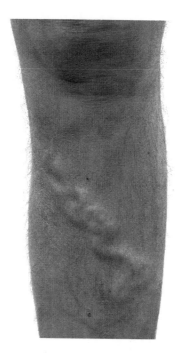

Varicose veins are dilated blood vessels, usually in the legs, which have lost tone in the valves that control blood flow. This swelling of the vascular structures occurs in about 15% of the population, and becomes more common with age (50% over age 50). Women are several times more likely to have this problem than men.

Varicosities are gravity dependent; they may be more common in people whose occupation requires constant standing. In a power-down setting, we will be spending more time on our feet by necessity. Therefore, we must plan to prevent, if possible, and treat varicose veins before they become serious.

Varicose veins are similar to but not the same as "**spider veins**". Spider veins are tiny vessels called capillaries and exist everywhere in your body. When they become varicose, they appear like little red or blue spider webs; you may find them on your legs, face, or just about anywhere. People with fair complexions seem to get more of them.

Classically, varicose veins are larger, blue, swollen, and stick out from the skin. They tend to look twisted or contorted. Varicosities cause the circulation to become less efficient. This causes pain and fatigue in the legs, and could lead to an inflammation known as "**phlebitis**".

You're more likely to get varicose veins if you:

- Are 50 years of age or older. The valves in your veins weaken as you age.
- Have a family history. If your mother had varicose veins, you are likely to get them as well.
- Are a woman. High levels of estrogen as seen during puberty, pregnancy, and while taking birth control pills increase your risk.
- Are obese. Extra weight puts pressure on the veins and causes them to dilate.
- Work in a profession that requires long periods of standing, lifting weights or sitting with your legs bent.
- Spend longs hours in the sun, especially if your complexion is fair. You may notice them first on your cheeks or nose.

Besides the discomfort and an unpleasing cosmetic appearance, varicose veins are usually not dangerous. Occasionally, however, you might see one of these complications:

Thrombophlebitis: a varicose vein on the surface of the skin can become inflamed; this is due to a blood clot which formed due to the poor circulation in the area. Symptoms include:

- Painful swelling
- Warmth to the touch
- Redness (sometimes along the line of the vein).
- Tender, hard nodules
- Itching
- Fever

Basic treatment involves moist warm compresses and anti-inflammatory medicine for discomfort and fever. Elevation of the affected extremity may be useful. Elastic support hose is helpful while performing activities of daily living. Although most cases of thrombophlebitis are not due to infection, antibiotics are occasionally needed. Cephalexin (Keflex) is known to have activity against Staphylococcus, the most common bacterial culprit.

As an aside, hemorrhoids are a type of superficial thrombophlebitis: See the section describing them later in the book.

Deep vein thrombosis (DVT): A blood clot that forms in a DEEP vein. The patient will experience a "full" or "firm" feeling, usually in the calf area. This will be accompanied by pain, heat, swelling, and redness as in superficial thrombophlebitis.

While many people may present with no symptoms at all, a DVT can be dangerous if the blood clot dislodges and makes it way to the lungs or other vital organs. Indeed, shortness of breath may be the only symptom noticed. In this circumstance, a blood clot may have already made it into the lung. This is referred to a "**pulmonary embolism**" and is possibly life-threatening. Other signs and symptoms may include breathlessness, chest pain, a fast heart rate, panting, and/or bloody phlegm.

In addition to compresses and pain relief, patients with deep vein thrombosis may require blood thinners; Salicin from the under bark of willows, poplars, and aspens is a natural alternative if the pharmaceuticals have run out. The amount given using this method will, however, always be uncertain. Each tree may have variable amounts of Salicin. Do not attempt this treatment on someone currently on medications such as Coumadin.

If your patient has varicose veins, have them stock up on compression stockings or support pantyhose while times are good. These will be unavailable in a collapse setting and neither will curative treatments like surgery, lasers, or chemical injections. If the resources are there to eliminate this issue in normal times, consider doing so. Encourage your patients at risk to:

- Exercise their legs to improve tone; this will provide support to the blood vessels.
- Avoid standing for long periods of time. Shift their weight from foot to foot often and take a short walk if they sit all day.

- Keep their weight down to avoid putting strain on their legs.
- Elevate their legs above the level of the heart for a half hour daily, and perhaps during sleep.
- Wear support stockings.
- Avoid wearing high heels for long periods (I doubt you'll be wearing high heels after a disaster).
- Eat a low-salt diet. Less salt consumption can help with the swelling that you see with varicose veins.
- Wear sunscreen; this will limit spider veins in people with fair complexions.

The herbal remedy most quoted to treat varicose veins is the horse chestnut (Aesculus hippocastanum. Horse chestnuts contain a substance called aescin, which appears to block enzymes that damage capillary walls. Make a tincture (grain alcohol-based mixture) with the herb and take 1 tablespoonful up to 3 times a day.

For external use only, rub a mixture of 4 parts witch hazel with 1 part tincture of horse chesnut and rub on affected varicosities.

SECTION 8

✦   ✦   ✦

OTHER IMPORTANT MEDICAL ISSUES

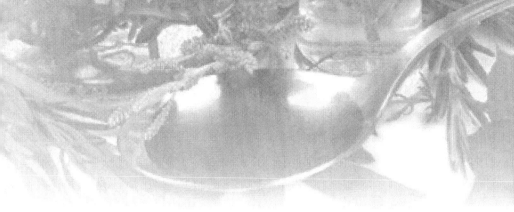

CPR IN AUSTERE SETTINGS

✚✚✚

Most medical books start off with a chapter on CPR (Cardio-Pulmonary Resuscitation), so you might wonder why this subject has not been given coverage so far in this volume. The answer is based on hard realities that we must confront in a survival scenario.

Although CPR (cardio-pulmonary resuscitation) is an important skill that everyone should know, there are fewer situations in a collapse scenario where CPR will return a victim to normal function. There are only a small number of circumstances where a patient goes from being a patient in need of resuscitation to a person who is back to normal.

CPR is best used as a stabilization strategy. You want to get the heart pumping and breathing supported so that you can get your patient as quickly as possible to a facility where there are ventilators, defibrillators, and other high technology. But what about a situation where this technology is no longer available?

There won't be cardiac bypasses for your patient who has had a heart attack. There won't be surgical suites for your patient with a shotgun blast to the abdomen or chest. The sobering truth is that many of these injuries will be "**mortal**" **wounds**. This means that death is the inevitable end result, no matter what you try to do. The poor prognosis for these people in hard times is tragic; it makes you truly appreciate the benefits of modern medicine.

There are still instances, however, where CPR may actually restore a gravely ill person to normal function. Airway obstruction with a foreign object can be dealt with by using the Heimlich maneuver. Environmental conditions such as hypothermia, heat stroke or smoke inhalation will oftentimes respond to resuscitative efforts with complete recovery. Severe anaphylactic reactions may require CPR until the patient responds to Epinephrine and resolves the attack. Rarer events such as lightning strikes or drowning may require resuscitation to revive the victim.

I chose not to put a large number of illustrations or write an entire course on how to do CPR in this book. There is no substitution for learning it in person by taking a hands-on course. I don't want you to think that you don't have to do this just because you read this book. Your responsibility as medic is to get training; this is mandatory for anyone that expects to be a caregiver in a long-term survival scenario.

Airway Obstruction

One situation where you can save a life by knowing how to perform a simple maneuver is in the case of an airway obstruction. This most commonly occurs as a result of a bite of food lodging in the back of the throat and cutting off respiration. This is a relatively common way to die, even in modern times, and it really shouldn't be.

If you see a conscious adult in sudden respiratory distress, ask quickly: Are you choking on something? If they can answer you, there is still air passing into their lungs. If it's a complete blockage, they will be unable to speak. They will probably be agitated and holding their throat, but they will hear you and (frantically) nod their head "yes". This is your signal to jump into action.

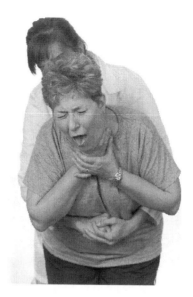

Tell the victim that you're there to help them and immediately get into position for the Heimlich maneuver, otherwise known as an "abdominal thrust" (see figure above). Get behind the victim and make a fist with your right hand. Place your fist above the belly button; then, wrap your left arm around the patient and grasp the right fist. Make sure your arms are positioned just below the ribcage. With a forceful upward motion, press your fist abruptly into the abdomen. You might have to do this multiple times before you dislodge the foreign body.

If your patient loses consciousness and you are unable to dislodge the obstructive item, place the patient in a supine position and straddle them across the thighs or hips. Open their mouth and make sure that the object can't be removed manually. Give several upward abdominal thrusts with the heels of your palms above the belly button (one hand on top of the other). Check again; you might have partially dislodged the offending morsel of food.

In old movies, you might see someone slap the victim hard on the back; this is unlikely to dislodge a foreign object and will waste precious time. An exception to this is in an infant: place the baby over your forearm (facing down) and apply several blows with the heel of your hand to the upper back.

An extreme method that can be used to open an airway is the "tracheotomy". This procedure, also called a cricothyroidotomy, involves cutting an opening in the windpipe below the level of an obstruction. Tracheotomy should be performed only when an airway obstruction completely prevents the ability to breathe after multiple Heimlich maneuvers have been attempted unsuccessfully.

To perform a tracheotomy, you will need a sharp blade and some sort of tube, such as a straw. Of course, a good first aid kit would be very helpful. Don't worry about antiseptics for now; you are performing this procedure because someone may die in the next few minutes.

The procedure goes as follows;

- Start at the Adam's apple. Move about 1 inch down the neck until you feel a bulge. This is the cricoid cartilage.
- Make a horizontal incision with your knife or a razor blade in the crease between the Adam's apple and the cricoid cartilage. This incision can be less than an inch long.
- Incise downward a half-inch deep or so. There shouldn't be a lot of blood.
- Below the incision, you'll see the greyish crico-thyroid membrane. Make an incision through it; this should allow passage of air into the lungs. Be careful not to cut too deeply.
- Place something hollow in the opening, to maintain a clear airway. A straw would do in a pinch. Try to get it a couple of inches down the windpipe; doing this makes it less likely to fall out.
- If the patient fails to breathe on their own, you may need to perform CPR, including rescue breaths through the tube you inserted.

I don't have to tell you that this is a dangerous procedure. A lot can go wrong, but the patient is dying and it may be your last resort. Only consider it when help is NOT on the way, and you have tried every other option first.

CPR in the Unconscious Patient

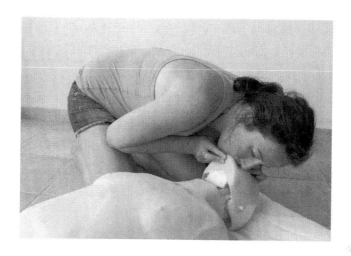

Rescue Breath(only if CPR-trained)

If you come across someone who is apparently unconscious, be certain to first verify their mental status. Simply ask them loudly: "Are you OK?" No answer? Grasp the person's shoulders and move them gently while continuing to ask them questions. If they are still unresponsive (which you should be able to determine in seconds), it's time to check their pulse and respirations. If they aren't breathing or no pulse is felt, it's time to start resuscitative efforts. Place your patient in a position so that they are lying flat on their back.

You will begin chest compressions by placing the heel of your hand in the middle of the chest; Place it, palm down, over the lower half of the breastbone at the level of the nipple. Place your other hand on top and interlace your fingers. Keeping yourself positioned directly above your hands (arms straight), press downward in such a fashion that the breastbone (also called the "sternum") is compressed about 2 inches. Allow the chest to recoil completely and then perform 30 compressions, at a rate of at least 100 compressions per minute.

This works well for adults but you would want less pressure in a child. Be certain to avoid the rib cage, as broken ribs are a common complication of the procedure.

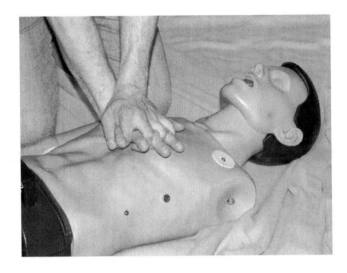

After 30 chest compressions, evaluate the victim for breathing and clear the airway. Look quickly inside the mouth for a foreign object. If there is none, place the patient's head in a position that will allow the clearest passage for air to enter the body. This is called the "**Chin-Lift**". Tilt the head back (unless there is evidence of a neck injury) and grasp the underside of the chin and lower jaw with one hand and lift. Using this method, the tongue and other throat structures are placed in a position that helps the patient take in oxygen. A useful medical item is a plastic "airway". There are both rigid oral and flexible nasal versions that help keep the airway open.

If you aren't trained in CPR, just continue compressions. If you DO know CPR, you may give 2 long breaths mouth-to-mouth (3-5 seconds between each one). These are called "rescue breaths". Pinch the nose closed to prevent the escape of air that needs to get into the lungs.

You can determine the effectiveness of your efforts by watching the patient's chest rise as you give the breaths. Continue giving 30 compressions, then 2 rescue breaths for 5 cycles or two minutes. Then, check your patient's status. If no luck, repeat the process all over again.

Many people are reluctant to perform rescue breaths due to concerns about contagious disease. If this is an issue, take a nitrile glove and cut the ends off of the two middle fingers. Place over the victim's mouth (cut glove fingers down) as you breathe for them. This provides a barrier that still allows air flow. Commercially-produced protective CPR masks are also available to keep with your first aid kit.

Another useful item for your medical supplies is a bag valve mask, otherwise known by the brand name "Ambu-Bag". This can be placed on the patient's mouth to form a seal through which you can ventilate them by pressing on an air-filled "bag". This provides pressure to force air inside the respiratory passages.

To review: if you are the lone resuscitator and have training, perform 30 compressions and then deliver 2 more breaths as before. Try for a compression rate of 80-100 beats per minute. Perform several cycles of the above; then re-evaluate the patient's pulse and respirations. If you don't have training, simply perform chest compressions at a rate of 100 per minute until a trained helper arrives. Once you have started CPR, don't stop until the patient has responded or it is clear that they will not.

After 30 minutes of CPR without result, the pupils of the patient's eyes will likely be dilated and will not respond to light. At this point, your patient has expired and you can cease your efforts. Some may feel this is not long; in truth, however, just a few minutes without oxygen is enough to cause irreversible brain damage. In a grid-down situation, you will not be equipped to provide long term chronic care to someone who no longer has brain activity.

There are units known as **defibrillators** available that, though quite expensive, may be useful in a cardiac arrest. These machines produce an electric shock to the heart and sometimes can restart a pulse that has stopped. If caused by a heart attack, a cardiac arrest without defibrillation will have a very low survival rate. It would be wise for your survival group to chip in and purchase a unit. "Home" defibrillators can be found online and are surprisingly easy to use:

Turn the unit on and connect the electrodes per the instructions. Place one electrode pad on the right chest about the nipple and below the collarbone. Place the other on the left chest outside the nipple and several inches below the armpit. The unit will analyze the heart rate (or lack of one) and tell you, believe it or not, whether a shock is necessary. If one is indicated, clear everyone away from the patient and press the button to activate the electric shock. Recheck vital signs and begin chest compressions as needed.

Let's say that you are successful in establishing a pulse and breathing in your unconscious patient. If you must, for some reason, leave them, position them so that they will not vomit and possibly aspirate stomach acid into the lungs. (see image below). This is known as the "**recovery position**".

In some cases, the actual injury or illness that caused unconsciousness may not be fatal, but the resulting regurgitation of stomach acid into the lungs ("**aspiration pneumonia**") will be. Many alcohol, pill or recreational drug overdoses cause death in this manner.

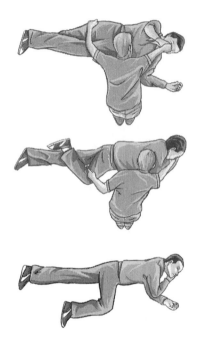

The Recovery Position

To achieve the recovery position:

- Kneel on one side facing the patient.
- Position the patient's arm (the one closest to you) perpendicular to the body.

- Flex the elbow.
- Position the other arm across the body.
- Bend the leg that is farthest from you up; reach behind the knee and pull the thigh toward you.
- Use your other arm to pull the shoulder farthest from you while rolling the body toward you.
- Maintain the upper leg in a flexed position so that the body is stabilized.

Although CPR will be of limited use when modern medical facilities are not available, it is still important to know. A survival community medic should not only be skilled in performing CPR, but should also teach it to every group member.

HEADACHE

Headaches are one of the most common medical symptoms that you will see in your role as medic. The brain matter itself doesn't have pain receptors; there are several structures around the brain, however, that do. Muscles, blood vessels, and sinuses are just some examples.

Many consider headaches to be, well, more of a headache than an actual danger, but headaches can be associated with a large number of medical conditions, not to mention traumatic injuries.

There are almost more causes for headaches than you can reasonably write down; in a collapse, however, common causes will be:

- Hunger
- Dehydration
- Stress
- Infections
- Fevers
- Elevated blood pressures
- Caffeine or Alcohol withdrawal
- Fumes

Headache pain is the interaction between the brain, blood vessels, and local nerves. Nerves associated with blood vessels and muscles are activated and send pain signals to the brain. Headaches that occur suddenly may be related to infection or colds/flus, but may be the herald of a life-threatening event such as a stroke. Ear and sinus infections are particularly likely to cause headaches.

Headache Types

Tension headache

By far, the most frequently-seen type of headache is the tension headache. This is caused by spasms of the muscles of the neck and head. Tension headache is usually seen bilaterally (on both sides) and/or the back of the head and neck. They may be related to stress, anxiety or depression, a head injury, or even just time spent with the head or neck in an abnormal position. Lack of sleep, teeth grinding, and poor posture are also factors.

Tension headaches may last a half hour or they can last a week. A sensation of pressure or tightening is the most common symptom. This type of headache may be improved by massaging the back of the neck and temples. Ibuprofen and Acetaminophen are old standbys as treatment. Identifying the situation that triggers the headache may help avoid future episodes.

Sinus Headache

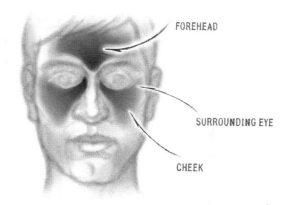

FOREHEAD

SURROUNDING EYE

CHEEK

SINUS HEADACHE

Sinus headaches are associated with constant pain in the front of the face. A **sinus** is an air-filled cavity in the bones of the skull. The forehead, cheeks or the bridge of the nose are the areas affected most by sinus infections; oftentimes, they may be one-sided, which will help you to make the diagnosis. Sudden head movement may intensify the pain.

Antibiotics may be helpful to treat the infections that can cause this type of headache. Amoxicillin (Fish-Mox Forte) 500mg three times a day for a week is a reasonable first choice. If you are allergic to Penicillin family drugs, consider Trimethoprim-Sulfamethoxasole (Bird-Sulfa) 160mg/800mg twice daily. Nasal decongestants such as Pseudoephedrine (Sudafed) may give some relief; so may sterile saline nasal rinses.

Migraines

The other common cause of headache is the migraine. The exact cause of migraines is uncertain. It is thought by some to be related to spasms in the blood vessels. Migraines may be genetic in nature, as they seem to run in families. Women are more susceptible than men.

A specific pattern of symptoms is seen in this variety of headache:

- Pain behind the eye (usually one-sided)
- Sensitivity to light, noise or odors
- Nausea and vomiting (causing loss of appetite or stomach discomfort)
- Vision changes (blurring, light and color phenomena)

Bed rest in the dark will be helpful here, as well as Ibuprofen and/or Acetaminophen. Some migraine medications use caffeine, and sometimes are effective. Teas and Coffee might be alternatives in an austere setting. If you are a chronic migraine sufferer, ask your physician for Sumatriptan (Imitrex), a strong anti-migraine medication, to stockpile.

Other headache causes

In women, hormonal changes may be responsible for headaches. Pregnancy, menopause, menstruation, and the use of birth control pills have all been implicated as risk factors. Cranberry juice and other natural diuretics may be helpful to limit swelling that may cause some headaches in these cases. Limiting pre-menstrual salt intake may also help.

Headache caused by dehydration will be rampant in a long-term survival situation. This variety will also present bilaterally and is commonly made worse by standing up rapidly from a lying position. These patients need fluids, which will gradually improve their symptoms.

Less common causes of headache would include an infection of the central nervous system called "**meningitis**". Along with headaches, meningitis presents with a stiff neck, fever, and possibly a rash. This condition may be caused by bacteria or viruses. Without modern medical facilities and labs, you could treat this condition with antibiotics and antivirals; expect variable results.

Uncontrolled high blood pressure or a burst blood vessel in the brain may cause a stroke (previously discussed elsewhere in this book). Besides the sudden onset of a severe headache, you will notice that your patient has lost strength in the arm and leg on one side; you will also note decreased motion on one side of the face and absent or slurred speech. Loss of vision in one eye is sometimes seen.

This condition, in a collapse, will be treated only with bed rest. There is often some improvement over the first 48 hours or so. Beyond this point, further recovery may be limited. This is one of the main reasons why it is so important for you as medic to treat all cases of high blood pressure.

Natural Headache Relief

If you would like a strategy to deal with a headache without drugs, try the following:

- Place an ice pack where the headache is.
- Have someone massage the back of your neck.
- Using two fingers, apply rotating pressure where the headache is.
- Lie down in a dark, quiet room. Get some sleep if at all possible. If your blood pressure is elevated, lay on your left side (pressure is usually lowest in this position).
- Track what you were doing or perhaps what you ate before the headache started; avoid that activity or food if possible.

A number of herbal remedies are available that might help headache. Feverfew is an herb that stops blood vessel constriction and is anti-inflammatory. This can be taken on a daily basis (1-2 leaves) for those with chronic problems (warning: Feverfew should not be ingested during pregnancy or nursing). Gingko Biloba has a similar action.

The pain of tension headaches can be relieved if you utilize herbs that have sedative and antispasmodic properties. Teas made from Valerian, skullcap, lemon balm, and passion flower have both. Herbal muscle relaxants may also help: rosemary, chamomile, and mint teas are popular options.

For external use, consider lavender or rosemary oil. Massage each temple with 1-2 drops every few hours.

EYE CARE

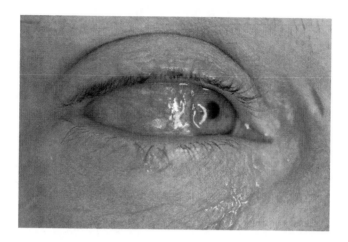

Conjunctivitis or "Pink Eye"

By picking up this book, you have demonstrated that you have excellent foresight. Unfortunately, that doesn't mean that you necessarily have excellent eyesight. Ask anyone on the street which of the five senses they would least be willing to sacrifice. They probably will tell you that their vision is the sense they would most want to preserve. Human beings aren't perfect, and one of our most common imperfections is that of being nearsighted (also known as "**myopia**") or farsighted (also known as "**hyperopia**").

Most of us correct our eye issues with eyeglasses or contact lenses. In a collapse setting, these vision aids become more precious than gold, but most people haven't made provision for multiple replacement pairs of contact lenses or spare eyeglasses.

Imagine what would happen in a collapse setting if your contact lenses dry out or one of your children steps on your glasses. I can't think of anything scarier than being on your own and not be able to see. Having a few pairs of reading glasses in your storage will be helpful as well; everyone reaches an age when eyesight naturally changes. It's important to know that neither contact lens nor eyeglasses will be manufactured in times of trouble.

Eye protection glasses are another required item. Many of us with perfect vision will be negligent about wearing eye protection when they chop wood or other chores likely to be part of normal off-grid living. Without eye protection, the risk of injury when performing strenuous tasks will be much higher.

Early in this book, I mentioned that you should deal with your medical issues BEFORE a societal collapse occurs. Bad eyesight might be one of those issues. One option you may not have considered is having your eyesight corrected to 20/20 with **LASIK** surgery. Lasik surgery uses pinpoint lasers to change the shape of your retina so that you are less near-sighted or farsighted. It has been routinely available for years now, and is one of the safest surgical procedures in existence.

The LASIK procedure for both eyes takes less than ten minutes from beginning to end, and the actual laser surgery usually takes less than 20 seconds for each eye. Your eyesight will improve almost immediately, and there is usually no downtime. At most, you might feel the sensation of a grain of sand in your eye for a few days. The procedure isn't cheap, but where else can you get such a tangible benefit (perfect vision) from your investment? I, myself, have had this procedure and recommend it highly to those with vision problems.

Most don't consider sunglasses to be a medical supply item, but they are. Even if you are just taking a hike outdoors, sunglasses provide eye protection from ultraviolet light. Ultraviolet (UV) light causes, over time, damage to the retinal cells which can lead to a clouding over of your eye's lenses (also called "**cataracts**"). This condition can only be repaired by surgery that will not be available in a collapse. Protection from ultra-violet (UV) light will help prevent long-term damage.

In cold weather conditions, failure to use sunglasses can cause a type of vision loss known as "**snow blindness**". Snow blindness is painful and dangerous in the wilderness, but, luckily, will go away on its own with eye patching. The truth of the matter is that, whenever you are doing chores or are outdoors, you should ask yourself why you SHOULDN'T have on your eye protection.

Infections of the Eye

There are various eye conditions that will be more common in a grid-down situation. The most common will be "**conjunctivitis**". Conjunctivitis is an inflammation which causes the affected eye to become red and itchy, and many times will cause a milky discharge (see photo at the beginning of this section). It can be caused by chemical irritation (soap in your eyes, for example), a foreign body, an allergy, or an infection.

This infection is also called "Pinkeye" and is highly contagious among children due to their rubbing their eyes and then touching other people or items. Studies have shown that people commonly touch their faces and eyes with their (often dirty) hands throughout the day. Observe any family member for a half hour and you'll see that this is true.

Irritated red eyes with tears may also be seen in allergic reactions, which can be treated with antihistamines orally or anti-histamine eye drops. Eye allergies can be differentiated from eye infections; they are less likely to have a milky discharge associated with them.

To avoid spreading the germs that can cause eye infections:

- Don't share eye drops with others.
- Don't touch the tip of a bottle of eye drops with your hands or your eyes because that can contaminate it with germs. Keep the bottle 3 inches above your eye.
- Don't share eye makeup with others.
- Never put contact lenses in your mouth to wet them. Many bacteria and viruses — maybe even the virus that causes cold sores — are present in your mouth and could easily spread to your eyes.
- Change your contacts often, the longer they stay in your eyes, the higher the chance is that your eye can get infected or even develop corneal ulcers.
- Wash your hands regularly.
- Any time you have an eye examination, ask the doctor if he/she has any samples of medicated eye drops to give you, in case of emergency.

Antibiotics like Doxycycline 100mg twice a day for a week (or less if improved) will relieve infectious conjunctivitis. Herbal treatment may also be of benefit. To treat pinkeye using natural products, pick one or more of the following methods:

- Apply a wet Chamomile or Goldenseal tea bag to the closed, affected eye, for 10 minutes, every two hours.
- Make a strong chamomile or Eyebright (*Euphrasia officinalis*) tea, let cool and use the liquid as an eyewash (using an eyecup) three to four times daily.
- Use 1 teaspoon of baking soda in 2 cups of cool water as an eyewash solution.
- Dissolve1 tablespoon of honey dissolved in 1 cup hot water; let cool and use as an eyewash.

Use the above tea, baking soda liquid or honey solution on gauze or cloth, and then apply a compress to affected eye for 10 minutes, every two hours. . For relief from the discomfort of conjunctivitis, a slice of cucumber over the eyes will be effective due to its cooling action.

Another common eye issue is called a "sty". A sty is essentially a pimple which has formed on the eyelid. It causes redness and some swelling and is generally uncomfortable. Warm moist compresses are helpful in allowing the sty to drain. Using Tobramycin antibiotic eye drops

will prevent worsening of this infection, which will usually resolve over the next few days. Any of the previously mentioned antibiotic or natural treatments for conjunctivitis can also be used.

Eye Trauma

The human body is truly a miracle of divine engineering. The conformation of your skull is such that your eyes are slightly recessed in bony sockets, which helps protect them from injury. Despite this, there are many different activities of daily living that can be traumatic to your eyes.

EYE CARE

Here are just a few of the ways you can injure your eyes:

- Accidents while using tools
- Spatter from bleach or other household chemicals
- Hedge clippers or lawn mowers
- Grease splatter from cooking
- Chopping wood
- Hot appliances near your face, such as curling irons or hair dryers

The list goes on and on; you could put your eye out by popping a cork on a bottle of champagne (if you could find champagne in a collapse). The grand majority of these injuries are avoidable with a little planning. Despite this, it is likely you will come upon an eye injury at one point or another.

The most important thing to do when anyone presents to you with eye pain is a careful examination. A foreign object is the most likely cause of the problem, and it's up to you to find it. Use a moist cotton swab (Q-tip) to lift and evert the eyelid. This will allow you to effectively examine the area. An amount of clean water can be used as irrigation to flush out the foreign object. Alternatively, touch lightly with the Q-tip to dislodge it.

After assuring that there is no foreign object still present, look at the "cornea". The cornea is a clear layer of tissue over the colored part of the eye (the 'iris") which exists for purposes of protection and to help with focusing. When this layer of tissue is damaged, it is called a "corneal abrasion". This type of injury may be caused by any of the things listed earlier; as well, people who wear contact lenses are especially at risk. The patient will probably relate to you that they feel as if there's a grain of sand in their eye.

After cleaning the eye out with water and using antibiotic eye drops (if available), cover the closed eye with an eye pad and tape. Ibuprofen is useful for pain relief. Over the next few days, the eye should heal.

For prevention of corneal damage, consider the following:

- Wear eye protection whenever you're performing any activity that could possibly cause an eye injury. (carpentry, target shooting, using power tools). Eye protection isn't just for you; it's for anyone who is close to you when you're doing these activities.
- When working in the yard, watch for low hanging branches; before mowing the yard, remove loose objects in your path. Make sure that your kids never point water under force (say, from a garden hose) at someone's face.
- Put in your contact lenses carefully; don't sleep in them.
- For kids (and adults, too), keep fingernails trimmed short.
- Use a grease shield when you're using your frying pan.

Occasionally, blunt trauma to the eye or even simple actions like coughing or sneezing may cause a patch of blood to appear in the white of the eye. This is called a subconjunctival hemorrhage or "**hyphema**", and certainly can be alarming to the patient. Luckily, this type of hemorrhage is not dangerous, and will go away on its own without any treatment.

If there is a loss of vision associated with the hyphema, however, there IS cause for concern. This is most likely after an episode of blunt trauma to the area. Evaluate this injury as described for abrasions.

Keeping the patient with the head elevated will allow any blood to drain to the lower part of the eye chamber. This strategy may help preserve vision. Cool compresses applied lightly to the affected eye are also recommended.

NOSEBLEEDS AND NASAL TRAUMA

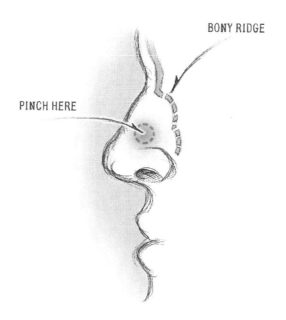

NOSE BLEED

It's a rare individual who has never had a nosebleed. The nose has many tiny blood vessels and is situated in a vulnerable position as it protrudes from the face. Nosebleeds can occur at any age, but are seen mostly in children and the elderly.

Nosebleeds can occur from outside causes, such as trauma to the face. It can also be caused by factors that affect the inside of the nose, such as excessive "picking" or irritation from upper respiratory infections. Environmental factors such as cold or dry climates may also play a role. In rare cases, underlying illness such as faulty blood clotting may be implicated as the cause.

To effectively stop a nosebleed:

- Sit upright with the head tipped slightly forward. Although you may have been taught to tilt your patient's head backward, this may just cause blood to run down the back of the throat.

- Breathe through your mouth.
- Spit out blood in the mouth and throat instead of swallowing it. Blood may irritate the stomach.
- Using your thumb and index finger, firmly pinch the soft part of the nose just below the bone. Push towards the face.
- Spray the nose with a medicated nasal spray such as oxymetazoline hydrochloride, 0.05 percent (Afrin) before applying pressure.
- Apply an ice pack to the side that is bleeding. Cold constricts the blood vessels and may help stop the bleeding.
- Apply pressure for 5-10 minutes. Be patient.
- Check to see if your patient's nose is still bleeding after 10 minutes. If still bleeding, hold it for 10 more minutes.
- Place a little petroleum jelly inside the nose.

In prolonged cases, a strip cut from Celox or Quikclot powder-impregnated gauze may be placed delicately with a blunt tweezers or Kelly clamp. Alternatively, the bleeding nostril can be flushed with sterile saline; then, gently introduce a thin strip of cloth drenched in epinephrine (from an Epi-pen or other anaphylactic shock kit) gently into the nostril. Do not remove the packing for several hours. Other commercial products such as Nasalcease or Woundseal are available and are thought to be effective; you consider them as medical storage items.

A natural hemostatic agent is geranium oil. A few drops on a strip of gauze could be placed in the bleeding nostril with good results in many cases.

Whether the bleeding is due to trauma or not, blowing the nose to eject blood and clots should be avoided, as it may restart the bleeding.

The "Broken" Nose

If there is a fracture, the patient will find that any pressure on the nose is very painful. Although it may be painful, an obvious deformity of the nose due to trauma can possibly be adjusted back into place.

Traumatic injury to the nose can result in damage to the cartilage. This may cause deformity and difficulty breathing due to swelling. Few major medical problems will result from this type of injury, but it is important to understand the best way to treat it.

First, you may choose to reduce the deformity by using both hands to straighten the cartilage. This may be appropriate as the broken nose, if deformed, will not straighten out by itself. Be aware that this may cause further damage.

You might consider taping the nose in its normal position. Then, place some ice wrapped in a cloth over the nose, for periods of 20 minutes throughout the day. This will be useful for the first 48 hours only, but will help reduce swelling and discomfort. Acetaminophen and Ibuprofen will also be helpful in this circumstance. Swelling in nasal passages may be improved with a nasal decongestant.

EARACHE

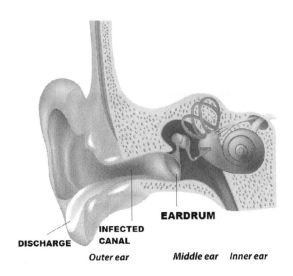

It's a rare parent who hasn't had to deal with this problem at one point or another. In some cases, it's a chronic problem that affects the quality of life of an otherwise healthy child. The most common symptom you'll see relating to the ear is pain, usually due to an infection.

The ear is divided into 3 chambers, the outer, middle and inner ear. Inflammation of the ear is called "**otitis**". The most common ear infections will be in the external and middle ear chambers.

The easiest way to prevent this is to carefully use cotton swabs moistened with rubbing alcohol to dry the ear canal after swimming or excessive sweating. Forceful use of a cotton swab, however, is to be avoided; it is, indeed, the next most common cause of ear pain. Normally, you shouldn't place anything in the ear canal sharper than, say, your elbow.

Ear Infections

Otitis Externa

Otitis Externa, also known as "**Swimmer's Ear**" is an infection of the outer ear canal, and most commonly affects children aged 4 -14 years old.

Cases peak during summer months, when most people go swimming. Bacteria will accumulate and multiply in water or sweat. Once caught in the ear canal, inflammation and discomfort ensue.

Symptoms of Otitis Externa include:

- Gradual development of an earache or, possibly, itching
- Pain worsened by pulling on the ear
- Ringing in the ears (**tinnitus**) or decreased hearing
- A "full" sensation in the ear canal with swelling and redness
- Thick drainage from the ear canal

Standard treatment may include a warm compress to the ear to help with pain control. An antibiotic/steroidal ear drop will be useful, and should be applied for 7 days. In order to get the most effect from the medicine, place the drops in the ear with the patient lying on their side. They should stay in that position for 5 minutes to completely coat the ear canal. Severe cases may be treated with oral antibiotics (such as Amoxicillin) and ibuprofen.

Otitis Media

The most common cause of earache is an infection of the middle ear, called "**otitis media**". Normally, the eardrum is shiny and grayish. When there is an infection in the middle ear canal, the eardrum will appear dull. This is because there is pus or inflammatory fluid behind it. Standard treatment often includes oral antibiotics and ibuprofen, especially in adults with the infection.

Otitis Media is most common, however, in infants and toddlers. This is why mothers are always cautioned against bottle or breast-feeding with their baby lying flat. You can expect it to present with one or more of the following:

- Pain, more so when lying down
- Difficulty sleeping, crying, and irritability
- fever
- loss of appetite
- Loss of balance

- Holding or pulling the affected ear
- Drainage of fluid from the affected ear
- Difficulty hearing from the affected ear

A number of natural remedies are available for earache. Follow this procedure:

- Mix rubbing alcohol and vinegar in equal quantities, or alternatively, hydrogen peroxide.
- Place 3-4 drops into affected ear.
- Wait 5 minutes; then, tilt head to drain out the mixture.
- Next, use either plain warm olive oil, or add 1 drop of any one of these essential oils to 2 ounces of the olive oil: tea tree, eucalyptus, peppermint, thyme, lavender, garlic, mullein.
- Warm the olive oil slightly and place 2-3 drops into the ear canal. This does not have to be drained or removed.
- A cotton ball with 2 drops of eucalyptus oil may be secured to the ear opening during sleep.

Some patients find a heat source soothing to a painful ear. If you are in a collapse situation, dip a sock or other absorbent material into heated water. Wring it out and place it on the outside of the affected ear.

Other ear problems

Inner ear canal issues often cause dizziness, also known as "**vertigo**". Oftentimes, it is caused by an inflammation known as **Otitis Interna**. These patients commonly feel nauseous as well as dizzy. Treatment with diazepam (Valium) or Dimenhydrinate (Dramamine) can help with symptoms. Amoxicillin (veterinary equivalent: Fish-Mox Forte) 500mg three times a day for 7 days is an appropriate antibiotic therapy if the otitis was caused by an infection.

Ear wax, also known as "**cerumen**" is a chronic problem for certain people. Cerumen is normal and protective in healthy ears. It traps dust particles before they can reach the ear drum.

Normally, people use cotton swabs to remove ear wax, but this method often pushes ear wax further in. Cleaning the opening of the ear canal with a twisted moist washcloth is safer.

When, for whatever reason, cerumen is lodged against the eardrum, it can affect hearing. Other symptoms include:

- Earache
- Hearing loss
- Itching
- Odor or discharge
- Ringing in the ear (also called "**tinnitus**")

Commercial ear rinses with special syringes are available for treatment. Standard home remedies involve a few drops of mineral or baby oil in the ear. This softens the wax, which can then be flushed out with 3% hydrogen peroxide. Some just use the hydrogen peroxide by itself.

Using an Otoscope

Evaluation of the ear canal is performed with a special instrument known as an "**otoscope**". Always hold the otoscope in the left hand if you're looking in the left ear, the right hand for the right ear. Holding the otoscope like you would a hammer seems to work best for me, as it allows me to gently rest my knuckles against the side of the head. Alternatively, you could hold the otoscope as you would a pencil.

The external ear canal is about 2-5cm long in adults, shorter in kids. In children, it's relatively straight; in adults, it is not, so you will need to pull the fleshy part of the ear (the "**pinna**") upwards and backwards to get a better view of the ear drum (also known as the "**tympanic membrane**").

If using the otoscope on a child, always start by explaining what you're doing, and that it might feel "weird", but shouldn't hurt. Choose an otoscope end attachment (called a "speculum") of appropriate size for a child. They often come in sets of different sizes.

Examine the normal ear first. This will allow you to see what the normal anatomy looks like and also will prevent your transferring the infection from the infected ear to the healthy one. Be sure to have the light at high intensity.

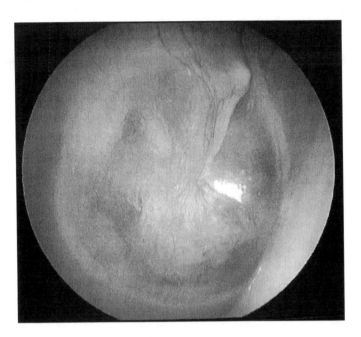

Normal Eardrum

You will first see the external canal wall. Is there redness or swellness compared to the normal ear? Is there debris, excessive wax, or even a foreign object? Don't be surprised if you see hair; this is normal.

Now look at the eardrum at the end of the canal. A normal eardrum will appear pearly gray, shiny, and generally transparent. A yellowish color to the eardrum usually indicates fluid behind it; in the worst cases, the eardrum will appear to bulge out towards you.

HEMORRHOIDS

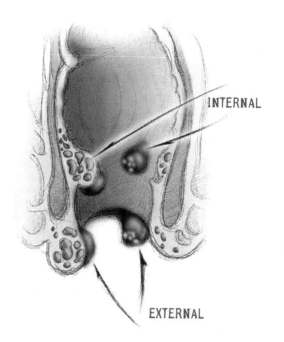

INTERNAL

EXTERNAL

HEMORRHOIDS

Hemorrhoids are painful, swollen veins in the lower portion of the rectum that often protrude from the anus. They are thought to be caused from pressure due to the human trait of standing on two legs; animals that walk on four legs rarely get them. Another likely cause a low fiber diet causing excessively hard stool. This causes straining during bowel movements which may increase the risk of hemorrhoids.

Hemorrhoids are extremely common during pregnancy and are usually asymptomatic unless they develop a clot ("**thrombosis**") and become inflamed. Once they become thrombosed, they cause a constant pain that will make it difficult to carry out activities of daily survival (or even sit down).

THE SURVIVAL MEDICINE HANDBOOK

Hemorrhoids may be internal or external. Symptoms of hemorrhoids include:

- Anal itching.
- Bleeding, usually seen on toilet tissue.
- Pain, worse in the sitting position.
- Pain during bowel movements
- Painful bumps near the anus.

Diagnosis is easily made simply by looking at the area. They will appear as a bluish lump at the edge of the anal opening. Some hemorrhoids develop inside the anal canal, and may be difficult to spot. A rectal exam will make the diagnosis in this case.

Hemorrhoids only require treatment when symptomatic. Treatments for hemorrhoids include:

- Mild corticosteroid creams such as Anusol-HC or wipes such as Tucks pads to help reduce pain and swelling
- Stool softeners to decrease further trauma to the inflamed tissue.
- Witch Hazel compresses to reduce itching.
- Warm water baths (known as "Sitz baths" to reduce general discomfort.

Even painful hemorrhoids will usually go away by themselves over a few weeks, but sometimes the discomfort is so severe that you may be required to remove the clot from the swollen vein. This is performed by incising the skin over the hemorrhoid and draining the clotted blood.

A scalpel may be used (preferably under local anesthesia) to incise the hemorrhoid after cleaning the area thoroughly with Betadine. Cut just deep enough to evacuate the clot. The patient should experience quick relief as a result Gauze pads should be placed at the site to absorb any bleeding. Be prepared to suture the incision site if the bleeding is heavy.

It should be noted that this procedure is not the best way to remove a hemorrhoid, as simple incision does not remove it in its entirety. It may come back at a later time. Modern procedures, such as placing bands around the hemorrhoid, are less traumatic and more permanent in their results, but will not be available in a collapse situation.

442 SECTION 8 *OTHER IMPORTANT MEDICAL ISSUES*

BIRTH CONTROL, PREGNANCY, AND DELIVERY

It's a rare individual that doesn't have a wife, girlfriend, mother, daughter or granddaughter that isn't of childbearing age (say 13 to 50 years old). Even if they aren't related to you personally, they could be in your survival group. Remember that, even if you have a daughter that's only 5 years old now, one day she will come of reproductive age.

In a collapse situation, society will be unstable and organized medical care will be spotty at best and nonexistent at worst. If we reach the point that we lose our access to modern healthcare, one of the least welcome events might be one that, for many families, is ordinarily considered a blessing: A pregnancy.

In a long-term survival situation, the normal view would be that we have the responsibility to repopulate the world. This is absolutely true further down the road, but first your family must survive. Until things settle down, a pregnancy and the possible complications that accompany it will be a burden.

So why is it important to prevent pregnancies in the early going of a societal collapse? The death rate among pregnant women (also known as the Maternal Mortality Rate) at the time of the American Revolution was about 2-4% PER PREGNANCY. Given that the average woman in the year 1800 could expect 6-10 pregnancies over the course of her reproductive life, the cumulative Maternal Mortality Rate easily approached 25 per cent. That means that 1 out of 4 women died due to complications of being pregnant, either early, during the childbirth, or even soon after a successful delivery.

If a major disaster occurs, women might face unacceptable levels of risk. There won't be either medicine or medical supplies in which to treat pregnancy and childbirth complications. Deaths may happen simply because there are no IV fluids or medications to stop bleeding or treat infection.

These tragedies would happen at a time when we will need every member of our survival group to be productive individuals. Growing food, managing livestock, perimeter defense, and caring for children will take the energy of all involved. When a pregnancy goes wrong, it takes away a valuable contributor from the survival family (sometimes permanently) and places an additional strain on resources and manpower.

Pregnancy Complications

Let's discuss some of the reasons that women could cease to become productive group members (or even die) during pregnancy or childbirth:

Hyperemesis Gravidarum

Simply put, this is medical-speak for excessive vomiting during pregnancy. Almost every woman will experience nausea and vomiting in the early stages. A small percentage of them, however, have an exaggerated response to the hormones of pregnancy that causes them to vomit so much that they become dehydrated. Since they can't maintain a reasonable fluid intake, intravenous hydration is required. As a practicing obstetrician for 25 years, it seemed to me that I always had someone in the hospital with this condition.

How many survival groups will have access to IV equipment and the know-how to institute IV fluid therapy? One of my hobbies is collecting old medical books, most of them from at least 100 years ago (in other words, where we will be medically if a collapse occurs). When these books discuss Hyperemesis Gravidarum, they relate death rates in 10% to 40% in severe cases!

Miscarriage

The human race is not perfect, and we don't always produce perfect pregnancies. Approximately 10% of all pregnancies end in miscarriage. When a woman miscarries, many times she will not pass all of the dead tissue relating to the pregnancy. On occasion, this tissue will become infected or cause excessive bleeding.

The treatment in this case would be something called a **dilatation and curettage** (D & C), which is a procedure that use scrapers called curettes to remove the retained tissue. This will stop the bleeding and prevent infection. Again, how may survival groups have the ability and knowledge to perform this procedure or have access to the antibiotics necessary to treat possible infection?

Hypertension

There is a condition known as Pregnancy-Induced Hypertension. When a woman reaches the last month of a pregnancy (usually her first baby), she might begin to have elevated blood pressures that cause extreme swelling (called edema). Normal pregnancy causes swollen ankles, but pregnancy-induced hypertension swells up the entire body, including the face. Left untreated, this condition leads to seizures and can be life-threatening. If a collapse situation happens, the only treatment available would be bed rest, which at best takes away a productive member of your group, and at worst may fail to prevent a worsening of the condition.

Childbirth Complications

Let's say the pregnancy itself was uncomplicated. The birth process, while usually perfectly natural and routine, could also present some dangers. Every childbirth, for example, involves some bleeding. It could be a little; it could be a lot. It could be caused by lacerations from the passage of the infant through the vaginal canal or from a stubborn **placenta** (afterbirth) that does not expel itself spontaneously.

When childbirth is associated with excessive bleeding, certain procedures and maneuvers are performed by trained midwives or obstetricians to stop the hemorrhage. When hemorrhage occurs and no trained individuals are present at the birth, the bleeding may not stop before major damage has been done to the mother.

In some cases, it's necessary to actually reach into a woman's uterus, grab the placenta and remove it. This procedure is performed when part of the placenta is "retained". If a portion of the placenta is "stuck" and not spontaneously expelled after birth, this tissue will prevent the uterus from contracting. Uterine contractions are the natural way that bleeding stops. Therefore, excessive bleeding may occur.

Of course, retained tissue could become infected, also. Does your group have the knowledge, equipment and medications that might be needed to safely get your women through childbirth?

Complications After Childbirth

Conditions in the delivery room after a societal collapse could be conducive to the development of infections, even if the delivery goes without a hitch. This was a major cause of maternal mortality before modern medical care and antibiotics became available.

Other problems may manifest themselves in the "**postpartum**" period, the first days to weeks after the baby is born. For example, a woman who has a hemorrhage during childbirth could be so weakened by anemia that she is unable to return to normal activities for a very long time.

I don't want everyone to think that all women will die during, or right after, their pregnancy. I'm only saying that not all survival groups have prepared to obtain the knowledge, resources, and ability to deal with the complications that could occur. Also, if people are rioting in the streets and your garden isn't doing so well yet, do you really need to add a newborn baby to your list of responsibilities?

How To Prevent Pregnancy

So, what's your plan? Even long-time Preppers haven't spent much time figuring out what birth control method they will use in a collapse situation. Have you included condoms or other birth control method in your bug-out bag? The majority have not, so congratulations if you did. That means you've thought about more than just beans and bullets.

It's important to have **condoms** in your storage, but condoms can break; even if they don't, they won't last forever. With spermicide, condoms expire after 2 years; without spermicide, perhaps at most 5 years. **Diaphragms**, another common method in which a woman places a rubber or latex barrier over her cervix, require chemical spermicides and will also become brittle over time.

Some women use IUDs (**intrauterine devices**) to prevent pregnancy. Some of these use hormones that wear off over time. They must be inserted into the body of the uterus, something best done by someone with experience to prevent injury.

Birth control pills are useful, but are difficult to get more than a few months' supply at any one time. Insurance companies tightly control when women can get their next pack of pills. Some offer 3 month's supply at a time, but you still have to wait until the end of those 3 months to get more. Even if you could get them, they cost a bundle if purchased outside of insurance plans. The cost of stockpiling several years' worth these can be difficult for the average person.

Natural Birth Control Methods

Some advocate the use of lemon or lime juice as a douche prior to intercourse. The high acid content is thought to be lethal to sperm. Others consider using a slice of lemon or lime as a "cap" in the vagina during the act of intercourse.

It's important to know that these methods are NOT effective if used after the sexual act, as multitudes of sperm have already entered the cervix and are well on their way to performing their duty . Be aware that some women will experience some irritation preventing pregnancy in this manner.

There is no commercial or even herbal contraceptive that is 100% effective and is guaranteed to have no side effects. Therefore, the best strategy is to predict, as accurately as possible, fertile parts of the cycle and plan to be abstinent or especially careful during these times.

To make these predictions, we will have to go back to a traditional form of birth control: **Natural Family Planning** (the modern version of the Rhythm Method). Although not as effective in preventing pregnancy as the Pill, it is up to 90% effective if implemented correctly. There is no need to put hormones into your system and no side effects. Natural Family Planning is a time-honored strategy to prevent pregnancy that fits in well with any collapse strategy.

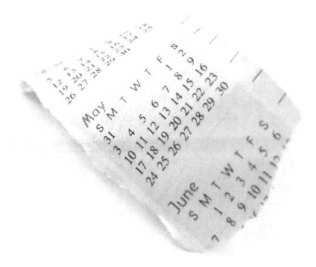

This method involves trying to figure out your fertile period and avoiding unprotected intercourse during that time. This method works best on women who have relatively regular cycles. Cycles are predictable if a woman releases an egg for fertilization (this is called "**ovulation**") on a regular basis.

If you or your partner has 28 day menstrual cycles, you can bet that ovulation is occurring. A pregnancy is likely in any couple having regular sexual relations. So likely, in fact, that 80-85% of couples can expect a pregnancy within the first year of a collapse situation if not careful. The egg will disintegrate in 24-48 hours, however, if not fertilized.

You can tell the day that you or your partner is ovulating by doing a little research. This involves, in part, taking your temperature with a thermometer daily for a cycle or two. There are actually special thermometers that are used for this purpose called **Basal Body Temperature** Thermometers, although I would think that any thermometer that goes up by 1/10 degree increments would suffice (e.g., 98.1, 98.2, 98.3 degrees Fahrenheit). Make certain to take temperatures daily at the same time, preferably before you get out of bed in the morning. This might be problematic during a survival situation, so consider performing this calculation PRIOR to a catastrophe.

When you ovulate, your basal body temperature goes up about half a degree and stays up until the next period. Make a graph or chart of the

BIRTH CONTROL, PREGNANCY, AND DELIVERY

daily temperatures and you'll see a pattern develop. Always count Day #1 as the first day of menstrual bleeding to start with. It should be noted that this method will work only with those women who have regular cycles.

Once you've done this for a few cycles, you will have a good idea about when you or your partner is at risk for getting pregnant. A common physical symptom that goes along with this: Many women will notice some one-sided discomfort in the lower abdomen when they ovulate.

Let's say that you or your partner has 28 day cycles and that the temperature rise occurs around day 14. You should avoid having unprotected sexual intercourse from about day 10 - day 18 (a few days prior and a few days after the likely day of ovulation). If ovulation occurs later, say day 16, just move the "danger" period over to day 12 - day 20. Ovulation may occur a couple of days earlier or later in any one cycle, so you want to have a margin of error in determining the time period eligible for fertilization.

Observing the cyclical changes in cervical mucus is a useful adjunct. The **cervical mucus method** is based on observation of the character of cervical mucus during the course of the menstrual cycle. Before ovulation,

To use this method, it's important to understand how cervical secretions change during a typical menstrual cycle. Generally, you'll see:

- Little or no cervical secretions for several days after each period.
- Sticky, thick secretions for the next few days.
- Copious clear and watery mucus as ovulation occurs.
- A thicker and less quantity of cervical secretions until the period ends.

Cervical mucus when not ovulating will be thick; spreading your fingers will cause it to snap. During ovulation, spreading two mucus-laden fingers will cause the watery mucus to stretch significantly before breaking.

As evaluating your cervical mucus involves placing your finger deep inside the vagina all the way to the cervix, make sure you have washed your hands thoroughly and have an ample supply of gloves. Nitrile gloves are preferable to avoid reactions in those women allergic to latex.

Performed correctly, the Natural Family Planning method is an effective and completely natural way to prevent pregnancy. In a collapse, it will allow you to decide when things are stable enough to bring a newborn into the world.

Pregnancy Care Basics

Despite all the best efforts made to prevent pregnancy, the best laid plans of mice and men sometimes go awry. Whether by accident or on purpose, you may find yourself responsible for the care of a pregnant woman. It will be important to know how to support that pregnancy and, eventually, deliver that baby.

In a survival situation, you won't have access to ultrasound technology to take a look at the fetus; whether it's a boy or a girl will once again become a mystery. Even twins might be a surprise.

Without prenatal mega-vitamins, babies will be smaller at birth. This may also not be so bad, since Caesarean Section will no longer available. It's less traumatic for the mother to deliver a 6 or 7 pound baby than a 10 pounder.

Despite all the possible complications that I mentioned in the previous section, pregnancy is still a natural process. It usually proceeds without major complications and ends in the delivery of a normal baby. Although your pregnant patient will not be as productive for the survival group as she would ordinarily be, she will probably still be able to contribute to help make your efforts a success. To make a pregnancy a success, the medic will need to have a little knowledge of the subject and an idea of how to deliver the fetus.

We are, of course, fortunate to have simple tests that can identify pregnancy almost before your miss a period. What if these tests are no longer available? You will have to rely on the following tried and true signs and symptoms to identify the condition:

- Absent menstruation
- Tender Breasts
- Nausea and Vomiting

- Darkening of the Nipples/Areola
- Fatigue
- Frequent Urination
- Backache

These symptoms, in combination, are indicative of pregnancy. The timing of each will be variable; some will be noticed earlier than others. It should be noted that this investigation will likely be necessary only in those women experiencing their first pregnancy. Once you have been pregnant, you will most likely know when it happens again.

Of course, as time goes on, the abdominal swelling associated with uterine and fetal growth will be undeniable. Stretch marks come later, as do hemorrhoids, backache, and varicose veins (all very common but not universal). These changes are part and parcel of the average healthy pregnancy. Most of the above will improve after the pregnancy is over, but may not disappear completely.

So, what's the due date? This is the question everyone will want answered once a pregnancy is identified. A human pregnancy lasts 280 days or 40 weeks from the first day of the last menstrual period to the estimated date of delivery. This used to be called the "estimated date of confinement" because, yes, they confined women to their beds as they approached it.

This date is simple to calculate if you have regular monthly periods. To get the **due date**, subtract 3 months and add 7 days to the first day of the last period. Example: If the first day of last menstrual period (LMP) is 9/7, then the due date is 6/14.

If the woman does not know when her last cycle started, you can still estimate the age of the pregnancy by physical signs. When you gently press on the woman's abdomen, you will notice a firm area (the uterus) and a soft area (the intestines). Identify the uppermost level of firmness, and you will able to estimate the approximate age of the pregnancy.

If the "lump" is peaking just over the pubic bone, you're at 12 weeks. Halfway between the pubic bone and the belly button is 16 weeks. At the belly button is 20 weeks. Each centimeter above the belly button adds a week, so have a measuring tape handy. A term pregnancy will measure 36-40 centimeters from the pubic bone to the top of the uterus.

Twins, as you might imagine, will throw all of these measurements out the window. They will occur in 1 in 60 births, more often if there is a family history. Don't worry about triplets: They occur in only 1 in 7,000 births, unless you use fertility drugs.

Once you have identified the pregnancy, you should make every effort to assure that your patient is getting proper nutrition. Deficiencies can affect the development of the fetus, so obtaining essential vitamins and iron through the diet will give the best chance to avoid complications. If you have stockpiled prenatal vitamins, use them.

Common early pregnancy issues will include **hyperemesis**, as described in the last section. Be sure to ask your physician for prescriptions for Zofran (ondansetron) and/or other anti-nausea medications to add to your stockpile. Hyperemesis will disappear in almost all women as they advance in the pregnancy. Dry bland foods, like crackers, are helpful in getting a woman through this stage. Ginger tea is a time-honored home remedy to decrease "**morning sickness**".

Another early pregnancy issue is the **threatened miscarriage**. This will be characterized by bleeding or spotting from the vagina, along with pain that simulates menstrual cramps. As 10% of pregnancies end in miscarriage and a higher percentage threaten to, this will be an issue that you must know how to deal with.

Other than placing your patient on bed rest, there will not be much you'll be able to do in this circumstance. Some of these pregnancies don't continue because the fetus is abnormal, and no amount of rest will stop many of these pregnancies from ending very early. The good thing is that a single miscarriage generally does not mean that future pregnancies will be unsuccessful.

Keep a close eye out for evidence of infection, such as fever or a foul discharge from the vagina. Women with these symptoms would benefit from antibiotic therapy.

Pregnant women should be evaluated periodically to see how the fetus is progressing. Besides verifying progressive growth in the size of the uterus, the fetal heartbeat should be audible via stethoscope at around 16-18 weeks, or much earlier if you have a functioning battery-powered fetal heart monitor (also called a Doppler ultrasound). These are available for sale online. Your exams should be more frequent as the pregnancy advances.

Weight gain is desirable during pregnancy; you should shoot for 25 pounds or so, total. Blood pressure should be taken regularly to rule out pregnancy-induced hypertension. Elevated blood pressures behoove you to place your patient on bed rest. Lying on the left side will keep her blood pressure at its lowest. Check for evidence of edema (swelling of the feet, legs and face) as well as excessive weight gain).

Delivery

As the woman approaches her due date, several things will happen. The fetus will begin to "drop", assuming a position deep in the pelvis. The patient's abdomen may look different, or the top of the uterus (the "**fundus**") may appear lower. As the neck of the uterus (**the cervix**) relaxes, the patient may notice a mucus-like discharge, sometimes with a bloody component. This is referred to as the "**bloody show**" and is usually a sign that things will be happening soon.

If you examine your patient vaginally by gently inserting two fingers of a gloved hand, you'll notice the cervix is firm like your nose when it is not ripe and soft like your lips when the due date is approaching. This softening of the cervix is called "**effacement**". As time goes on, the sides of the cervix will thin out until they are as thin as paper.

Dilation of the cervical opening will be slow at first, and speed up once you reach about 3-4 cm. At this level of dilation, you will be able to place two (normal-sized) fingertips in the cervix and feel something firm; this is the baby's head. Frequent vaginal exams are invasive, however, and not necessary in most cases.

Contractions will start becoming more frequent. To identify a contraction, feel the skin on the soft area of your cheek, and then touch your forehead. A contraction will feel like your forehead. False labor, or Braxton-Hicks contractions, will be irregular and will abate with bed rest, especially on the left side, and hydration. If contractions are coming faster and more furious even with bed rest and hydration, it may just be time to have a baby! A gush of watery fluid from the vagina will often signify "**breaking the water**", and is also a sign of impending labor and delivery. The timing will be highly variable.

The delivery of a baby is best accomplished with the help of an experienced midwife or obstetrician, but those professionals will be hard to find in a collapse situation. If there is no chance of accessing modern medical care, it will be up to you to perform the delivery.

To get ready for delivery, wash your hands and then put gloves on. Then, set up clean sheets so that there will be the least contamination possible. Tuck a sheet under the mother's buttocks and spread it on your lap so that the baby, which comes out very slippery, will land onto the sheet instead of landing on the floor if you lose your grip on it. Place a towel on the mother's belly; this is where the baby will go once it is delivered. It will be very important to dry the baby and wrap it in the towel, as newborns lose heat very quickly. Newborns are also susceptible to infection, so avoid touching anything but mother and baby if you can.

As the labor progresses, the baby's head will move down the birth canal and the vagina will begin to bulge. When the baby's head begins to become visible, it is called "**crowning**". If the water has not yet broken (which can happen even at this late stage), the lining of the bag of water will appear as a slick gray surface. Some pressure on the membrane will rupture it, which is okay at this point. It might help the process along.

To make space, place two gloved fingers along the edge of the vagina by the "**perineum**". This is the area between the vagina and anus. Using gentle pressure, move your fingers from side to side. This will stretch the area somewhat to give the baby a little more room to come out.

With each contraction, the baby's head will come out a little more. Don't be concerned if it goes back in a little after the contraction. It will make steady progress and more and more of the head will become visible. Encourage the mother to help by taking a deep breath with each contraction and then pushing while slowly exhaling.

On occasion, a small cut is made in the bottom of the edge of the vagina to make room for the baby to be delivered. This is called an "**episiotomy**". I discourage this if at all possible, as the cut has to be sutured afterward. I always make this decision as the head is crowning; I will only perform an episiotomy if I believe a very large, jagged tear will occur that would damage the anal sphincter or rectum.

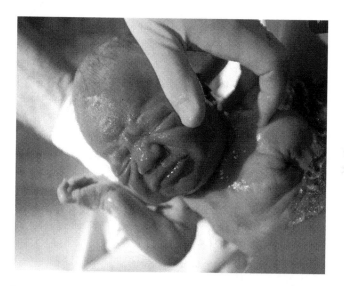

As the baby's head emerges, it will usually face straight down or up, and then turn to the side. The cord might appear to be wrapped around its neck. If this is the case, gently slip the cord over the baby's head. In cases where the cord is very tight and is preventing delivery, you may choose to doubly clamp it and cut between. This will release the tension and make delivery easier.

Next, gently hold each side of the baby's head and apply gentle traction straight down. This will help the top shoulder out of the birth canal. Occasionally, steady gentle pressure on the top of the uterus during a contraction may be required if the mother is exhausted. Many times, however, little if any help will be needed for the baby to deliver, (especially in a woman who has had children before). Once the shoulders are out, the baby will deliver with one last push. The mother can now rest.

Put the baby immediately on the mother's belly and clean out its nose and mouth with a bulb syringe. It will usually begin crying, which is a good sign that it is a vigorous infant. Spanking the baby's bottom to get it to cry is rarely needed, and is more of a cliché than anything else. A better way to stimulate a baby to cry is to rub the baby's back.

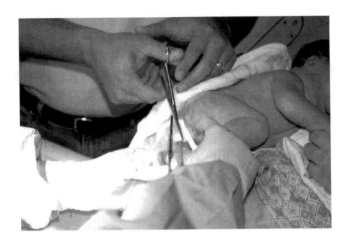

Dry the baby and wrap it up in a small towel or blanket. At this point, you may clamp the cord twice (2 inches apart) with Kelly or Umbilical clamps, and cut in between with a scissors. There is no hurry to perform this procedure. By the way, delivery kits are available online with everything you need, including drapes, clamps, bulb syringes, etc.

Once the baby has delivered, it's the placenta's turn. Be patient: In most cases, the placenta will deliver by itself in a few minutes. Pulling on the umbilical cord to force the placenta out is usually a bad idea. Breaking the cord due to excessive traction will require your placing your hand deep in the uterus to extract it. This is traumatic and can introduce infection. You can ask the mother to give a push when it's clear the placenta is almost out.

If traction is necessary for some reason, place your fingers above the pubic bone and press as you apply mild traction. This will prevent the uterus being turned inside out (a potentially life-threatening situation) if the placenta is stubborn. A moderate amount of bleeding is not unusual after delivery of the afterbirth.

Once the placenta is out, examine it. The "fetal" surface is grey and shiny; turn it inside out and you will see the "maternal" surface, which look like a rough version of liver. The fetal surface is separated into compartments called "**cotyledons**". If a portion of the placenta remains inside, you may have to extract it manually.

The uterus (the top of which is now around the level of the belly button) contracts to control bleeding naturally. In a long labor, the uterus may be as tired as the mother after delivery, and may be slow to contract. As a result, this may cause excessive bleeding. Gentle massage of the top of the uterus (known as the "fundus") will get it firm again and thus limit blood loss. You may have to do this from time to time during the first 24 hours or so after delivery.

Monitor the mother closely for excessive bleeding over the next few days. In normal situations, the bleeding will become more and more watery as time progresses. This is normal. Also, keep an eye out for evidence of fever, foul discharge or other issues.

Place the baby on the mother's breast soon after delivery. This will begin the secretion of "**colostrum**", a clear yellow liquid rich in substances that will increase the baby's resistance to infection. Suckling also causes the uterus to contract; this is also a factor in decreasing blood loss.

It should be noted that there are different schools of thought regarding some of the above. Remember that your goal is to have an end result of a healthy mother and baby, both physically and emotionally.

ANXIETY AND DEPRESSION

If we ever find ourselves in the midst of a societal upheaval, it goes without saying that we will experience epidemics of both anxiety and depression. The stress of living off the grid will be (for most) a wrenching emotional roller-coaster. As such, an effective medic will have to be skilled in identifying those with the condition, and doing everything possible to support and treat the patient.

The stability of your survival community is dependent on the stability of its members. Be mindful of group dynamics, and work to foster a sense of common purpose and caring. Those medics who can accomplish this goal will have the most well-adjusted and stable patient population.

Anxiety

It is a rare individual who will not experience significant anxiety when deprived of the benefits of modern civilization. Anxiety is really a hodgepodge of related symptoms, so sufferers may present to you quite differently from one another. The symptoms may be mostly emotional, mostly physical or some combination of both. Here are the various things you may notice:

Emotional Symptoms:

- Irrational fear
- Difficulty concentrating
- Jumpiness
- Extreme pessimism
- Irritability
- Mental paralysis/Inability to act
- Inability to stand still

Physical Symptoms:

- Shortness of breath
- Palpitations (rapid pulse)
- Perspiration

- Upset stomach/diarrhea
- Tremors/tics/twitches
- Tense muscles
- Headache
- Insomnia

Acute anxiety attacks, also known as "**panic attacks**", may occur without warning and are characterized by intense feelings of fear and impending doom. Panic attacks are usually short-lived but severe enough that a person may feel what they believe to be physical chest pain. These patients, usually young adults, will appear to be hyperventilating and may complain of chest pain or feeling faint. Patients with panic attacks have some classic complaints:

- Chest pain
- Choking sensation
- Feeling they are in a unreal or surreal environment
- Feeling the walls close in on them ("claustrophobic")
- Nausea or strange "pit of the stomach" feelings
- Hot flashes (sensations of heat and flushing)

Panic attacks may last an hour or more in severe cases, but a single episode will usually resolve without medication. Despite this, the most successful treatment of frequent attacks appears to come from a combination of medications/supplements (both anti-anxiety and anti-depressant) and behavioral therapy.

Unless your patient had a history of anxiety problems pre-collapse, you won't have stockpiled many anti-anxiety medications like Xanax. As such, you should look to your medicinal herb garden for plants that may have an effect. Alternative therapies include massage therapy combined with herbs such as Valerian, Kava, Lavender, Chamomile, and Passionflower. Any herb with a mild sedative effect might be of use.

Essential oils used as aromatherapy may also be helpful:

- Bergamot
- Cypress

- Geranium
- Jasmine
- Lavender
- Rose
- Sandalwood

Essential oils of lavender, frankincense, geranium, and chamomile are versatile and can be used as direct inhalation therapy or for topical use. Just rub the oil between your hands and bring them up to your nose and slowly inhale. For topical use, a 50/50 mixture of essential oil with a carrier oil (such as olive) will be beneficial when applied on temples, neck and shoulders twice a day.

A multitude of teas are known to be especially helpful in people with anxiety disorders. The following are all reported to have a calming effect and help with sleep:

Catnip
Valerian root
Fennel
Passionflower
Ginseng
Lemon balm
Mullein
Peppermint
Lavender
Verbena

Drink the tea warm with honey, 1 cup three times daily, as needed.

Perhaps most importantly, you will have to treat your anxious patient with good counseling technique. When you have an honest conversation with your anxious group member, listen calmly and attentively. Ask them to tell you exactly what they're worrying about, and then have them write those concerns down on paper. Sometimes just the act of acknowledging their fears and seeing them in black and white will result in an improvement of the condition. Your validation and support will also earn you something very important: Trust.

There will items on their list that relate to the uncertainty of their current situation. Inform them that there is always some uncertainty in life, both in good times and bad times. Try to convince them that dwelling on those issues will not make things any less uncertain, but WILL prevent them from functioning normally.

Convince your patient to set aside just a short part of their day to concentrate on their worries with their list in hand. Keep that time period limited, say 20 minutes or so, and then have them resolve to think less of their fears the rest of the day.

Work to improve your patient's quality of life. You can do this by:

- Assuring good nutrition
- Reducing substances such as nicotine, caffeine, and alcohol
- Encouraging exercise and constructive activities
- Promoting rest breaks and good sleep habits
- Instituting sessions for relaxation therapy (meditation, massage, and deep breathing are examples)

Depression

Many people with anxiety disorders also suffer from depression. Since depression makes anxiety worse (and vice versa), it's important to have strategies to treat both conditions. In a collapse, things may be so bad that everyone is depressed to one degree or another.

This response to the strain of a survival situation is understandable, and is referred to as "**situational depression**". Their circumstances are what have made them depressed, not some misfiring of neural cells in their brain as in some other cases. Some depression is cyclical, relating to, for example, a woman's menstrual cycle or the time of the year. Like anxiety, there are a number of symptoms that are commonly seen in various combinations:

- Feelings of hopelessness or inadequacy
- Apathy
- Change in Appetite
- Weight loss or gain

- Irritability (especially common in men)
- Exhaustion
- Reckless behavior
- Difficulty concentrating on tasks
- Aches and pains (without clear physical cause)

Severe cases of depression are marked by inability to get out of bed in the morning and even thoughts of suicide. Various medications known as "**antidepressants**" are available on the market; these include Prozac, Zoloft, and Paxil, among others.

Unfortunately, they will be unlikely to be in your medical supplies unless a member of your group already suffers from chronic depression. As such, you must look to alternatives.

Vitamin supplements like B12, Folic Acid, Tryptophan, and Omega-3 antioxidants may be effective in some sufferers. St. John's Wort has been used with some success, but is not to be used on pregnant women or children. As with anxiety, you, as healthcare provider, will have to depend on your counseling skills to aid your patient.

In situational depression as will be seen in a collapse situation, you would return to many of the techniques used to treat anxiety:

- Assuring good nutrition
- Reducing substances such as nicotine, caffeine, and alcohol
- Encouraging exercise and constructive activities
- Promoting rest breaks and good sleep habits
- Instituting relaxation techniques (meditation, massage, deep breathing)

Additionally, it will be especially important to make sure your people cultivate supportive relationships with each other. People who are depressed often feel very alone. You must work to foster a sense of community; this with provide strength to your emotionally weakened members.

Make sure to accentuate the positive, even in the little things. Encourage each member of your group to share their feelings with the

ANXIETY AND DEPRESSION

others. Group meetings for this purpose will encourage communication and bonding in the survival group. Incorporate these meetings as a regular event in your community.

You might have read about **Post-Traumatic Stress Syndrome** (PTSD). This condition affects many who are exposed to stressful events like sexual assault, combat, or natural disasters. Relapses are common and can last for years.

Oftentimes, the patient will re-experience traumatic events mentally; they may become agitated and, sometimes, uncontrollable. Anger, insomnia, decreased work performance, and apathy are common manifestations. Although anxiety is a component of PTSD, anti-anxiety medications do not seem to help as much as anti-depressants. Follow the treatment guidelines previously discussed for depression.

The success of your survival group will depend greatly on your ability to spot emotional issues before the situation deteriorates. Once out of control, these conditions will damage the cohesion necessary to succeed in an adverse environment. Close observation and quick intervention are skills as important to develop as any specific technical skill in a collapse.

SLEEP DEPRIVATION

As a practicing obstetrician in the early part of my medical career, I can tell you that delivering babies at 4 a.m. is not conducive to a good sleep pattern. Lack of sleep is called "**sleep deprivation**", and can be an acute or chronic condition. In a survival situation, you can imagine the many reasons why you might suffer from not enough sleep: Unfamiliar environments, increased responsibilities, fatigue from strenuous activities, and just plain old stress will combine to greatly increase the incidence of this medical issue.

Sleep deprivation can significantly impair your brain's function. There are significant negative effects on alertness and performance which are likely due to a decrease in activity in certain areas of the brain involved in higher thought processes. As a result, you may become incapable of putting events into the proper perspective and taking appropriate action.

This makes you a poor addition to a survival group. It stands to reason that many car crashes and industrial accidents are, at least in part, caused by lack of sleep. Indeed, the National Highway Traffic Safety Administration confirms that over 100,000 serious traffic accidents a year are caused by sleeping at the wheel. The British Medical Journal equates 17-21 hours without sleep as the equivalent of a blood alcohol level of .05 – .08%.

When you don't get enough sleep, healing is delayed and the increased amount of muscle activity (from not resting) leads to the equivalent of physical overexertion. In a 2004 study that evaluated the performance of medical residents, those getting less than 4 hours of sleep made twice the medical errors that residents who slept 7-8 hours a night. As I can tell you from personal experience, very few residents have the luxury of 7-8 hours of sleep on a regular basis. This is especially dangerous: Chronically sleep-deprived individuals often don't realize that they are functioning at an impaired level.

In addition to what's happening in your brain, the failure to get 7-8 hours of sleep every night causes many of the following signs and symptoms:

- Irritability
- Depression
- Tremors
- Bloodshot, puffy eyes
- Headaches
- Confusion
- Memory loss
- Muscle aches
- Hallucinations and other psychotic symptoms
- Ill effects on control of diabetes and high blood pressure
- Blackouts (also called "microsleeps")
- Weight loss or gain

Actual brain damage has been documented in a number of studies, the most prominent being the one performed by the University of California in 2002. Using animal subjects, it showed that non-rapid eye movement sleep (deep sleep) is necessary for turning off brain chemicals called "**neurotransmitters**" and allowing their receptors to replenish.

The lack of deep sleep impairs mood and decreases learning ability. Deep sleep is also important to allow natural enzymes to repair damage caused by "**free radicals**", molecules responsible for aging and tissue damage. The study also found that lack of rapid eye movement sleep (dreaming) worsens depression. Depressed patients have depleted amounts of neurotransmitters in the brain, and sleep deprivation worsens this condition.

The treatment of sleep deprivation depends on the cause. The best start is to consider a concept we'll call "**sleep hygiene**". Sleep hygiene is adjusting your behavior to maximize the amount of restful sleep you get. Consider:

- Adhering to a standard bedtime (and wakeup time)
- Making your environment as comfortable as possible
- Avoiding Nicotine, Caffeine, and Alcohol before going to bed.

- Exercising regularly, but not before going to bed
- Eliminating as much light as possible in the room at bedtime
- Staying away from heavy foods for at least 2 hours before going to sleep
- Keeping your mind clear of stressful issues at bedtime

As you can imagine, some of this may be difficult in collapse scenarios, so do your best now to improve your sleep hygiene beforehand. Of course, there are many sleep aids, prescription and over-the-counter that might help. Prescription sleep aids include:

- triazolam (Halcion)
- lorazepam (Ativan)
- temazepam (Restoril)
- zolpidem (Ambien
- zaleplon (Sonata)
- eszopiclone (Lunesta)

In addition, many antidepressants and pain meds have sedative effects. All of the aforementioned medications should be used, if at all, with the utmost caution, due to the potential for addiction and abuse (some more than others).

Sleeping pills should never be used by those with airway obstruction issues like sleep apnea. It may prevent them from waking up to breathe. "CPAP" equipment, which keep the airway open by air pressure, are more appropriate in these patients, but will likely be difficult to use in an austere environment.

Over the counter sleep aids include the old standby Diphenhydramine, found in medications like Benadryl and Sominex. Usually, this medicine is used for allergic reactions; the 50 mg. dose is more effective in inducing sleep, but sometimes leads to drowsiness the next day and other side effects. Another antihistamine with sedative effects is Doxylamine, also known as Unisom. Other products like Melatonin may be helpful, but work best in those with documented low levels of the chemical naturally. Be aware that many drugs taken by adults will have the opposite effect on children. Instead of becoming sleepy, they may become agitated.

A better alternative to start with would be some form of natural sleep aid. Some of the common alternative remedies for sleeplessness include the following, usually made into teas:

- Chamomile
- Kava Root
- Lavender
- Valerian Root
- Catnip

Good nutrition is important for general health, but some foods are also thought to be helpful in promoting a good night's sleep. They contain sleep-inducing or muscle-relaxing substances like melatonin, magnesium, or tryptophan:

- Oatmeal – melatonin
- Milk – tryptophan
- Almonds – tryptophan and magnesium
- Bananas – melatonin and magnesium
- Whole wheat Bread – helps release tryptophan

Yoga, massage, meditation, sound machines, and even acupuncture are also alternative methods of dealing with sleep deprivation. Consider making some lifestyle changes now, so that you will be rested and prepared for whatever these uncertain times send your way.

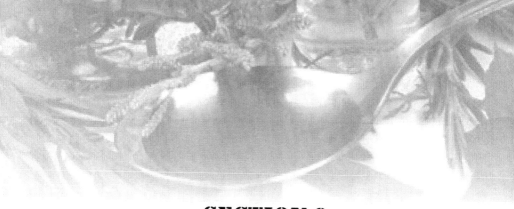

SECTION 9

✛ ✛ ✛

MEDICATIONS

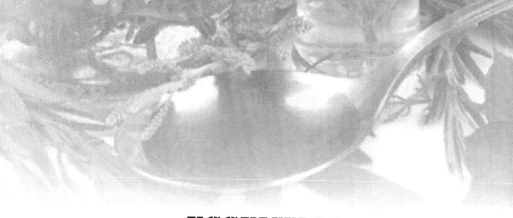

ESSENTIAL
OVER-THE-COUNTER DRUGS

O ver the counter (OTC) medications deal with a wide variety of problems; indeed, many of them were once only available by prescription. These drugs are widely available, and easy to accumulate in quantity. As such, they are ideal for the survival medic's cache of medical supplies.

The Physician's Desk Reference puts out a guide to OTC medications with descriptions, images, risks, benefits, dosages, and side effects. Consider this book for your survival medical library; it is widely available.

Given the complexity of manufacturing pharmaceuticals, most OTC drugs will be nearly impossible to produce after a collapse. Even aspirin, the oldest manufactured drug, won't be available (at least not in a form you'd recognize).

Let's put together a list of what you absolutely must have in quantity as part of your medical supplies. The medications will be listed by their generic names, with U.S. brand names in parenthesis where applicable. Adult doses are also listed. In no particular order, they are:

- **Ibuprofen 200mg** (Motrin, Advil):
  A popular pain reliever, anti-inflammatory, and fever reducer. This medication is useful for many different problems, which makes it especially useful as a stockpile item. It can alleviate pain

from strains, sprains, arthritis, and traumatic injury. As well, it can help reduce inflammation in the injured area. Ibuprofen is also useful in reducing fevers from infections. The downside to Ibuprofen is that it can cause stomach upset. Ibuprofen can be used 1 or 2 every 4 hours, 3 every 6 hours, or 4 every 8 hours.

- **Acetaminophen 325mg** (Tylenol):
Another popular pain reliever and fever reducer, it can be used for all of the problems that you can take Ibuprofen for, with the added benefit of not causing stomach irritation or thinning the blood. Unfortunately, it has no significant anti-inflammatory effect. This drug is excellent for treatment of pain and fevers in children at lower doses. Tylenol comes in regular and extra strength (650mg); adults take 1-2 every 4 hours.

An Aside: Patients with heat stroke receive little benefit from efforts to reduce their body core temperature with Ibuprofen or Acetaminophen; these drugs work best when the fever is caused by an infection, and don't work as well when infection is not involved.

- **Aspirin, 325mg:** If you have Ibuprofen and Acetaminophen in your medical storage, why consider Aspirin? Aspirin has been around since the late 19th century as a pain-reliever, fever reducer, and anti-inflammatory, but it has blood thinning properties as well. It may be all we have to help those with medical issues that require the use of anti-coagulants. It is also useful to treat older folks with coronary artery disease. If you suspect someone of having a heart attack, have them chew an adult aspirin immediately. 1 baby aspirin (81mg) daily may help prevent coronary artery disease.
The ingredient in Aspirin can also be obtained by chewing on a cut strip of the under bark of a willow, aspen or poplar tree. Take 2 adult aspirin every 4 hours for pain, fever, and inflammation. In a collapse situation, higher doses may be appropriate to replace drugs like Coumadin, but have not been fully researched. Watch for stomach upset.

- **Loperamide, 2mg** (Imodium): There's a high likelihood of food and water contamination issues in a collapse situation, so this medication is essential as an anti-diarrheal. By slowing intestinal motility, less water loss will occur from the body. This decreases the chance of developing dehydration, a known killer in austere settings. With diarrheal disease, you often have nausea and vomiting, so you will also want to have:

- **Meclizine 12.5, 25, 50mg** (Antivert): Mecilizine is a medication that helps prevent nausea and vomiting. Often used to prevent motion sickness, Meclizine also helps with dizziness, and tends to act as a sedative as well. As such, it may have uses as a sleep aid or anti-anxiety medication. Take 1 25mg tablet 1 hour before boarding or 50-100mg daily in divided doses for dizziness, anxiety or sleep.

- **Triple Antibiotic Ointment** (Neosporin, Bacitracin, Bactroban): In situations where we are left to fend for ourselves, we'll be chopping wood and performing all sorts of tasks that will expose us to risk of injury. When those injuries break the skin, it puts us in danger of infections which could lead to a life threatening condition. Triple antibiotic ointment is applied at the site of injury to prevent this from happening. It should be noted that triple antibiotic ointment won't cure a deep infection; you would need oral or IV antibiotics for that, but using the ointment immediately after an injury will give you a good chance at preventing it. Apply 3-4 times a day.

- **Diphenhydramine 25mg, 50mg** (Benadryl): An antihistamine that alleviates the itching, rashes, nasal congestion and other symptoms of allergic reactions. It also helps drain the nasal passages in some respiratory infections. At the higher 50 mg dose, it makes an effective sleep aid. Use 25mg every 6 hours for mild reactions, 50mg every 6 hours for severe reactions, anxiety or sleep. Diphenhydramine also comes in an ointment for skin eruptions.

- **Hydrocortisone cream** (1%): Highly useful for rashes, this cream is used for various types of dermatitis that causes redness, flakiness, itching, and thickening of the skin. It's a mild steroid which reduces inflammation and, as such, the various symptoms of allergic dermatitis, eczema, diaper rash, etc. Apply 3-4 times a day to affected area.

- **Omeprazole 20-40mg, Cimetidine 200-800mg, Ranitidine 75-150mg** (Prilosec, Tagamet, Zantac, respectively): In a situation where we may be eating things we're not accustomed to, we may have issues with stomach acid. The above antacids will calm heartburn, queasiness, and stomach upset. Calcium Carbonate (Tums) or Magnesium sulfate (Maalox) is also fine in solid form. These medications are also useful for acid reflux and ulcer disease.

- **Clotrimazole, Miconazole cream/powder** (Lotrimin, Monistat vaginal cream): Infections can be bacterial, but they can also be caused by fungus. Common examples of this would be Athlete's foot, vaginal yeast infections, ringworm, and jock itch. These conditions, which will be just as common in times of trouble as they are now, if not more. Apply clorimazole twice a day externally or miconazole once daily intravaginally. Some vaginal creams come in different strengths. In some, the whole treatment course is over in one day; in others, 3 days or a week.

- **Multivitamins:** In a societal collapse, the unavailability of a good variety of food may lead to dietary deficiencies, not just in calories but in vitamins and minerals. Vitamin C deficiency, for example, leads to Scurvy. To prevent these issues, you should have plenty of multivitamins, commercial or natural, in your medical storage.
  You won't necessarily have to take these on a daily basis; many multivitamins give you MORE than you need if taken daily. In most cases, you'll just excrete what your body can't absorb. In a collapse, once a week would be sufficient to prevent most problems.

The good news is that you can probably obtain a significant amount of all of the above drugs for a reasonable amount of money. To retain full potency, these medications should be obtained in pill or capsule form; avoid the liquid versions of any of these medicines if at all possible.

When storing, remember that medications should be stored in cool, dry, dark places. A medicine stored at 90 degrees will lose potency much faster than one stored at 50 degrees.

Over the counter drugs are just another tool in the medical woodshed; accumulate them as well as prescription drugs such as antibiotics. Essential oils, herbal supplements, and medical equipment are also important. With a good stockpile, you'll have everything you need to keep it together, even if everything else falls apart.

PAIN MEDICATIONS

Being an old and cranky individual (some find it charming, I like to think), I frequently complain about my various aches and pains. It stands to reason that minor issues with discomfort now will be multiplied by the increased workload demands of a power-down situation. To get a feel for what I am talking about, try lugging a full 5 gallon bucket of water from your local natural water source to your home a few times.

Sprains, strains, and worse will be part and parcel of any long-term survival situation. Therefore, any person who hasn't considered providing for pain issues in times of trouble is not medically prepared. It's a good idea to have a working knowledge of the actions and uses of various pain medications.

Pain is extremely variable; it can be sharp, dull, throbbing or numbing. It can be major or minor, and might or might not be a sign of something serious. It can be made better or worsened by various factors; as such, the exact same injury in two different individuals may elicit different levels of pain.

If we characterize pain by the kind of damage that it is caused by, we can group it into two or perhaps three categories. Pain is most commonly caused by tissue damage ("nociceptive" pain). The damage may be due to trauma or may be due to disease, such as tissue destruction from cancer. Even certain medical treatments such as radiation may cause tissue damage that could lead to pain. This type of pain is often described as "sharp", "stabbing", "achy", or worsens with movement ("it only hurts when I laugh").

Another category is pain caused by nerve damage ("neuropathic" pain). Nerves transmit pain signals from the damaged area to the brain. If the nerve is damaged, the sensation you feel may be very different from what you would expect. This is called a "**paresthesia**". You might feel burning where there is no reason, for example. You might even feel pain in a limb that is no longer there, due to amputation.

This type of pain is more likely to be chronic than pain from tissue damage. Besides burning, this type of pain can be described as prickling, "pins and needles", or similar to an electric shock.

The third type of pain is "psychogenic", or "all in the mind". Although fear, depression, anxiety and other emotions may play a part in someone's pain, there is most often some physical origin. Never dismiss a group member's complaints of pain without fully evaluating them by physical exam.

Pain medications are used to, well, relieve pain. Pain relief is referred to as **"analgesia"**. As pain is variable, there are many different types of drugs available that have different mechanisms of action:

Non-steroidal anti-inflammatories: Also known as NSAIDS, these drugs act to decrease inflammation and fever as well as pain. The most popular NSAIDs are Ibuprofen and Aspirin; Naproxen is another other NSAID available without a prescription. For quick relief from pain, the shorter acting Ibuprofen or Aspirin is superior to Naproxen. Naproxen may not have an effect until you have taken a couple of doses, but works well for long-term relief.

These drugs are especially useful in injuries associated with swelling or other signs of inflammation. There are various prescription versions of NSAIDS on the market, such as Meclomen, Ponstel, Toradol, and many other U.S. brands. Are they better than the non-prescription versions? Despite pharmaceutical company claims to the contrary, there is no proven evidence that these expensive medications are much more effective. Your experience may vary. Long-term use of NSAIDS is associated with bleeding and other symptoms related to the gastrointestinal tract.

Acetaminophen: This drug relieves pain by changing the body's sensitivity to things that cause pain (its "pain threshold"), and also lowers fever. This drug is often as effective as NSAIDs for pain and has fewer side effects (unless you have liver disease). Acetaminophen has no anti-inflammatory action, however; therefore, it may be less effective than NSAIDs for some conditions.

Steroids: Corticosteroids exert their effect upon pain by a very strong anti-inflammatory action. The most common steroids used for inflammation are Prednisone and Cortisone. They can be taken orally or are sometimes injected directly into damaged and inflamed joints. Long-term use of steroids is associated with a whole gamut of side effects and must be used with the utmost caution.

Muscle Relaxants: Drugs that relax tense and damaged muscles and also have a sedative effect. A common one is cyclobenzaprine (Flexeril). These are especially helpful for back strains or other injuries that cause muscle spasms.

Opioids: Narcotics are used for pain in severe cases, and act by modifying pain signal transmission in the brain. If you have had surgery, you likely have been given these medications for pain relief during recovery.

Opioids and other drugs are classified in "schedules" by the U.S. government. The lower the number, the more restricted the substance. These categories relate to the tendency to cause addiction, be unsafe, or have no legal medical use. Besides the risk of addiction, narcotics have a strong sedative as well as analgesic effect, and must be used with extreme caution during manual work or driving a vehicle.

The categories are as follows:

SCHEDULE 1 (CLASS 1) DRUGS are illegal to possess because they have no accepted medical use, high abuse potential, and clearly unsafe. Heroin is a good example.

SCHEDULE 2 DRUGS (CLASS 2) DRUGS have a high potential for abuse and dependence but have an accepted medical use, although the addictive potential is high. These drugs include opioids and barbiturates. Meperidine hydrochloride (Demerol) falls into this category.

SCHEDULE 3 (CLASS 3) DRUGS have a lower potential for abuse than drugs in the first two categories, accepted medical uses, and mild to moderate possible addiction. These drugs include many steroid, hydrocodone, and codeine-based drugs. Vicodin (hydrocodone and acetaminophen) qualifies to be included here.

SCHEDULE 4 (CLASS 4) DRUGS have a lower abuse potential than Schedule 3 Drugs, accepted medical uses, and less potential for addiction. These include many sedatives and anti-anxiety agents such as Diazepam (Valium) and Alprazolam (Xanax).

SCHEDULE 5 (CLASS 5) DRUGS have a low abuse potential, accepted medical use, and little potential for addiction. These consist primarily of preparations containing limited quantities of narcotics or stimulant drugs for cough, diarrhea, or pain. Lomotil (diphenoxylate/atropine), an anti-diarrheal, is a classic example.

Anti-anxiety and anti-depressant agents: Drugs such as Xanax or Prozac may have an effect on pain by relieving "psychogenic" factors such as anxiety or depression; this allows the patient to better deal with their pain issues. They work by adjusting level of certain chemicals in the brain tissue.

Anti-Seizure Medication: Some anti-convulsant drugs, such as Tegretol, used for epilepsy are useful to calm damaged nerves, and are possible options for "neuropathic" pain described earlier.

Combination Drugs: Some pain medications are combinations of different drugs. Percocet, for example, is Acetaminophen and Oxycodone (an opioid). Some are used alternatively during the day; An NSAID may be prescribed between doses of an opioid.

Most of these drugs are by prescription only, and it will be unlikely that you'll be able to stockpile large quantities of any but the non-prescription versions. As such, it will be important to know about all the natural alternatives you have for pain relief

NATURAL PAIN RELIEF

In a long-term survival situation, your limited supplies of the above medicines will eventually run out. This leaves you with natural alternatives from products that you can grow yourself or, perhaps, find in your environment. Although it's true that you can't be certain of the exact amount of pain relief you will experience, you also are less likely to have major side effects, as well. Let's discuss some of these alternatives:

Capsaicin: This is an ingredient in chili peppers and decreases pain sensation by deactivating nerve receptors on the skin. This is especially helpful for headache, muscle ache, and arthritis sufferers and those with neuropathic pain. The most pain relief occurs after using a capsaicin ointment for a month or so. Commercial Capsaicin can be found easily on the internet.

Salicin: Salicin is the original ingredient in the first pharmaceutical, Aspirin, and has been manufactured since the 19th century. Found in the bark of Willow, Aspen, and Poplar trees, Salicin can give pain relief by chewing on strips of under bark (not outer bark) and making a tea. Like Aspirin, Salicin will help reduce fever, as well.

Arnica: A natural anti-inflammatory, this substance reduces swelling and, therefore, discomfort from injuries to joints and muscles.

Methylsulfonyl-methane (MSM): Derived from sulfur, this substance helps slow down degeneration from joint disease, especially when combined with Glucosamine and Chondroitin. Over the course of time, osteoarthritis sufferers often report significant pain relief. It works by decreasing transmission of pain nerve impulses, and is very popular in Europe.

Curcumin: The herb Turmeric contains this substance, which increases the body's defense against inflammation, thereby decreasing pain.

Fish Oil: Filled with omega-3 fatty acids, fish oil reduces inflammation by releasing chemicals called prostaglandins when digested. It also blocks the production of inflammatory chemicals in the body. Commonly recommended in those with coronary artery disease, larger doses (2000-4000mg/day) are shown in several studies to give significant pain relief from various joint and immune disorders. Be aware that high doses of fish oil can thin the blood.

Ginger Root: A tea made of ginger root is thought to decrease inflammation and provide pain relief.

Boswellia: This herb from India produces certain acidic compounds that are touted as useful for chronic pain, and is said to decrease inflammation. Used long term, Boswellia is thought to provide as much pain relief as many NSAIDS.

Quercitin: Flavinoid compounds found in various plants, such as onions, may decrease inflammation. Quercitin can also be found in red wine. Some researchers believe that vegetarian diets limit the amount of pain experienced by those who adhere to them.

S-adenosylmethionine (Sam-e): An amino acid, Sam-e seems to reduce inflammation and increase neurotransmitters in the brain that increase the sensation of well-being. Taking this supplement long-term seems to give the best likelihood of obtaining pain relief.

Olive Oil: A compound in olive oil known as Oleocanthal works in the same way as many NSAIDS to relief discomfort. Use the "extra virgin" variety.

Hops: Isooxygene, an ingredient found in hops, has anti-inflammatory effects; some studies find it comparable to Ibuprofen. Hops may cause a worsening of depressive symptoms in some patients.

Cherries: If eaten when slightly unripe, cherries have antioxidant properties. An ingredient known as Anthocyanin is thought to exert an anti-inflammatory response and may be helpful for various joint diseases.

Many of the above substances are available in supplements that you can find online, many times in combination with each other. The results with regards to pain relief will be variable from patient to patient.

What if your patient is in more than slight pain? For major discomfort, here are some well-known (and usually, illegal) substances:

Opium: Derived from the seed pods of poppies, this highly addictive compound exerts significant pain-killing effects. This plant is the source of popular heavy pain medicines such as morphine and codeine. Heroin is another very potent product of the poppy plant.

Cocaine: A well-known derivative of the coca plant from South America, cocaine has natural anesthetic properties and was a popular painkiller for dental procedures not so very long ago. Some local anesthetics like Novocain and Procaine imitate the effect if cocaine. Growing this is also very, very, illegal.

Curare: Another South American plant, the Pareira vine, contains the compound Curare, which was used by natives on their arrow and spear points to paralyze their prey. This drug is still used today by anesthesiologists to paralyze respiratory action so that they can more easily perform intubations for surgery. Without medications to reverse the effect, the paralysis effect leads to death.

Besides all of the above, consider alternative methods such as aromatherapy, massage, inhalation therapy, Yoga, and Acupuncture. These options have been used for treatment of pain and many people have reported significant relief.

Be open to every strategy available to deal with a medical issue; there are a lot of tools in the medical woodshed, and you should take advantage of any method to keep your family healthy in uncertain times.

STOCKPILING MEDICATIONS

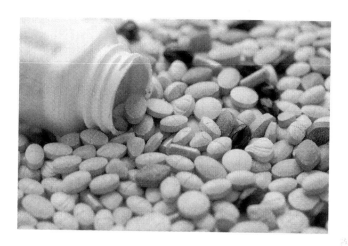

Accumulating medications for a possible collapse may be simple when it comes to getting Ibuprofen and other non-prescription drugs. It will be a major issue, however, for those who need to stockpile prescription medicines; most people don't have a relationship with a physician who can or will accommodate their requests. Antibiotics are one example of medications that will be very useful in a collapse situation. Obtaining these drugs in quantity will be difficult, to say the least.

The inability to store antibiotic supplies is going to cost some poorly prepared individuals their lives in a collapse situation. There will be a much larger incidence of infection when people have to fend for themselves and are injured as a result. Any strenuous activities performed in a power-down situation, especially ones that most of us aren't accustomed to, will cause various cuts and scratches. These wounds will very likely be dirty. Within a relatively short time, they can begin to show infection, in the form of redness, heat, and swelling.

Treatment of such infections at an early stage improves the chance that they will heal quickly and completely. However, many rugged individualists are most likely to "tough it out" until their condition worsens and the infection spreads to their blood. This causes a condition known as sepsis; the patient develops a fever as well as other problems that could eventually be life-threatening. The availability of antibiotics would allow the possibility of dealing with the issue safely and effectively.

The following advice is contrary to standard medical practice, and is a strategy that is appropriate only in the event of societal collapse. If there are modern medical resources available to you, seek them out.

Antibiotic Options

Small amounts of medications can be obtained by anyone willing to tell their doctor that they are going out of the country and would like to avoid "Travelers' Diarrhea". If you choose this route, ask them for Tamiflu for viral illness before every flu season, and Amoxicillin, Doxycycline and Metronidazole for bacterial/protozoal disease.

This approach is fine for one or two courses of therapy, but a long term alternative is required for the survival caregiver to have enough antibiotics to protect a family or survival group. Thinking long and hard for a solution has led me to what I believe is a viable option: Aquarium antibiotics.

For many years, my hobby was tropical fish. I also have kept parrots for many years. Currently, we are growing tilapia as a food fish in an aquaculture pond. After years of using aquatic medicines on fish and avian medicines on birds, we decided to evaluate these drugs for their potential use in collapse situations. They seemed to be good candidates: All were widely available, available in different varieties, and didn't require a medical license to obtain them.

A close inspection of the bottles revealed that the only ingredient was the drug itself, identical to those obtained by prescription at the local pharmacy. If the bottle says FISH-MOX, for example, the sole ingredient is Amoxicillin, which is an antibiotic commonly used in humans. There are no additional chemicals to makes your scales shiny or your fins longer.

I understand that you might be skeptical about considering the use of aquarium antibiotics for humans in a collapse. Those things are for fish, aren't they? Yet, a number of them seem to come in dosages that correspond to pediatric or adult human dosages. Indeed, some ONLY come in human dosages.

Why should this be? Why should a 1 inch long guppy require the same dosage of, say, Amoxicillin (aquatic version: FISH-MOX FORTE) as a 180 pound adult human? I was told that it was due to the dilution of the drug in water. However, at the time of this writing, there are few instructions that tell you how much to put in a ½ gallon fishbowl as opposed to a 200 gallon aquarium.

Finally, my "acid test" was to look at the pills or capsules themselves. The aquatic or avian drug had to be identical to that found in bottles of the corresponding human medicine. For example, when I opened a bottle of FISH-MOX FORTE and a bottle of Human Amoxicillin 500mg, I found:

- Human Amoxicillin 500mg: Red and Pink Capsule, with the letters and numbers WC 731 on it
- FISH-MOX FORTE: Red and Pink Capsule with the letters and numbers WC 731 on it.

Logically, then, it makes sense to believe that they are manufactured in the same way that human antibiotics are. Further, it is my opinion that they are probably from the same batches; some go to human pharmacies and some go to veterinary pharmacies.

This is not to imply that all antibiotic medications meet my criteria. Many cat, dog, and livestock antibiotics contain additives that might even cause ill effects on a human being. Look only for those veterinary drugs that have the antibiotic as the SOLE ingredient.

Here is a list of the products that meet my criteria and that I believe will be beneficial to have as supplies and are discussed in the next section:

- FISH-MOX (Amoxicillin 250mg)
- FISH_MOX FORTE (Amoxicillin 500mg)
- FISH-CILLIN (Ampicillin 250mg)
- FISH-FLEX (Keflex 250mg)
- FISH-FLEX FORTE (Keflex 500mg)
- FISH-ZOLE (Metronidazole 250mg)
- FISH-PEN (Penicillin 250mg)
- FISH-PEN FORTE (Penicillin 500mg)

- FISH-CYCLINE (Tetracycline 250mg)
- FISH-FLOX (Ciprofloxacin 250mg)
- FISH-CIN (Clindamycin 150mg)
- BIRD BIOTIC (Doxycycline 100mg) - used in birds but the antibiotic is, again, the sole ingredient
- BIRD SULFA (Sulfamethoxazole 400mg/Trimethoprin 80mg) also used in birds

These medications are available without a prescription from veterinary supply stores and online sites everywhere. They come in lots of 30 to 100 tablets for less than the same prescription medication at the local pharmacy. If you so desired, it appears that you could get as much as you need to stockpile for a collapse. These quantities would be close to impossible to obtain even from the most sympathetic physician.

Of course, anyone could be allergic to one or another of these antibiotics, but it would be a very rare individual who would be allergic to all of them. There is a 10% chance for cross-reactivity between Penicillin drugs and Keflex (if you are allergic to penicillin, you could also be allergic to Keflex). For penicillin-allergic people, there are suitable safe alternatives. Any of the antibiotics below should not cause a reaction in a patient allergic to Penicillin-family drugs:

- Doxycycline
- Metronidazole
- Tetracycline
- Ciprofloxacin
- Clindamycin
- Sulfa Drugs

This one additional fact: I have personally used some (not all) of these antibiotics on my own person without any ill effects. Whenever I have used them, they have been undistinguishable from human antibiotics in their effects.

Having said this, I do NOT recommend self-treatment in any circumstance that does not involve the complete long-term loss of access to modern medical care. This is a strategy to save lives in a post-calamity scenario only.

Finding Out More

Antibiotics are used at specific doses for specific illnesses; the exact dosage of each and every medication in existence is beyond the scope of this handbook. It's important, however, to have as much information as possible on medications that you plan to store, so consider purchasing a hard copy of the latest Physician's Desk Reference. This book comes out yearly and has just about every bit of information that exists on a particular drug. Online sources such as drugs.com or rxlist.com are also useful, but you are going to want a hard copy for your library. You never know when we might not have a functioning internet.

The Desk Reference has versions that list medications that require prescriptions as well as those that do not. Under each medicine, you will find the "**indications**", which are the medical conditions that the drug is used for. Also listed will be the dosages, risks, side effects, and even how the medicine works in the body. It's okay to get last year's book; the information doesn't change a great deal from one year to the next.

Antibiotic Overuse

It's important to understand that you will not want to indiscriminately use antibiotics for every minor ailment that comes along. In a collapse, the medic is also a quartermaster of sorts; you will want to wisely dispense that limited and, yes, precious supply of life-saving drugs. You must walk a fine line between observant patient management (doing nothing) and aggressive management (doing everything).

Liberal use of antibiotics is a poor strategy for a few reasons:

- Overuse can foster the spread of resistant bacteria, as you'll remember from the salmonella outbreak in turkeys in 2011. Millions of pounds of turkey meat were discarded after 100 people were sent to the hospital with severe diarrheal disease.

- Potential allergic reactions may occur that could lead to anaphylactic shock (see the section on this topic earlier in this book).
- Making a diagnosis may be more difficult. If you give antibiotics BEFORE you're sure what medical problem you're actually dealing with, you might "mask" the condition. In other words, symptoms could be temporarily improved that would have helped you know what disease your patient has. This could cost you valuable time in determining the correct treatment.

You can see that judicious use of antibiotics, under your close supervision, is necessary to fully utilize their benefits. Discourage your group members from using these drugs without first consulting you.

Other Medicines

For medications that treat non-infectious illness, such as cholesterol or blood pressure drugs, you will also need a prescription. These medications are not available in aquarium supply houses, so how can you work to stockpile them?

You may consider asking your physician to prescribe a higher dose than the amount you usually take. Many drugs come in different dosages. If your medicine is a 20 milligram dosage, for example, you might ask your doctor to prescribe the 40 mg dosage. You would then cut the medication in half; take your normal dosage and store the other half of the pill. It's very important to assure your physician that you will continue to follow their medical advice and not take more medicine than is appropriate for your condition. Your success in having your request granted will depend on the doctor.

Others have managed to obtain needed prescriptions by indicating that they are traveling for long periods of time out of the country or telling their physician some other falsehood. I can't recommend this method, because I believe that dishonesty breaks the bond of trust between doctor and patient.

Consider having a serious discussion with your healthcare provider. Describe your concerns about not having needed medications in a disaster situation. You don't have to describe the disaster as a complete societal collapse; any catastrophe could leave you without access to your doctor for an extended period.

Alternative therapies such as herbal supplements and essential oils should be stockpiled as well. Honey, onion, silver, and garlic have known antibacterial actions; be sure to integrate all medical options, traditional and alternative, and use every tool at your disposal to keep your community healthy. If you don't, you're fighting with one hand tied behind your back.

Remember that traditional medicines and even essential oils will eventually run out in a long term collapse. Begin your medicinal garden now and get experience with the use of these beneficial plants. There is a learning curve, and you don't want to go through it in tough times.

I would like to take a second to voice my concern over the apparently indiscriminate use of antibiotics in livestock management (what I call Agri-Business) today. 80% of the antibiotics manufactured today are going to livestock, such as cattle and chickens. Excessive antibiotic use is causing the development of resistant strains of bacteria such as Salmonella, which can cause a type of diarrheal disease in humans. Recently, 36 million pounds of turkey meat were destroyed due to an antibiotic resistant strain of the bacteria. Over 100 people wound up in the hospital as a result of eating contaminated food.

Consider patronizing those farmers who raise antibiotic-free livestock; this will decrease the further development of resistant bacteria, and thus the antibiotics you've stockpiled will be more effective.

If we ever find ourselves without modern medical care, we will have to improvise medical strategies that we perhaps might be reluctant to consider today. Without hospitals, it will be up to the medic to nip infections in the bud. That responsibility will be difficult to carry out without the weapons to fight disease. Accumulate equipment and medications and never ignore avenues that may help you gain access to them.

HOW TO USE ANTIBIOTICS

There are many antibiotics, but what antibiotics accessible to the average person would be good additions to your medical storage? When do you use a particular drug? In this section, we'll discuss antibiotics (all available in veterinary form without a prescription) that you will want in your medical arsenal:

- **Amoxicillin** 250mg/500mg (FISH-MOX, FISH-MOX FORTE)
- **Ciprofloxacin** 250mg/500mg (FISH-FLOX, FISH-FLOX FORTE)
- **Cephalexin** 250mg/500mg (FISH-FLEX, FISH-FLEX FORTE)
- **Metronidazole** 250mg (FISH-ZOLE)
- **Doxycycline** 100mg (BIRD-BIOTIC)
- **Ampicillin** 250mg/500mg (FISH-CILLIN, FISH-CILLIN FORTE)
- **Sulfamethoxazole** 400mg/Trimethoprim 80mg (BIRD-SULFA)
- **Clindamycin** 150mg (FISH-CIN)
- **Azithromycin** 250mg (Aquatic Azithromycin)

There are various others that you can choose, but these selections will give you the opportunity to treat many illnesses and have enough variety so that even those with Penicillin allergies will have options.

Other than allergies, there are other times when a particular antibiotic (or other drug) should not be used. Many medications, for example, are not recommended for use during pregnancy. Sometimes, this is because lab studies have shown birth defects in animal fetuses exposed to the drug. Other times, it is because no studies on pregnant women or animals have yet been performed.

There are additional circumstances where a particular medication should not be used. There may be warnings about mixing one drug with another because there may be a dangerous interaction between them. For example, taking the antibiotic Metronidazole (Fish-Zole) and drinking alcohol will make you vomit. Some drug interactions may cause the effect of one of them to become stronger or weaker. A certain medicine, for example, may decrease the effect of another when taken together. As well, you may wish to avoid some drugs due to their side effects.

You cannot be expected to know everything regarding every medication. You should, however, know quite a bit about drugs that you could expect to use in a survival situation. This information is freely available; you just have to spend some time absorbing it.

It should be noted that different physicians may use a specific antibiotic for different purposes and to treat a variety of infections. There is always some variance when you receive opinions about treatment from different caregivers. Some will not agree with everything you see written in this book.

Amoxicillin

Let's discuss how to approach the use of antibiotics by using an example. Amoxicillin (veterinary equivalent: FISH-MOX, FISH-MOX FORTE, AQUA-MOX): comes in 250mg and 500mg doses, usually taken 3 times a day. Amoxicillin is the most popular antibiotic prescribed to children, usually in liquid form. It is more versatile and better absorbed and tolerated than the older Pencillins, and is acceptable for use during pregnancy. Ampicillin (Fish-Cillin) and Cephalexin (Fish-Flex) are related drugs.

Amoxicillin may be used for the following diseases:

- Anthrax (Prevention or treatment of Cutaneous transmission)
- Chlamydia Infection (sexually transmitted)
- Urinary Tract Infection (bladder/kidney infections)
- Helicobacter pylori Infection (causes peptic ulcer)
- Lyme Disease (transmitted by ticks)
- Otitis Media (middle ear infection)
- Pneumonia (lung infection)
- Sinusitis
- Skin or Soft Tissue Infection (cellulitis, boils)
- Actinomycosis (causes abscesses in humans and livestock)

- Bronchitis
- Tonsillitis/Pharyngitis (Strep throat)

You can see that Amoxicillin is a versatile drug. It is even safe for use during pregnancy, but all of the above is a lot of information. How do you determine what dose and frequency would be appropriate for which individual? Let's take an example: Otitis media is a common ear infection often seen in children. Amoxicillin is often the "**drug of choice**" for this condition. That is, it is recommended to be used FIRST when you make a diagnosis of otitis media. The drug of choice for a particular ailment can change, over time, based on new scientific evidence.

Before administering this medication, however, you would want to determine that your patient is not allergic to Amoxicillin. The most common form of allergy would appear as a rash, but diarrhea, itchiness, and even respiratory difficulty could also manifest. If you see any of these symptoms, you should discontinue your treatment and look for other options. Antibiotics such as Azithromycin or Sulfamethoxazole/Trimethoprim (Bird-Sulfa) could be a "**second-line**" solution in this case.

Once you have identified Amoxicillin as your treatment of choice to treat your patient's ear infection, you will want to determine the dosage. As Otitis Media often occurs in children, you might have to break a tablet in half or open the capsule to separate out a portion that would be appropriate. For Amoxicillin, you would give 20-50mg per kilogram (2.2 pounds) of body weight (20-30mg/kg for infants less than four months old). This would be useful if you have to give the drug to a toddler less than 30 pounds.

A common older child's dosage would be 250mg and a common maximum dosage for adults would be 500 mg three times a day. Luckily (or by design), these dosages are exactly how the commercially-made aquatic medications come in the bottle. Take this dosage orally 3 times a day for 10 to 14 days (twice a day for infants). All of the above information can be found in the Physician's Desk Reference.

If your child is too small to swallow a pill whole, you could make a mixture with water (called a "**suspension**"). To make a liquid suspension, crush a tablet or empty a capsule into a small glass of water and drink it; then, fill the glass again and drink that (particles may adhere to the walls of the glass). You can add some flavoring to make it taste better.

Do not chew or make a liquid out of time-released capsules of any medication; you will wind up losing some of the gradual release effect and perhaps get too much into your system at once. These medications should be plainly marked "Time-Released".

You will probably see improvement within 3 days, but don't be tempted to stop the antibiotic therapy until you're done with the entire 10-14 days. Sometimes, you'll kill most of the bacteria but some colonies may persist and multiply if you prematurely end the treatment. This is often cited as a cause of antibiotic resistance. In a long-term survival situation, however, you might be down to your last few pills and have to make some tough decisions.

Ciprofloxacin

A useful option is Ciprofloxacin (veterinary equivalent: FISH-FLOX). Ciprofloxacin is an antibiotic in the fluoroquinolone family. It kills bacteria by inhibiting the reproduction of DNA and bacterial proteins. This drug usually comes in 250mg and 500mg doses.

Ciprofloxacin (brand name Cipro) can be used for the following conditions:

- Bladder or other urinary infections, especially in females
- Prostate infections
- some types of lower respiratory infections, such as pneumonia
- Acute sinusitis
- Skin infections (such as cellulitis)
- Bone and joint infections
- Infectious diarrhea
- Typhoid fever caused by Salmonella
- Inhalational Anthrax

In most cases, you should give 500mg twice a day for 7-14 days, with the exception of bone and joint infections (4-6 weeks) and Anthrax (60 days).

You can get away with 250mg doses for 3 days for most mild urinary infections. Generally, you would want to continue the medication for 2 days after improvement is noted.

Unlike Amoxicillin, many antibiotics may not be safe for use in certain situations. For example, Ciprofoxacin has not been approved for use during pregnancy. Among its side effects, Cipro has been reported to occasionally cause weakness in muscles and tendons. It may also cause joint and muscle complications in children, so it is restricted in pediatric use to the following conditions:

- Urinary tract infections and pyelonephritis due to E. coli (the most common type)
- Inhalational anthrax

In children, the dosage is measured by multiplying 10mg by the weight in kilograms (1 kg = 2.2 lbs.). The maximum dose should not exceed 400mg total twice a day, even if the child weighs more than 100 pounds. Ciprofloxacin should be taken with 8 ounces of water.

Cephalexin

Cephalexin (veterinary equivalent: Fish-Flex, Fish-Flex Forte) is an antibiotic in the Cephalosporin family. It is different from but cross-reactive with the Penicillin family; this means that a percentage of Penicillin-allergic patients will also be allergic to Cephalosporins.

Cephalexin works by interfering with the bacteria's cell wall formation. This causes the defective wall to rupture, killing the bacteria. This antibiotic is useful in the treatment of:

- Cystitis (bladder infections)
- Otitis Media (ear infections)
- Pharyngitis (sore throats)
- Skin or Soft Tissue Infection (i.e., infected cuts)
- Osteomyelitis (infections of the bone)
- Prostatitis (prostate infections)
- Pyelonephritis (kidney infections
- Upper Respiratory Tract Infection

Cephalexin is also used as a preventative before surgical procedures in people who are at risk for heart valve infections. It is also one of the few antibiotics which is thought to be safe to use during pregnancy.

Cephalexin is marketed in the U.S. under the name Keflex.

To use this medication, you would normally give 250mg (Fish-Flex) or 500mg (Fish-Flex Forte) every 6 hours for 7-14 days. Severe bacterial infections may require an additional week of treatment. Infections of the bone (osteomyelitis) are particularly dangerous and require 4-6 weeks of therapy.

Pediatric dosages are calculated using 12.5 to 25 mg per kilogram of body weight orally every 6-12 hours (don't exceed adult dosages).

Doxycycline

Another useful antibiotic in a collapse would be Doxycycline (veterinary equivalent: Bird-Biotic). Doxycycline is a member of the Tetracycline family, and is also acceptable in patients allergic to Penicillin. It inhibits the production of bacterial protein, which prevents its reproduction. Doxycycline is marketed under various names, including Vibramycin and Vibra-Tabs.

Doxycycline is an extraordinarily versatile drug. Indications for its usage include the following:

- E. Coli, Shigella and Enterobacter infections (diarrheal disease)
- Chlamydia (sexually transmitted disease)
- Lyme disease
- Rocky Mountain spotted fever
- Anthrax
- Cholera
- Plague
- Gum disease (severe gingivitis, periodontitis)
- Folliculitis (boils)
- Acne and other inflammatory skin diseases, such as hidradenitis (seen in armpits and groins)
- Some lower respiratory tract (pneumonia) and urinary tract infections

- Upper respiratory infections caused by Strep
- Methicillin-resistant Staph (MRSA) infections
- Malaria (prevention)
- Some parasitic worm infections (kills bacteria in their gut needed to survive)

In the case of Rocky Mountain spotted fever, doxycycline is indicated even for use in children. Otherwise, doxycycline is not meant for those under the age of eight years. It has not been approved for use during pregnancy.

The recommended Doxycycline dosage for most types of bacterial infections in adults is 100 mg to 200 mg per day for 7-14 days. For chronic (long-term) or more serious infections, treatment can be carried out for a longer time. Children will receive 1-2mg per pound of body weight per day. For Anthrax, the treatment should be prolonged to 60 days. As prevention against malaria, adults should use 100mg per day.

Although antibiotics may be helpful in diarrheal disease, always start with hydration and symptomatic relief. Prolonged diarrhea, high fevers, and bleeding are reasons to consider their use. The risk is that one of the most common side effects of antibiotics is....diarrhea!

Azithromycin

Another antibiotic available in an aquatic equivalent is Azithromycin 250mg. Azithromycin is a member of the macrolide (Erythromycin) family and can be found also as "Aquatic Azithromycin". It works by stopping the growth and multiplication of bacteria. I prefer it to aquatic Erythromycin powder (Fish-Mycin) as Azithromycin is available in a capsule; thus, it is more easily administered.

Azithromycin can be used to treat various types of:

- Bronchitis
- Pneumonia
- Ear infections
- Skin infections
- Throat infections (some)

- Sinusitis
- Tonsillitis
- Typhoid fever
- Gonorrhea
- Chlamydia
- Whooping cough
- Lyme Disease (early stages)

Azithromycin is taken 250mg or 500mg once daily for a relatively short course of treatment (usually five days). The first dose is often a "double dose," twice as much as the remainder of the doses given. This method of taking the drug is known in the U.S. as a "Z-Pack".

For acute bacterial sinusitis, azithromycin way be taken once daily for three days. If you are taking the 500mg dosage and have side effects such as nausea and vomiting, diarrhea, or dizziness, drop down to the lower dosage. Azithromycin is not known to cause problems in pregnant patients.

Clindamycin

Clindamycin (Fish-Cin) is part of the family of drugs called Lincomycin antibiotics. It, like Azithromycin, works by slowing or stopping the growth of bacteria. It works best on bacteria that are **anaerobic**, which means that they thrive in the absence of oxygen. It can be used to treat:

- Acne
- Dental infections
- Soft tissue (skin, etc.)
- Peritonitis (inflammation of the abdomen)
- Pneumonia and lung abscesses
- Uterine infections (such as after miscarriage or childbirth)
- Blood infections
- Pelvic infections
- MRSA (Methicillin-resistant Staph. Aureus infections)
- Parasitic infections (Malaria, Toxoplasmosis)
- Anthrax

Clindamycin is given in 150mg or 300mg doses every 6 hours with a glass of water. It should be used with caution in individuals with a history of gastrointestinal disease as it can cause diarrhea during treatment. Sometimes, a very serious "colitis" (infection of the intestine) can develop. This drug is, like Azithromycin, pregnancy category B, which means that no ill effects have been determined in animal studies. With most drugs, testing cannot be done ethically on pregnant humans, so very few drugs are willing to say that any medicine is completely safe during pregnancy.

Ciprofloxacin, Clindamycin, Doxycycline, and Azithromycin are acceptable for use in patients with Penicillin allergies. This is not to say that you might not have a different allergy to one or the other, however.

Metronidazole

Metronidazole (aquatic equivalent: Fish-Zole) 250mg is an antibiotic in the Nitroimidazole family that is used primarily to treat infections caused by anaerobic bacteria and protozoa.

"Anaerobes" are bacteria that do not depend on oxygen to live. "Protozoa" have been defined as single-cell organisms with animal-like behavior. Many can propel themselves from place to place by the means of a "flagellum"; a tail-like "hair" they whip around that allows them to move.

Metronidazole works by blocking some of the functions within bacteria and protozoa, thus, resulting in their death. It is better known by the U.S. brand name Flagyl and usually comes in 250mg and 500mg tablets. Metronidazole is used in the treatment of these bacterial diseases:

- Diverticulitis (intestinal infection seen in older individuals)
- Peritonitis (infection due to ruptured appendix, etc.)
- Some pneumonias
- Diabetic foot ulcer infections
- Meningitis (infection of the spinal cord and brain lining)
- Bone and joint infections
- Colitis due to Clostridia bacterial species (sometimes caused by taking Clindamycin!)
- Endocarditis (heart infection)

- Bacterial vaginosis (common vaginal infection)
- Pelvic inflammatory disease (infection in women which can lead to abscesses) – used in combination with other antibiotics
- Uterine infections (especially after childbirth and miscarriage)
- Dental infections (sometimes in combination with amoxicillin)
- H. pylori infections (causes peptic ulcers)
- Some skin infections

And these protozoal infections:

- Amoebiasis: dysentery caused by Entamoeba species (contaminated water/food)
- Giardiasis: infection of the small intestine caused by Giardia Species (contaminated water/food)
- Trichomoniasis: vaginal infection caused by parasite which can be sexually transmitted

Amoebiasis and Giardiasis can be caught from drinking what appears to be the purest mountain stream water. Never fail to sterilize all water, regardless of source, before drinking it.

Metronidazole is used in different dosages to treat different illnesses. Here are the dosages and frequency of administration for several:

- Amoebic dysentery: 750 mg orally 3 times daily for 5-10 days. For children, give 35 to 50 mg/kg/day orally in 3 divided doses for 10 days (no more than adult dosage, of course, regardless of weight).
- Anaerobic infections (various): 7.5 mg/kg orally every 6 hours not to exceed 4 grams daily.
- Clostridia infections: 250-500 mg orally 4 times daily or 500-750 orally 3 times daily.
- Giardia: 250 mg orally three times daily for 5 days. For children give 15 mg/kg/day orally in 3 divided doses (no more than adult dosage regardless of weight).
- Helicobacter pylori (ulcer disease): 500-750mg twice daily for several days in combination with other drugs like Prilosec (Omeprazole).

- Pelvic inflammatory disease (PID): 500 mg orally twice daily for 14 days in combination with other drugs, perhaps doxycycline or azithromycin.
- Bacterial Vaginosis: 500mg twice daily for 7 days
- Vaginal Trichomoniasis: 2 g single dose (4 500mg tablets at once) or 1 g twice total.

Like all antibiotics, Metronidazole has side effects which you can review by picking up a Physician's Desk Reference or going to drugs.com or rxlist.com. One particular side effect has to do with alcohol: drinking alcohol while on Metronidazole will very likely make you vomit. Metronidazole should not be used in pregnancy. but can be used in those allergic to Penicillin.

Sulfa Drugs

Sulfamethoxazole 400mg/Trimethoprim 80mg (avian equivalent: Bird-Sulfa) is a combination of medications in the Sulfonamide family. This drug is well-known as its U.S. brand names Bactrim and Septra. Our British friends may recognize it by the name Co-Trimoxazole.

Sulfamethoxazole acts as an inhibitor of an important bacterial enzyme. Trimethoprim interferes with the production of folic acid in bacteria, which is necessary to produce DNA. The two antibiotics together are stronger in their effect than alone (at least in laboratory studies).

Sulfamethoxazole 400mg/Trimethoprim 80mg is effective in the treatment of the following:

- Some upper and lower respiratory infections (chronic bronchitis and pneumonia)
- Kidney and bladder infections
- Ear infections
- intestinal infections caused by E. Coli and Shigella bacteria
- skin and wound infections
- Traveler's diarrhea
- Acne

The usual dosage is one tablet twice a day for most of the above conditions in adults for 10 days (less in traveler's diarrhea).

The recommended dose for pediatric patients with urinary tract infections or acute otitis media is 8 mg/kg trimethoprim and 40 mg/kg sulfamethoxazole per 24 hours, given in two divided doses every 12 hours for 10 days. Remember that 1 kilogram equals 2.2 pounds. This medication is contraindicated in infants 2 months old or younger.

In rat studies, the use of this drug was seen to cause birth defects; therefore, it is not used during pregnancy. Sulfamethoxazole 400mg/ Trimethoprim 80mg is well known to cause allergic reactions in some individuals. These reactions are almost as common as seen in Penicillin allergies.

Ampicillin

Ampicillin (veterinary equivalent: Fish-Cillin) is a member of the penicillin family. It interferes with the ability of bacteria to make cell walls. Ampicillin can be used to treat a number of infections:

- Respiratory tract Infections (bacterial bronchitis)
- Throat infections
- Ear infections
- Cellultis
- Meningitis
- Urinary tract infections
- Typhoid fever (Salmonella)
- Dysentery (Shigella)

Ampicillin is usually given to adults in doses of 500mg 4 times a day for 7-10 days. A common pediatric dosage formula is 6.25 to 12.5 mg/ kg every 6 hours (maximum 2 to 3 g/day). Ampicillin is acceptable for use during pregnancy. Like most antibiotics, it has stronger effect in intravenous form, and can be used IV in some cases of septicemia (blood infection) and endocarditis (heart infection).

Anti-Fungal Drugs

Not every medication you use to treat infection will kill bacteria. Viruses and fungi can also cause infection, and you will have to stockpile these drugs as well. Common fungal infections like Ringworm, Athlete's Foot, and Jock Itch will be rampant in wet climates or in situations where you might not be able to change socks or underwear often.

Therefore, it makes sense to keep some antifungal medication around as well. **Clotrimazole** (Lotrimin) is a good choice here, as it comes in cream or powder, and doesn't require a prescription. Medications like **Miconazole** (Monistat) would be useful for vaginal yeast infections. There is an oral tablet as well called **Fluconazole** (Diflucan), which may be more convenient than creams or powders, but requires a prescription.

Like some antibiotics, some anti-fungal drugs come in veterinary equivalents. **Ketoconazole** is a common anti-fungal that can be obtained in its aquatic version (Fish-Fungus 200mg). It kills certain fungi by interfering with the formation of the fungal cell membrane. Ketoconazole is best taken by itself, as there are many medicines that interact with it to cause ill effects. In rare cases, Ketoconazole may cause liver dysfunction.

Ketoconazole Tablets are indicated for the treatment of **systemic** (throughout the body) fungal infections. It is only used for local infections when severe and the previously-mentioned anti-fungal medications fail. In other words, stick with the other anti-fungals if at all possible. Ketoconazole is used for:

- Systemic candidiasis (same fungus as in vaginal infections)
- Oral thrush (mouth infections, usually in infants)
- Candiduria (fungus in the urine)
- Fungal lung infections (various species)

Ketoconazole Tablets should not be used for fungal meningitis; it penetrates poorly into the cerebral-spinal fluid.

Anti-Viral Drugs

Finally, anti-viral medications will be useful as well. Many of the infections, especially respiratory, that we assume to be bacterial in nature are more likely to be viral. Antibiotics have no significant effect on viruses; despite this, many patients will demand an antibiotic prescription from their doctors as soon as they feel the first symptom. This overuse is one of the reasons that antibiotic resistance is growing.

One of the most popular anti-viral influenza drugs is called Tamiflu (**Oseltamvir**). Tamiflu gives effective relief against symptoms of influenza and decreases the amount of time your patient would be sick. It can be taken upon exposure to the infection, even before symptoms have begun. If the drug is taken early enough, it might even prevent the illness altogether. Taken in the first 48 hours of a flu-like syndrome, it may decrease the severity and duration of symptoms.

The adult preventative dose of Tamiflu is 75mg once daily for 10 days. To treat symptoms, take 75mg twice a day for 5 days. For children, follow the above regimen in the following doses:

- 15 kg (33 lbs.) or less: 30 mg dosage
- 16-23 kg (34-51 lbs.): 45 mg dosage
- 24-40 kg (52-88 lbs.): 60 mg dosage
- Above 40 kg (89 lbs. or more): adult dosage

Tamiflu will not have much effect if taken after the first 48 hours of flu symptoms. Also, it is not proven to be effective against anything other than influenzas. Despite this, it is wise to obtain prescriptions for every member of your family at the beginning of every flu season.

Other anti-viral drugs such as Acyclovir or Famcyclovir are usually used to treat herpes-virus related conditions, such as:

Shingles (painful skin eruption)
Adults: 800 mg every 4 hours for 5 to 10 days
Children under 40 kg (and older than 2 years):
20 mg/kg 4 times a day for 5 days.

Varicella (chickenpox)
Adults: 800 mg 4 times a day for 5 days
Children under 40 kg (and older than 2 years):
20 mg/kg orally 4 times a day for 5 days

Oral/genital Herpes (Herpes Simplex)
Adults: 200 mg every 4 hours for 10 days OR 400 mg 3 times a day for 7-10 days
Children under 40 kg (and older than 2 years):
40 to 80 mg/kg a day in 3 to 4 divided doses for 5 to 10 days. Max dose: 1 g per day

Don't forget that natural products such as Garlic and Honey have significant properties against certain infections. Garlic, for example, is thought to have anti-bacterial, anti-fungal, and anti-viral effects. Many people report significant antibacterial/antiviral effect with colloidal silver, as well. Before there were antibiotics, there was silver; it is still used in topical creams to prevent infection.

EXPIRATION DATES

A question that I am asked quite often and to which my answer is, again, contrary to standard medical recommendations (but appropriate where modern medical care no longer exists) is: "What happens when all these drugs I stockpiled pass their expiration date"? The short answer is: In most cases, not very much.

Since 1979, pharmaceutical companies have been required to place expiration dates on their medications. But what do they signify? Officially, the expiration date is the last day that the company will certify that their drug is fully potent. Some believe this means that the medicine in question is useless or in some way dangerous after that date.

This is a false assumption, at least in the vast majority of those medicines that come in pill or capsule form. Expiration dates pertain to the strength of the medication in question. You will not grow a third eye in the middle of your forehead or be poisoned simply because the drug has "expired".

An exception to this was thought to be Tetracycline. A (disputed) report of kidney damage after taking expired Tetracycline was published in the Journal of the American Medical Association in 1963. Since that time, the formulation for the drug has changed, and I could find no similar recent reports in the medical literature. I did, however, find a study that used Doxycycline, a member of the Tetracycline family, in dialysis patients without ill effects. I personally prefer Doxycycline over Tetracycline as it is a newer generation drug, and might have less resistance issues.

About 25 years ago, the U.S. military commissioned a study regarding expiration dates. They had over one billion dollars worth of medications stockpiled and were faced with the challenge of destroying huge quantities every 2 years or so. The results were featured in the Wall Street Journal (3/29/00). The study was conducted by the Food and Drug Administration.

The results revealed that 90% of medications tested were acceptable for use 8-15 years after the expiration date. The FDA tested over 100 medications, prescription and non-prescription, and continues to study the issue today. The exceptions were mostly in liquid form (some pediatric antibiotics, insulin, among others). These lose their potency very soon after the date on the package. One sign of this is a change in the color of the liquid, but this is not proof one way or another.

Recently, a program called the Shelf Life Extension Plan evaluated a number of FEMA-stockpiled medications; these were mostly antibiotics that had been stockpiled for use in natural disaster that had passed their expiration dates. They found that almost all medications in pill or capsule form were still good 2 to 10 years after their expiration dates. The conclusion of the study states:

"The SLEP data supports the assertion that many drug products can be extended past the original expiration date....".

It also states that these extensions may vary from drug to drug.

Even more incredibly, Researchers at the University of California San Francisco School of Pharmacy found cases of 14 different medications in a retail pharmacy in their original, unopened packaging. These cases were labeled with expiration dates 28-40 years old.

The scientists used high-tech methods to measure the amounts of the active ingredients in the drugs. When analyzed, 12 of the 14 active ingredients persisted in concentrations that were 90% or greater of the amount indicated on the label. These results were conclusive enough for inclusion in the prestigious journal "Archives of Internal Medicine" (October 2012).

As a result of all these findings, even the government has changed their stance on expiration dates. During a recent flu epidemic, a 5 year extension was issued for the use of expired Tamiflu, a drug used to prevent and treat Swine Flu and other influenzas.

Surprisingly, few other extended use authorizations have been approved or, at least, publicized for the other medications, even though such information would be helpful for millions of people preparing for tough times. Another disturbing fact: The information from the study is not usually available to the general public, as the website that originally published it now requires a special access code to enter. Despite this, you can try to access a back copy of *The Journal of Pharmaceutical Sciences*, Vol.

95, No. 7, July 2006, where you will find a summary of the SLEP data. Most college medical libraries carry the journal. Here is the abstract, a short description of the study and its conclusions:

ABSTRACT: The American Medical Association has questioned whether expiration dating markedly underestimates the actual shelf life of drug products. Results from the shelf life extension program (SLEP) have been evaluated to provide extensive data to address this issue. The SLEP has been administered by the Food and Drug Administration for the United States Department of Defense (DOD) for 20 years.

This program probably contains the most extensive source of pharmaceutical stability data extant. This report summarizes extended stability profiles for 122 different drug products (3005 different lots). The drug products were categorized into five groups based on incidence of initial extension failures and termination failures (extended lot eventually failed upon re-testing).

Based on testing and stability assessment, 88% of the lots were extended at least 1 year beyond their original expiration date for an average extension of 66 months, but the additional stability period was highly variable. The SLEP data supports the assertion that many drug products, if properly stored, can be extended past the expiration date. Due to the lot-to-lot variability, the stability and quality of extended drug products can only be assured by periodic testing and systematic evaluation of each lot.

A PDF file of the entire study is also available online, at least at the time of this writing, at: http://ofcaems.org/ds-Stability_Profiles.pdf

The SLEP data found most of the failures among drugs that were in liquid form. Medications in pill or capsule form lasted the longest. It is true that the strength of a medication could possibly decrease over time, so it is important that your supplies are stored in a cool, dry, dark place. The effective life of a drug usually is in inverse relation to the temperature it is stored at. In other words, a drug stored at 50 degrees Fahrenheit will last longer than one stored at 90 degrees Fahrenheit. Storing in opaque or "smoky" containers is preferable to clear containers. Humidity will also affect medications, and could even cause mold and mildew to form, especially on natural remedies such as dried herbs and powders.

Planning ahead, we must consider all alternatives in the effort to stay healthy in hard times. Don't ignore any option that can help you achieve that goal, even expired medicine. I encourage everyone to conduct their own study into the truth about expiration dates; come to your own conclusions after studying the facts.

AN OPEN LETTER TO DOCTORS ABOUT MEDICAL PREPAREDNESS

In this book, I recommended a frank discussion with your current physician about the importance of being medically prepared for emergency situations, both short and long term. Many, however, will not know how to broach the subject, in fear of being ridiculed by the medical establishment.

Therefore, I have written a letter specifically meant for healthcare providers to introduce them to the concerns of our community. This is a letter that any person concerned about disaster situations can present to their physician. It addresses issues associated with the possible inadequacy of emergency medical response in situations such as the aftermath of a major storm or other disasters. Feel free to present it to your family physician if you think it would be beneficial to have them better understand preparedness issues.

To my fellow physicians:

I am a Fellow of both the American College of Surgeons and the American College of OB/GYN, recently retired, and I am writing this letter in an effort to inform you about the importance of improving the level of medical preparedness in your patient population.

We live in uncertain times, and more and more people are becoming concerned about what would happen in the event of a major disaster. From tornadoes to wildfires to national emergencies, there are circumstances where medical personnel may be overwhelmed by the number of victims requiring medical aid. In these situations, many of your patients will be unable to reach you. They may find themselves as the sole resource available to care for sick or injured members of their families.

In the aftermath of Hurricane Katrina in 2005, disaster medical assistance teams (DMATs) were formed from many areas in the country and converged upon New Orleans. They were immediately overwhelmed by the number of victims requiring medical help. In such a scenario, it stands to reason that your patients would benefit from a concerted effort on your part to help them be prepared to deal with likely problems they would face.

In an era of high technology, we may have expectations that our resources will always be sufficient to meet our emergency needs. Recent history has proven otherwise, and it may be time for us, as physicians, to increase the amount of education we provide for our patients; in this way, they can function as assets to their family if you or emergency medical personnel are not available.

Few medical offices provide information regarding the types and quantities of medical supplies that are recommended for the average household. These are my suggestions: Consider your area's likely needs for the disasters that might befall it, and print lists of items that you would advise your patients to have in their homes. As well, provide resources for classes that your patients can take so that they will have the medical education necessary to deal with possible emergencies during these events.

Direct them to sites recommended by the federal government for emergency preparedness, such as www.ready.gov; they will find free informational booklets that will help to increase their chances of surviving natural calamities and other disasters.

For your individual patients, especially those with chronic medical problems, you might consider providing the opportunity for them to keep a supply of needed medications by offering them an extra prescription to fill. In this manner, you can assure that your patients will have enough medicine to get them through situations which prevent them from contacting you in times of trouble.

I'm not asking you to abandon your responsibility by throwing prescriptions at them; I am simply suggesting that they would benefit from having some extra supplies available to deal with unforeseen circumstances. Also, consider listing recommended over-the-counter medications that would be useful to have on hand.

Our purpose as physicians is to improve the health of our people while doing no harm. Many doctors dedicate their entire lives to this purpose, and we must work to preserve the well-being of our patients in bad times as well as good times. The worst nightmare of your patients is the inability to reach you in a major disaster; help them become better prepared to deal with medical emergencies with education, compassion, and understanding.

Thank you for all you do to keep your patients healthy, and for your time and attention in reading this letter.

Joseph Alton, M.D., F.A.C.S., F.A.C.O.G.

This letter is available to print out at: www.doomandbloom.net.

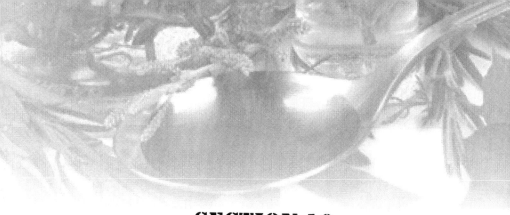

SECTION 10

✚ ✚ ✚

REFERENCES

Certainly, you have accumulated a reasonable amount of medical supplies to prepare you for the role of survival medic. If you have been prudent, you have taken emergency courses offered by your municipality and availed yourself of other hands-on teaching resources. Now, it is time to build your survival print and video libraries.

This book has taken an unusual route in assuming that no modern medical care or facilities will be available to you. Although we have attempted to be comprehensive in our approach, there is still much to learn. In power-down situations, you should have a number of printed medical books that you can refer to in times of trouble. In this section, we have given you a list that will be welcome assistance in your efforts to keep your people healthy.

While you have power, you should also avail yourself of the many resources available on the internet. For many procedures, there is no substitute to seeing something done in real time, such as placing a cast. Make every effort to download how-to videos on various medical subjects. No prepared individual should be without a source of power in hard times, so have a solar cell or other method to give you the ability to review these when you need them.

Arm yourself with an arsenal of medical knowledge. We refer to our library constantly to stay current on the options available to us, and so should you.

PRINT REFERENCES

I mentioned earlier that some reference books will be necessary for any aspiring medic. A printed medical library will still be there in a collapse situation, even if the internet, television, and other media are not. There are many good written resources for handling medical problems; these are but a few. The following books will be good additions to every medic's library:

Stedman's Medical Dictionary
(a must for any medic)

Gray's Anatomy for Students
(yes, the television show's title was taken from this book)

The Physician's Desk Reference
(comes out yearly, tells you indications, dosages, and risks of just about every medicine)

The Merck Manual
(good pocket reference on many common medical problems)

The Mayo Clinic Family Health book
(exhaustive and thorough with lots of photos)

Clinical Physiology Made Ridiculously Simple
by Stephen Goldberg, M.D. (all the basics on how the body works)

American College of Emergency Physicians First Aid Manual
(excellent first aid book)

Where there is No Doctor
by David Werner (third-world medicine)

Where there is no Dentist
by Murray Dickson (third-world dentistry)

A Comprehensive Guide to Wilderness and Travel Medicine
by Eric Weiss, M.D. (helpful pocket version)

Wilderness Medicine
by William W. Forgey, M.D. (outdoor survival)

Encyclopedia of Herbal Medicine
by Andrew Chevallier (talks about how medicinal plants work; information on every herb)

Prescription for Herbal Healing
by Phyllis A. Balch, CNC (extensive herbal remedy book)

Essential Oils Desk Reference
by Essential Science Publishing (exhaustive listings with photos)

Best Remedies
by Mary L. Hardy, M.D. and Debra L. Gordon (plain English home remedies for 100 different medical problems; excellent integrative medical reference)

Principles of Surgery
by Schwartz et al (for the very, very ambitious)

Tactical Medicine Essentials
by the American College of Emergency Physicians (for really high-risk situations)

Varney's Midwifery or **Varney's Pocket Midwife**
(you never know when you'll need it)

If you have all these books in your medical library, you will have as much information at your fingertips as you'll need to keep your loved ones healthy in times of trouble.

VIDEO RESOURCES

One of the best resources available to information seekers is the online video. This phenomenon has placed a veritable library at your fingertips with regards to medical information. Even better than a library, you can actually see important medical procedures being performed, such as in my video "How to Suture with Dr. Bones". They range from a short blurb of a minute or so to a full one hour medical school lecture. The next few pages are essentially an entire second book filled with medical knowledge.

I have endeavored to find a representative video for just about every subject that I cover in this book. Different sources are listed, so that you can see the many options available for health information in all fields. The source is listed in parentheses after the title of the video, along with a short comment. Search YouTube.com for the title EXACTLY as listed. If more than one video exists with the same title, look to see what the source is.

I have to say that I don't agree with everything said on every video; do your own research and make you own decisions. The important thing to remember is that these sources are interested in what is relevant in today's modern world. Many of them end with "and head for the hospital" or "see your doctor as soon as possible". Few if any are considering a societal collapse in their presentations, so be forewarned. In any case, the following videos will provide you an excellent base of knowledge from which to move forward:

7.Medical Interview -Review of Systems (by tvmariel) (One of various videos, it shows a doctor conducting an interview with a patient before an exam. Watch as many as you can.)

01.Physical Exam-Introduction & Vital Signs (by tvmariel) (Just one of many videos , it shows a doctor performing portions of the physical exam. Watch them all.)

Survival Medicine Gauze by Nurse Amy
(by drbonespodcast) (Review of all the different dressing materials)

What Are Essential Oils (Anyway)? (by kennethgardner)
(I can't verify all the claims made here; do you own research and decide for yourself.)

Using Colloidal Silver (by Chris Hyslop)
(All about how to use this alternative)

The Dangers of Colloidal Silver (by pogue972)
(A story about a man with argyria.)

Jacket Stretcher Wilderness First Aid Paul Tarsitano 1 of 3
Rope and Stick Stretcher Paul Tarsitano 2 of 3
Tarp Stretcher Wilderness First Aid Paul Tarsitano 3 of 3
(all by pault1960)
(3 videos by an expert in improvised patient transport)

Carrying the Injured (1933) (by wellcomefilm)
(Amazing old video with various patient carry techniques)

Extremities Lift and Carry (Pocket Tools Training - NCOSFM) (by ncosfm)
(Quick how-to for 2-man carry)

Blanket Drag (Pocket Tools Training – NCOSFM (by ncosfm)
(Another video in an excellent series)

FIREMAN CARRY COACH
(by lesmillsspartan)
(How to perform a one-man carry)

Lice-Mayo Clinic (by mayoclinic)
(Treatment basics)

Bed Bug Basics (by orkincommercial)
(Insect specialist discusses bedbugs)

How To Remove A Tick (by tickEncounter)
(Step-by-step procedure)

Mt. Everest Dental Extraction at Base Camp (by cristenhfdg)
(Tooth extraction in an austere environment)

How to INSTANTLY CURE A TOOTHACHE at home remedy (by askmydentisttv)
(Dentist teaches you how to make temporary filling cement)

Respiratory Infection Health Byte (by livestrong)
(Basics of upper and lower respiratory infections)

Signs of Dehydration - and How to Prevent It (by nsipartners)
(Identifying water loss)

How To Treat Diarrhea (by howcast)
(General information)

First Aid Tips : How to Treat Food Poisoning (by ehow)
(Basic information on first steps)

How To Recognize the Symptoms Of Appendicitis (by howcast)
(How to differentiate from other problems)

Appendectomy (Stab Appendectomy) by Dr. Irfan Ahmad Nadeem (by ianadeem)
(Performed under local anesthesia; appendix pops out at 3:50 mark)

Kidney Infection Health Byte (by livestrong)
A Health Byte: Urinary Tract Infection (by livestrong)
(Basics on urinary and kidney issues)

How to Treat Heatstroke (by howcast)
(Just what the title says.)

Hypothermia Treatment Scenario (by remotemedical)
(Actual wilderness video)

Health and Safety Abroad: Altitude Sickness (by HTHworldwide)
(Signs to look for)

First Aid - Minor wounds standard care (by businessrecovery)
(Basics)

Blister Treatment/ Survival Medicine By Nurse Amy (by drbonespodcast)
(simple ways to treat a blister.)

First Aid - Severe bleeding (by businessrecovery)
(Step by step)

How to Treat Gunshot & Knife Wounds (by sootch00)
(Just in case)

The Emergency Bandage (aka The Israeli Bandage) (by PerSysMedical)
(Best trauma bandage)

Quikclot Combat Gauze training (by wingmanusn)
(hemostatic agents in action)

Quikclot Demonstration (by peacemakerdill)
(Not for the squeamish)

How to Suture With Dr. Bones (by drbonespodcast)
(Learn how to put stitches into a pig's foot.)

How to Staple Skin with Dr. Bones (by drbonespodcast)
(Learn how to put staples into a pig's foot.)

Surgical Debridement (by nucleusanimation)
(Removing dead tissue from a wound)

Adventure Medical Preventing and Treating Blisters (by jamestowntv)
(Treatment process using certain brand name items)

First Aid Tips: How to Treat a Burn in the Wilderness (by ehow)
(Fire captain discussing burn injuries in the wild)

Burns: Classification and Treatment (by nucleusanimation)
(All the degrees and basic treatment explained)

How To Treat a Snakebite (by howcasst)
(step by step recommendations)

Black Widow spider bite - Day 3 (by varvelle)
(Classic appearance shown)

Be Safe from Anaphylaxis-Mayo Clinic (by Mayo Clinic)
(Important information)

Dermatology Treatments : How to Diagnose Skin Rashes (by ehowhealth)
(Some common skin rashes explained)

Abdominal wall cellulitis (by theedexitvideo)
(Example of cellulitis and abscess drainage procedure)

Symptoms of Tension vs. Migraine Headache (by fyinowhealth)
(List of symptoms of each)

Sprains and Strains (by universityhospitals)
(Quick overview)

Sprains Fractures and Dislocations (by uctelevision)
(Full 1 hour medical school lecture with lots of great info- early portion includes an easy quiz)

Symptoms and Treatments of Hypothyroidism (by mercola)
(Discussion of this common thyroid condition)

Diabetes Overview (by answerstv)
(Comprehensive discussion)

Understanding High Blood Pressure (HBP #1) (by healthguru)
(All the facts in plain English)

Chest pain vs. heart attack - ask the doctor (by wptvnews)
(Different causes of chest pain)

Dr. Oz - What causes acid reflux? (by sistagirl488deleted)
(TV doctor describes how it occurs)

Understanding Epilepsy (Epilepsy #1) (by healthguru)
(Why seizures happen)

Understanding Arthritis (Arthritis #1) (by healthguru)
(Osteoarthritis and rheumatoid arthritis overview)

Healthbeat - Kidney Stones (by koattv)
(Advice to avoid recurrences)

Gallstones Health Byte (by livestrong)
(Causes, types, symptoms)

How To Perform the Heimlich Maneuver (Abdominal Thrusts) (by howcast)
(Excellent demonstration)

CPR Training Video New 2010 / 2011 Guidelines - Preview Safetycare Cardiopulmonary Resuscitation (by safetycareonline)
(Excellent preview but not a substitute for a full course)

Eye Care & Vision Problems : How to Get Rid of Bloodshot Eyes (by ehowhealth)
(Discussion of eye allergies)

Conjunctivitis - Pink Eye (by drmdk)
(Question and answer session with an eye doctor)

Anterior Nasal Packing.MPG (by ausafakhan)
(Good procedure to know)

Ears 101 : How to Relieve an Ear Ache (by ehowhealth)
(Common infections and treatment)

Prenatal Care: Early Pregnancy Visits (by marchofdimes)
(Explains prenatal care and shows an actual visit)

Baby delivery (by saalie100)
(Typical hospital delivery – note an episiotomy is performed, which I don't recommend unless absolutely necessary. Also, cord does not have to be cut immediately and the baby should be placed on mother's stomach almost immediately for bonding purposes)

Anxiety Overview (by answertv)
(All the basics)

Signs, Symptoms, and Treatment of Depression (by nimhgov)
(Again, all the basics)

START Triage Basics (by unmcheroes)
(Excellent video on mass casualty event triage)

Trephining a nail to drain subungual haematoma (by travellerj)
(Treating a nailbed injury)

The Effects of Sleep Deprivation (by roperstfrancis)
(Personal story of a sleep deprivation patient)

Fish Antibiotics in a Collapse by Dr. Bones (by drbonespodcast)
(Alternative options for stockpiling antibiotics)

Expiration Dates and The Truth by Dr. Bones (by drbonespodcast)
(What expiration dates really mean)

GLOSSARY OF MEDICAL TERMINOLOGY

ABRASION: area of skin scraped off down to the dermis

ABSCESS: collection of pus and inflamed tissue

ACID REFLUX: Pain and burning caused by stomach acid traveling up the esophagus

ADRENALINE: name for epinephrine outside the U.S.

AIRWAY: breathing passage

ALLERGY: exaggerated physical reaction to a substance

AMNIOTIC FLUID: liquid inside the pregnant uterus

AMBU-BAG: CPR breathing unit (brand name)

ANAEROBE: organism that doesn't require oxygen to survive

ANALGESIA: pain relief

ANAPHYLAXIS::   hypersensitivity to a substance due to antibodies after an initial exposure

ANAPHYLACTIC SHOCK: life-threatening organ failure as a result of hypersensitivity to a substance

ANGINA: heart pain caused by lack of oxygen

ANTIBIOTIC: substances that kill bacteria in living tissue

ANTIBODY: substances produced by the body that respond to toxins

ANTICOAGULANT: substances that stop clotting

ANTIEMETIC: substances that stop vomiting

ANTIHISTAMINE:	drugs that relieve minor allergies
ANTIINFLAMMATORY:	substances that limit inflammation
ANTISEPTIC:	anything that limits the spread of germs on living surfaces
ANTISPASMODIC:	decreases blood vessel constriction
ANTIVENIN:	substance that inactivates snake or insect venom
ANTIVIRAL:	substances that kill viruses
APPENDICITIS:	inflammation of the appendix
ARTERY:	blood vessel that carries oxygen to the tissues
ARTHRITIS:	inflammation of the joints
ASCITES:	fluid accumulation in the abdomen
ASPHYXIANT:	substance that deprives the body of oxygen
ASPIRATION:	inhalation of fluids into the airways
ASTHMA:	shortness of breath caused by a narrowing of airways, often due to an allergic reaction
ASYMPTOMATIC:	without signs or symptoms
ATHEROSCLEROSIS:	blockage of the coronary arteries
AVULSION:	tissue torn off by trauma
BAG VALVE MASK:	CPR breathing apparatus
BANDAGE:	wound covering
BETADINE:	iodine antiseptic solution
BILE:	fluid found in the gall bladder

B.R.A.T. DIET:	diet used to treat dehydration consisting of bananas, rice, applesauce and dry toast
BRONCHITIS:	inflammation of the airways
BRONCHUS:	main respiratory airway
BRUISE:	injury that does not break the skin but causes bleeding due to damaged blood vessels
CAPILLARY:	tiny blood vessel that connects arteries to veins throughout the body
CARDIAC:	relating to the heart
CARTILAGE:	fibrous connective tissue found in various parts of the body, such as the joints, outer ear, and larynx.
CATARACT:	a clouding of the lens of the eye
CELLULITIS:	inflammation of soft tissues
CHIN-LIFT:	CPR technique that improves airflow
CHOLECYSTITIS:	inflammation of the gall bladder
CHOLELITHIASIS:	gall stones
CIRRHOSIS:	chronic liver damage
CLOSED FRACTURE:	broken bone that does not break the skin
COLLAPSE SITUATION:	circumstance where modern medical care no longer exists for the long term
COLOSTRUM:	early breast milk rich in antibodies
CONCUSSION:	loss of consciousness caused by trauma to the cranium
CONJUNCTIVITIS:	inflammation of the eye membrane
CORNEA:	clear covering over the iris

COSTOCHONDRITIS:	chest pain caused by inflammation of the rib joints
COTYLEDONS:	segments of the placenta
CPR:	cardio-pulmonary resuscitation
CROWNING:	late stage of labor when the baby's head start to emerge from the vagina
CURETTAGE:	scraping dead pregnancy tissue from the uterus after a miscarriage
CYANOSIS:	blue color caused by lack of oxygen
DEBRIDEMENT:	removal of dead tissue from a wound
DEHYDRATION:	loss of body water content
DERMATITIS:	inflammation of the skin
DERMIS:	deep layer of the skin
DIABETES:	disease in which the body fails to produce enough Insulin to control blood sugar levels (type 1) or is resistant to the Insulin it produces (Type 2)
DIAGNOSIS:	Identification of a medical condition
DILATION:	the act of making more open
DISCHARGE:	drainage from a surface or wound
DISINFECTANT:	substance that kills germs on non-living surfaces
DISLOCATION:	traumatic movement of a bone out of its joint
DISTAL:	away from the torso
DIURETIC:	substance that increases urine flow
DRESSING:	wound covering
DRUG OF CHOICE:	best drug for a particular illness

DUODENUM: part of the bowel after the stomach

DYSENTERY: dangerous diarrheal disease

ECLAMPSIA: seizures caused by elevated blood pressures during a pregnancy

ECTOPIC PREGNANCY: pregnancy that implants outside of the womb

EDEMA: fluid accumulation

ELAPID: family of venomous "coral" snakes

ELECTROLYTES: elements found in body fluids

ENDEMIC: native to an area or species

EPIDERMIS: superficial layer of the skin

EPILEPSY: convulsive disorder

EPINEPHRINE: hormone used to treat severe allergic reactions (known as adrenaline outside the US)

EPISTAXIS: bleeding from the nose

ERYTHEMA: redness due to inflammation

ESOPHAGUS: tube that runs from the back of the mouth to the stomach

ESSENTIAL OILS: highly concentrated liquids of various mixtures of natural compounds obtained from plants.

EXPECTORANT: substance that loosens congestion

FRACTURE: a broken bone

FROSTBITE: frozen tissue, usually in extremities

GALL BLADDER: organ near the liver that stores bile

GANGRENE: death of tissue due to lack of circulation

GASTROENTERITIS: inflammation of the stomach/intestine

GINGIVITIS: inflammation of the gums

GLAND: organ that produces hormones

GLUCOSE: blood sugar

GRAND MAL SEIZURE: generalized convulsion in epileptics

GRANULOMA: nodule formed by immune system's attempt to wall off an infection or a foreign object

HEARTBURN: chest pain caused by stomach acid

HEAT STROKE: symptoms caused by overheating

HEIMLICH MANEUVER: action taken to remove foreign object from the airways

HEMOGLOBIN: red blood cell component that carries oxygen to the tissues

HEMORRHAGE: blood loss

HEMORRHOID: varicose vein near the anus

HEMOPTYSIS: coughing up blood

HEMOSTATIC AGENT: substance that stops bleeding

HEPATITIS: inflammation of the liver

HERNIA: weakness in the body wall

HESITANCY: difficulty starting a urine stream

HISTAMINES: substances formed in allergies that cause physical symptoms

HIVES: bumpy red rash caused by allergies

HORMONE: substance produced by a gland that affects body functions

HYDRATION: addition of water to the system

HYGIENE:	cleanliness as health strategy
HYPEROPIA:	farsightedness
HYPERTENSION:	high blood pressure
HYPERTHERMIA:	heat stroke or heat exhaustion
HYPERTHYROIDISM:	condition caused by high thyroid levels
HYPHEMA:	bleeding into the white of the eye
HYPOGLYCEMIA:	low blood glucose levels
HYPOTHERMIA:	syndrome caused by heat loss
HYPOTHYROIDISM:	condition caused by low thyroid levels
IMMOBILIZATION:	prevention of movement
IMMUNITY:	protection against a disease
IMPETIGO:	skin infection with weeping sores
INFARCTION:	death of heart tissue due to lack of oxygen
INFLAMMATION:	reaction to injury characterized by redness, swelling, discharge, pain and heat
INFLUENZA:	viral respiratory illness
INTEGRATED CARE:	treatment using different medical methods
INTOXICATION:	state of being poisoned
INTRAVENOUS:	inside the vein
IRIS:	colored portion of the eye
IRRIGATION:	forceful application of fluid to a wound to clean out debris, blood clots, and dead tissue
IRRITANT:	substance that causes inflammation of tissue

ISCHEMIC:	lacking oxygen due to circulatory failure
JAUNDICE:	yellowing of the skin and eyes due to liver malfunction
KETOACIDOSIS:	life-threatening condition related to failure of blood glucose control
KILOGRAM:	2.2 pounds
LACERATION:	penetration of both skin layers by injury
LARYNX:	the voice box
LASIK:	laser surgery to correct vision
LETHARGY:	extreme fatigue or drowsiness
LIGAMENT:	supportive tissue that connects bones
LITER:	0.264 gallons
LOCALIZED:	isolated to an area
LYMPHATICS:	drainage system for body fluids
MASS CASUALTY INCIDENT:	more victims than available help
MENINGITIS:	inflammation of the brain/spinal cord
MENSTRUATION:	periodic blood flow from the uterus
MIGRAINE:	headaches caused by vascular Spasms
MISCARRIAGE:	early pregnancy loss
MOLESKIN:	protective material for blisters
MYOPIA:	nearsightedness
NEUROLOGIC:	pertaining to the nervous system
OPEN FRACTURE:	broken bone that pierces the skin

OPTHALMOSCOPE: instrument used to look into the eyes

OTITIS: inflammation of the ear

OTOSCOPE: instrument used to look into ear canal

OVARY: female organ that produces eggs

PALPATION: to feel with the hands

PALPITATIONS: sensation of dread caused by a rapid heart rate

PATHOGEN: something that causes disease

PEDIATRIC: pertaining to children

PELVIC: pertaining to the bones that provide support for legs and spine

PEPTIC: relating to stomach acid

PERCUSSION: to tap on the body to identify hollow and solid areas; for example, when searching for a tumor.

PERINEUM: area between the vagina and anus

PERIOSTEUM: outside lining of the bone

PETIT MAL SEIZURE: epilepsy characterized by loss of awareness without generalized convulsive behavior

PHARYNX: the throat

PHLEBITIS: inflammation seen in varicose veins

PHLEGM: mucus discharge from the respiratory tract

PIT VIPER: snake in the rattlesnake family

PNEUMONIA: an infection of the lungs

PNEUMOTHORAX: free air in the lung cavity affecting breathing

POST-ICTAL STATE:	semi-conscious state after experiencing a grand mal seizure
POTABLE:	safe to drink
PRE-ECLAMPSIA:	pregnancy-induced hypertension
PROGNOSIS:	likely outcome of a medical condition
PRONE:	lying face down
PROPHYLAXIS:	preventative measures
PROXIMAL:	closer to the torso
PROTOZOA:	microscopic organisms that sometimes act as parasites
PULMONARY:	relating to the lungs
PRESSURE POINTS:	areas where pressure on blood vessels stops bleeding to distal areas
PRURITIS:	itchiness
PULMONARY:	relating to the lungs
PUS:	inflammatory discharge caused by the body's response to infection
PYELONEPHRITIS:	inflammation of the kidney
QUADRANT:	body area divided into quarters
REBOUND:	pain elicited by pressing, then made worse by releasing the pressure on a part of the body
REFLUX:	acid traveling up the esophagus
RELAPSE:	recurrence of a disease's symptoms
RENAL:	relating to the kidneys
RESPIRATORY:	relating to breathing

RHYTHM METHOD: method of determining fertile periods by tracking menstrual cycles

SALINE: salt water solution used for IV fluids and irrigating wounds

SEBORRHEA: oily, itchy rash on scalp and face

SEDATION: to relax or put to sleep

SEIZURE: convulsion

SHOCK: life-threatening syndrome caused by multiple organ failure or malfunction

SOFT TISSUE: muscle, tendons, ligaments, skin, fat

SPRAIN: damage to a ligament caused by hyperextension

SPHYGNOMANOMETER: instrument used to measure pressure

STERILE: free of germs

STERNUM: breastbone

STETHOSCOPE: instrument used for listening to heart, lungs, and for evaluating blood pressure

STRAIN: damage to a muscle or tendon

STROKE: brain hemorrhage with paralysis

SUBCUTANEOUS: under the skin

SUPINE: lying face up

SUSPENSION: a drug mixed in a liquid

SUTURE: wound closure with needle and thread

SYNDROME: collection of symptoms

SYSTEMIC: condition affecting the entire body

TACHYCARDIA: elevated heart rate

TENDON:	connection of a muscle to a bone
THERMOREGULATORY:	related to body temperature
TINCTURE:	plant extract made by soaking herbs in a liquid (such as water, alcohol, or vinegar) for a specified length of time, then straining and discarding the plant material.
TINNITUS:	ringing in the ears
TOURNIQUET:	item that uses pressure to stop bleeding from a wound
TRACHEOTOMY:	procedure meant to open an airway when no other method is possible
TRAUMA:	injury caused by impact
TREPHINATION:	drilling a hole into a nail to expel blood
TRIAGE:	to sort by priority
TUMOR:	a growth in or on the body
TYMPANIC MEMBRANE:	eardrum
ULCER:	damage to the wall of the skin, stomach or intestine due to pressure, acid or disease
ULTRAVIOLET:	invisible light waves that damage skin or eyes
UMBILICAL:	relating to the "belly button"
URGENCY:	sudden desire to urinate
URTICARIA:	allergic rash
UTERUS:	womb
VARICES:	enlarged and dilated veins
VASCULAR:	relating to blood vessels

VEIN: blood vessel that carries de-oxygenated blood back to the lungs

VERTIGO: dizziness

WHEEZING: high pitched noises heard while breathing during an asthma attack

INDEX

bacterial resistance, 69
bacterial vaginosis, 186
bactroban antibiotic ointment, 268
bag valve mask, for cpr, 419
baking soda,
  as toothpaste, 128
  in acid reflux, 387
  in burns, 320,
  in Dakin's solution, 278
  in pinkeye, 430
  in rehydration solution, 160
  paste, 254, 332, 335
balm, 68
bandages, 273
  butterfly, 280
  compression, 348
  in snake bite, 329
  wet-to-dry, 279
bedbugs, 337-341
bee sting, 331-2
benadryl (diphenhydramine), 473
  and dermatitis, 405
  and insect stings/bites, 238, 249,
    254,332,
  as sleep aid, 466
benzalkonium chloride, 56
  in animal bites, 324
betadine (tincture of iodine), 56
  as antiseptic for blocks, 290, 295
  as radiation protection, 260
  as wound irrigation, 273, 278
  in wounds, 268, 312, 361
  in tick bites, 123
bilirubin gallstones, 400
biological warfare, 261-4
bird-biotic (doxycycline), 490
bird-sulfa (sulfamethoxazole/
trimethoprim), 490
birth control, 443, 447-50
bites

animal, 323-6
snake, 327-30
insect, 199-200, 331-41
black tea treatment, burns, 319
black widow spiders, 333-5
bladder infection, 179-181
blanket hypothermia wrap, 212
blanket pull for transport, 106
blindness, snow, 428
blisters, 306-9
  in second-degree burns, 317
  in smallpox, 264
  in spider bites, 334
Blocks, nerve, 287-294
blood loss, 270-6, 354
  during delivery, 457
blood pressure, 87
  how to take, 374-5
body temperature, 87-8
  in heat stroke, 204-5
  in hypothermia, 208-10
  in ovulation, 448
boils, 193-4
braxton-hicks contractions, 453
broken nose, 434-5
bronchi, 144
bronchitis, 144-6
brown recluse spider, 334-5
brucella, 324
bruises, 267-8
burns, 315-22
  radiation, 257
  smoke inhalation, 225

C

c.o.l.d. strategy, 210
caffeine, for migraine, 424
calendula, 81
  in allergies, 238
  in burns, 320

in rabies, 326
in radiation sickness, 257
fault, earthquake, 235
fels-naptha soap, 253
fennel, 148, 460
fever, 87
  drugs for, 471-2
  herbs for, 82, 148
  in appendicitis, 174
  in biological warfare, 262-4
  in childhood seizures, 388-9
  in diarrheal disease, 158-9
  in heat stroke, 206
  in kidney infections, 180
  in liver disease, 183
  in malaria, 199-200
  in pelvic infections, 177
  in respiratory infections, 144-7
  salicin for, 148
feverfew, 82
finger blocks, 292-4
fireman's carry, 105-6
fire ant bites, 336-7
fire resistance, 222-3
fires, 221-6
first responder course, 46-7
fishhooks, 310
fish-cillin (ampicillin), 485
fish-cycline (tetracycline), 486
fish-flex (cephalexin), 485
fish-flox (ciprofloxacin), 486
fish-mox (amoxicillin), 485
fish-pen (penicillin), 485
fish-zole (metronidazole), 485
flagyl (metronidazole), 498-9
fluid replacement, 160-2
flukes, 125
food poisoning, 168-9
forceps, dental extraction, 140-1
forceps, for suturing, 281, 293
foreign object, in airway, 414-6

foreign object, in eye, 431
four F's of gallstones, 400-1
fracture, 353
  bone, 353-359
  dental,   134-6
  nasal, 434-5
  rib, 358-9
  skull, 342-4
  vs. sprain, 348-9
frankincense, 78
frequency, of urination, 179
frostbite, 213-4
Fujita tornado scale, 228
fundus, uterine in childbirth, 453, 457

G
gall bladder, 397, 400
gall stones, 400-402
gangrene in frostbite, 213
gangrene and amputation, 360
garden, medicinal, 80-85
garlic, 82, 489
  as wound antiseptic, 269
  in diarrhea, 162
  in respiratory illness, 148
  in urinary infections, 181
  in vaginal infections, 187
geranium, 77
  as insect repellant, 200
  in minor wounds, 268-9
  oil for strains, 350
gila monster, 330
ginger, 82
  in allergies, 239, 244-5
  in colds, 150
  in abdominal cramps, 162
  in morning sickness, 452
  in pain relief, 481
gingivitis, 130
gingko biloba, 83

neosporin ointment, 268
neti pot, 240
neurodermatitis, 405
nifedipine, for altitude
sickness, 220
nits, 118
nix, treatment for lice, 120
nosebleeds, 434-5
nuclear family medical bag, 58-60
nylon, as suture material, 283

O
oils, essential, general, 71-79
ointments, 68
omega-3 fatty acids, 480
omeprazole (prilosec), 474
ondansetron (zofran), 161, 452
open fracture, 353-5
open letter to physicians, 509-11
oral rehydration solution, 160-2
oregano, 78. 132, 269
oseltamivir (tamiflu), 502-4
in influenza, 145
osteoarthritis, 392-3
osteomyelitis, bone infection, 191,
354, 394
otitis, 436
externa, 436-7
media, 437-8
otoscope, 439-440
overuse, of antibiotics, 487-8
ovulation, 448-9

P
pack-strap carry, 107
pain medications, 473-9
pain relief, natural, 480-2
palpation, in physical exam, 89
pancreas, in diabetes, 370
pandemics, 3, 42, 146

panic attacks, 243, 459
paracord, 106
paresthesia, 248, 476
pathogen, 155
patient advocacy, 109-11
patient transport, 105-8
peak flow meter, 243
pedialyte, rehydration, 160
pelvic inflammatory disease, 177-8
peppermint, 76, 84
as insect repellant, 200
for lice, 121
in anxiety, 460
in colds and flu, 148-50
in diarrheal disease, 162
in insect stings, 332
in ear issues, 438
in wound care, 269
peptic ulcer, 385-6
pepto-bismol (bismuth), 161, 387
percussion, in physical exam, 89
perfusion, 94, 97
permethrin, 120
personal carry med kit, 57-8
pharyngitis, 144-145
phlebitis, 408-410
physical exam, 86-90
pillow splint, 356-7
pinkeye, eye infection, 429-30
pinna, ear, 439
pinworms, 125-6
pit vipers, 327-9
placenta, delivery, 445, 456
plague, 261-3
plumeria, 126
pneumonia, 143-6, 263, 420
pneumothorax, 358-9
poison ivy, 252-4
poison oak, 252-4
poison sumac, 252-4

INDEX

orthopedic, 346-360

nasal, 433-5

traumatic suture needle, 283

trench foot (immersion foot), 213

trephination, nail, 313-4

triage, 92-104

trichomoniasis, 186

triple antibiotic ointment, 194, 268, 279, 473

tsunami, 235

tubal pregnancy, 176-7

tuberculosis, 16, 324

tularemia, 324

turmeric, 85

in asthma, 245

in gallstones, 401

in joint disease, 396

in pain relief, 480

in spider bites, 335

typhoid fever, 159

typhus, 339

U

ultraviolet radiation, 155-6

eye damage, 428

in sterilizing water, 155

umbilical cord, 456

upper respiratory infection, 144-6

ureter, 179, 398

urgency, of urination, 179

urinary infections, 179-81

uva ursi, 181

V

vaginitis, 186-7

vaginosis, bacterial, 186

valerian, 85

for sleep, 467

in anxiety, 384, 459-60

in high blood pressure, 378

in seizure disorders, 390

in tension headache, 426

varicose veins, 407-10

as hemorrhoids, 441-2

vegetation management, in fires, 221

vermox (mebendazole), 126

vicryl, suture material, 283, 286

Video references, 517-523

vinegar, 169, 186-7, 396, 399

viruses, 56, 143-7, 167

and contact lenses, 429

in liver disease, 182-5

mosquito-borne, 200

rabies, 324-6

smallpox, 264

drugs against, 502-4

vision, 33, 388, 427-8

vital signs, 86-88

vitamin b12, 390, 405

vitamin c, 41-2, 147, 181, 378

W

warfare, biological, 261-4

wasp stings, 331-2

water moccasins, 327

west nile virus, 200

wheezes, in asthma, 241-3

wildfire preparedness, 221-6

wind chill, 209

wintergreen, 78, 239, 350

witch hazel, 82

as antiseptic, 269

for lice, 121

in blisters, 309

in burns, 319

in hemorrhoids, 442

in varicose veins, 410

worms, parasitic, 124-6

wormwood, 126

553

CONTACTS

DOCTOR: _____

DENTIST: _____

FIRE DEPT: _____

POLICE: _____

GROUP MEDIC: _____

GROUP MEMBERS: _____

_____

_____

_____

_____

_____

_____

_____

_____

_____

_____

_____

_____

_____

_____

_____

_____

NOTES

NOTES

NOTES

NOTES

NOTES

MEDICAL KITS FOR
THE SURVIVAL MEDIC

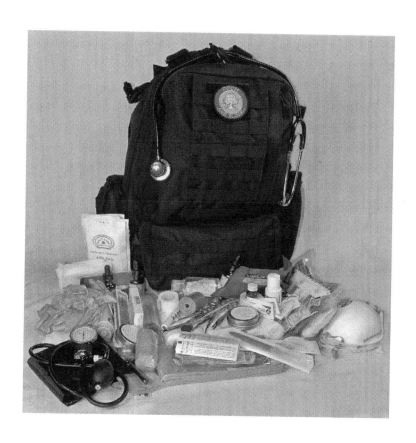

ENTIRE LINE OF MEDICAL KITS
AVAILABLE AT WWW.DOOMANDBLOOM.NET

28698555R00328

Made in the USA
San Bernardino, CA
04 January 2016